THE SCIENCE BEHIND CRANIAL ELECTROTHERAPY STIMULATION

Second Edition

THE SCIENCE BEHIND CRANIAL ELECTROTHERAPY STIMULATION

Second Edition

A complete annotated bibliography of 126 human and 29 experimental animal studies, plus 31 reviews and 2 meta-analyses, a current density model of CES, side effects and follow-up tables, all indexed and cross-referenced.

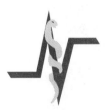

Daniel L. Kirsch, Ph.D., D.A.A.P.M., F.A.I.S.

with a prologue and epilogue by Pierre L. LeRoy, M.D., F.A.C.S.
and an introduction by Ray B. Smith, Ph.D., M.P.A.

Medical Scope Publishing Corporation
Edmonton, Alberta, Canada
2002

THE SCIENCE BEHIND CRANIAL ELECTROTHERAPY STIMULATION
SECOND EDITION

ISBN: 0-9684219-0-3

Disclaimer

This book is for informational purposes only. It is not intended to diagnose, prevent, or treat any disease and should not be considered as a substitute for consultation with a licensed health care professional. While side effects from cranial electrotherapy stimulation (CES) are rare, individual reactions may occur. Also not all CES devices are alike, so care should be taken to read the specific instructions provided with CES devices prior to use of any CES device.

Medical Scope Publishing Corporation
1015 Hooke Road
Edmonton, Alberta T5A 4K5 CANADA
(780) 456-9547
email: info@scopecom.com

Printed in Canada

ACKNOWLEDGEMENTS

There are so many people to thank that I had to divide them into three categories; those who actually studied CES, those who stood fast against the evil forces of government tyrants who were hell-bent on removing CES from the American pharmaceutical industry's competition, and of course, those who helped with this book.

First of all I must applaud the courage of those physicians and psychologists that began the journey into CES research in the 1960s. Technology was not dominating our lives back then so one can only imagine that their reference must have been limited to shock therapy (which CES most certainly is not!) and images of Frankenstein. Of all those whose work appears in these pages none can compare to psychiatrist Saul H. Rosenthal who virtually alone described the qualitative experiences of CES. Without doubt, experimental psychologist Ray B. Smith taught us the most about CES, and established the true foundations of CES science as a labor of love. Other great contributors are psychologists Michael Heffernan, Mary Ellen O'Connor, Stephen J. Overcash, and Marshall D. Voris; physicians Eric Braverman, Allen Childs, and Margret A. Patterson; and dentists Elliott J. Alpher, Michael Lerner, and Reid Winick among many others. With these are the thousands of forward-thinking clinicians who use CES in daily practice to provide their patients with a far safer, and usually much more effective alternative to drugs.

CES would no longer exist in the United States if not for the brave efforts of Electromedical Products International, Inc. (EPII) led by President Tracey B. Kirsch. She alone had the courage to stand up against the Food and Drug Administration who broke their own rules every step of the way in an incredibly biased attempt to deprive Americans of this therapy. Mrs. Kirsch was assisted in this task by attorneys Jonathan W. Emord of Emord and Associates, Larry R. Pilot, Ann M. Begley and Daniel Jarcho of McKenna & Cuneo, and Harry G. Preuss, M.D., Professor of Medicine and Pathology at Georgetown University Medical Center and science consultant to EPII. But this heroic effort also required the support of dozens of legislators who asked the FDA to explain themselves. The Honorable Joe Barton, Chair of the FDA Oversight Committee being most notably among them. Over 100 physicians, dentists, psychologists, therapists, and patients also helped by lobbying legislators to keep CES available to Americans.

Finally, the preparation of this book was encouraged and helped along the way by many people, but no one put more effort into, or stayed up more nights, editing, crunching numbers for the post marketing survey, and helping to lay out this book than my close colleague, Richard A. Floyd, Vice President of Electromedical Products International, Inc. Mr. Floyd could rightfully take a place as the fourth author.

To all those who use CES, I salute you for contributing to a humane therapy that has saved some lives, and certainly improved the quality-of-life of millions of people worldwide. We could all use a little CES from time-to-time. Its use should be mandated for government bureaucrats.

This book is dedicated to my beautiful and brilliant daughter,
Gabrielle Electra Kirsch, born February 13, 2000,
and to her mother and my darling wife, Tracey Burke Kirsch, who used CES faithfully
throughout her pregnancy and as the sole therapeutic modality for delivery.
These women taught me the true meaning of love.

Daniel L. Kirsch, Ph.D., D.A.A.P.M., F.A.I.S.
Mineral Wells, Texas

CONTENTS

1

PROLOGUE

*"The time has come," the Walrus said, "to talk of
many things, of shoes and ships-and sealing wax
of cabbages and kings, and why the sea is boiling
hot and whether pigs have wings."*

Lewis Carroll, *Through the Looking Glass*

This text reviews research and clinical data on an eclectic scope of historical research for practicing health professionals, concerning advances in cranial electrotherapy stimulation (CES). CES is the application of extremely low levels of electricity applied to the brain for the treatment of a wide range of psychiatric and medical disorders.

Unquestionably, the greatest event in human and medical history is the evolution of the human brain, for without its development the history of mankind would be vastly different. What happens when the brain's adaptive responses fail? It does not take much to offset the complex balance and harmonious relationships within the brain causing psycho-pathological and somato-autonomic syndromes to develop. These cerebral dysfunction's have been the precipitators of an epic quest for medicinal, behavioral, and interventional surgical therapies intended to rectify what are now thought to be complex centrally mediated electro-chemical disorders.

Unfortunately, all our reparative attempts to date have had their respective concomitant risks and complications. Accordingly, we must continue to search for new ways to accomplish better, more efficacious therapy that addresses these problems. Preferably ones that actually lead to healing.

Cranial electrotherapy stimulation offers a remarkable contribution towards this endeavor, and represents a significant advancement in neural science since it is based on sound, non-invasive neurophysiological principles long established in the world's published literature.

This volume elucidates a cogent, new approach to the treatment of a wide variety of related neuro-psychological disorders, moving from former mysticism to a modern rational approach for treatment. The path of discovery has been long.

For example, in antiquity in 46 AD, Scribonius Largus, physician to the Roman Emperor, noted the beneficial analgesic effect of the Torpedo, an electric eel.

The advances continued as Leo Galvani demonstrated that focused, man-made static electrical energy could influence neurophysiology in his classic experiments in the 1700s.

Later Pierre Bertholon described treatment benefits in his prophetic 1780 scholarly work, *The electricity of the human body in states of health and disease.*

Meanwhile, Duchenne of Boulogne demonstrated that electrical forehead stimulation induced effects for a variety of ailments while the patient's feet were immersed in seawater, an electrolyte media.

This book summarizes the latest information available in which the science and technology of CES therapy for mental and physical conditions is evaluated. We are indebted to all those who have contributed to the general fund of knowledge in CES.

These modern wonders build on prior contributions from such recognized basic science greats as Andre Ampere in France, Michael Faraday and Gilbert in England, Volta in Italy, Tesla in Yugoslavia and others whose work in understanding electricity has led to, and enabled, our present focus on neuro-electro-chemistry.

Basic science contributions in physics, chemistry and bioengineering have moved our analytical and therapeutic advances from nano to pico technology.

While progress concurrently moved from macro to micro-resolution new discoveries emerged to provide a better understanding of complex neurophysiological events, specifically those related to pain, behavior, and emotions.

This work follows correlative contributions by classic neuroanatomists and physiologists such as Charles Sherrington of England who published the Integrated Nervous System, Ranson and Clark in the United States on comparative neuroanatomy; Monnier of Switzerland and Iago in Scotland on specific receptor physiology, John Eccles of the United States and Wall in England who published their findings associated with pain and related temperature spinothalamic pathways, Abel-Fessard in France on the medial thalamus, and John Leibskind of the United States among many others who provided the foundation for behavioral scientists to bridge the poorly-understood emotional/physical gaps notably in the areas of anxiety, depression, insomnia and pain management. Ronald Melzack of Canada for promulgating the spinal gate control theory with Wall, psychologist Leibskind for periaquaducts interacting with Arnoff and Fordyce of the United States, and others who have continued to elucidate remarkable new understanding of the mind and body dilemma in the management of dysfunctional states linking pain to suffering and aberrant behavioral patterns, all emphasized by John Bonica, et al.

Applying these researchers' understandings to advances in biomedical engineering, Roger Avery and Don Mauer, neurosurgeons Charles Ray, Charles Burton, Giancarlo Barolot, Norman Shealy and others pursued development of electrical devices for implantation into human spinal cords. Then, further advances were made in electrical systems applicable for safe patient care for a variety of indications including regional pain syndromes especially when stress and adjustment reactions co-exist.

Neurosurgeon-physiologists Horsely, Clark, Speigel, Wyces, Cooper and others have further pioneered deep, central brain stimulation, and the modulation of efferent driven extra-pyramidal disorders connecting spinal-thalamic pathways, relaying them to the higher thalamic cortical centers. We do these things to lessen human suffering and to answer questions such as how do we link trembling to pain?

However, the definitive proximal central synaptic relays still remain elusive. More recent contributions by Abel Fessard in classic anatomic and electrochemical research of deep brain thalamic nuclear centers based on the prior works of neuroanatomist Schultenbrand and neurosurgeons Walker, Bailey and others, expanded our understanding between acute and chronic pain networks relaying over the neo- and paleo-spinal tracts, which are relatively new terms proposed by Kruger.

Clinical neurosurgical contributions by Ben Crue, William Sweet, Hasabuchi, John Loeser, and others made major contributions in our current understanding of the central neurophysiology of complex pain. Central versus peripheral schools of thought are still rigorously debated. Other research groups improved our understanding of the long-known but not well understood emotional limbic lobe function with connections, now providing limbic-somatic and autonomic pathways helping to better explain the somatic, emotional, behavioral, and autonomic interconnections. Emotional systems are evaluated by clinical methods of assessing somatic and autonomic responses.

Evaluation methods are also improving. For example, structured abnormalities imaged by CAT and MRI tests and dynamic PET scans are now correlating anatomic abnormalities with emotional responses. Autonomic neuro-vascular physiologic dysfunction is now documented by thermal infrared imaging.

How can we further improve patient care based on this impressive accumulating database? In the past medications, psychotherapy, behavior modification and selective invasive neuro-interventional approaches have been employed to treat a constellation of related regional pain syndromes frequently associated with psychological distress, anxiety, depression and insomnia. These trends are shifting now, from destructive neurosurgical procedures to less invasive or minimally invasive pain modulation techniques and now electrical procedures largely due to technological progress. For example, the use of linear accelerators and the gamma knife, direct photon beams of energy to destroy selective targets, all contributes to advancing the rapidly emerging field of electromedicine.

Steven Stahl of the University of California has described recent advances in pharmacodynamics identifying approximately 12 new classes of compounds, modulating six relays, and influencing three neurotransmitter systems. Understanding noradrenergic compounds, dopamine, and seratonin have significantly improved the psychodynamics of depression associated with pain management in clinical medicine but they still do not address the complex analgesic pathways. A major advance is accomplished by external noninvasive bioelectric systems categorized under the title of cranial electrotherapy stimulation.

Now, new advances in electrochemical modulation by a growing group of investigators, such as Alpher, Brotman, Gibson, Heffernan, Overcash, Rosenthal, Smith, Voris and others described in this text demonstrate that CES, sometimes also called Alpha Stimulation, is clinically efficacious. Why the name Alpha Stimulation? Because it changes the basic brain wave electrical rhythms while producing other physiologic changes such as modulating pain syndromes without being invasive. Cranial electrotherapy stimulators have passed all reasonable scientific requirements for risk/benefit ratios and are now clearly suitable for clinical application.

We are indebted to Dr. Daniel L. Kirsch for dedicating his professional efforts at compiling this text. Based on his pioneering concepts and extensive medical experiences he has brought together the efforts of published world contributors that are described in this publication which has also correlated with my own clinical experience and thermographic findings.

Dr. Ray B. Smith will review in more detail the history and science of CES in his introduction. Your responsible commentary is invited.

Pierre L. LeRoy, M.D., F.A.C.S., C.C.E.
Director, Delaware Pain Clinic
Neurosurgical Associates, P.A.
Newark, Delaware, USA

2

INTRODUCTION

> He ought not to risk his reputation by presenting to the learned body anything which appeared so much at variance with established knowledge, and withal so incredible.
>
> The British Royal Society
> re: Jenner's lecture on smallpox vaccination[1]

At the beginning of every book on electromedicine there is a brief history of the use of electricity to cure physical and/or emotional ailments of mankind, dating back to early Greek practices. Since this book is being authored by Dr. Daniel Kirsch, a pioneering inventor of microcurrent treatment for pain, it can simplify matters to quote from his Alpha-Stim® 100 Owner's Manual, now printed in six languages:

> "The application of electromedical currents is not a new concept. Ancients recognized the therapeutic value of naturally occurring electrical phenomena long before William Gilbert defined electricity in 1600. Both Aristotle and Plato refer to the Black Torpedo (electric ray fish), prescribed in 46 AD by the physician Scribonious Largus for the relief of a variety of medical conditions from headaches to gout... In the 1800s dentists reported excellent results using crude electrical devices for pain control.
> "...One hundred years ago, electrical devices were in widespread use to manage pain and 'cure' everything from cancer to impotency. Because of the unrefined early electrical technologies... this form of therapy fell into disrepute by the medical profession in the early part of the 20th century..."[2]

It is interesting that by the end of the 1700s a British surgeon, Charles Kite, had invented and was using an electrical cardiac defibrillator creating a storm of protest from the Christian community saying that this was reviving the dead and therefore the work of the devil. The treatment was soon abandoned, but now electrical defibrillators are back again. They are widely found in ambulances, emergency treatment rooms in hospitals, and in post surgery intensive care units, among other places. Their use is no longer tainted with the occult or an alleged association with mesmerism, which disbanded their earlier use. Bringing the otherwise dead back to life with a defibrillator is no longer the work of Satan, but of good, 20th century scientific medicine.[3]

A precursor to the modern transcutaneous electric nerve stimulator (TENS) was on the market by 1850. In that device, the patient held in one hand a metal handle which was attached to the generator by a wire and placed the other metal piece against the painful area on the body. The therapist turned a crank on the box which generated electrical current. That treatment had disappeared by the end of the 1800s, only to be revived after Melzack and Wall published their Gate Control theory of pain, causing TENS to reenter the U.S. market in the 1970s. TENS devices are now widely used in American medicine.[4]

Also in the 1800s an electric belt was manufactured that went around many parts of the patient's body, from his head, down his abdomen and back, around his arms to his hands, and down around his legs to his feet. Small batteries were attached at regular intervals that provided electrical stimulation along the entire belt. That invention was dismissed as a fraud. We now apply stimulation to similar points with acupuncture needles or microcurrent stimulator probes.[5]

In 1816 Berlioz published an early report on the potentiating effect of electroacupuncture,[6] and in 1825 Sarlandiere reported his use of electroacupuncture in treating gout, rheumatism and stress.[7] Fifty years later, in the U.S., Cohen reported one of the first uses of electricity in tumor surgery.[8]

In 1985, Robert O. Becker, M.D. wrote about his very intricate and involved scientific investigations that led to the use in the 1980s of electrical stimulation to stimulate healing in broken bones. That was seen as an incredible breakthrough until one of Becker's research assistants discovered that they had been beaten to this discovery by 150 years. Becker recounts:

> "Back in 1812, Dr. John Birch of St. Thomas' Hospital in London used electric shocks to heal a nonunion of the tibia. A Dr. Hall of York, Pennsylvania, later used direct current through electroacupuncture needles for the same purpose, and by 1860 Dr. Arthur Garratt of Boston stated in his electrotherapy textbook that, in the few times he'd needed to try it, this method had never failed."[9]

Becker began his research in an effort to understand bone regrowth in fractures. He did this by studying the regeneration process in salamanders. In an earlier study in 1909, an American researcher named Owen E. Frazee found that if he passed electrical currents through the aquarium water in which larval salamanders lived he could speed up their limb regeneration process.[10] That was one of the seminal lines of research that was to lead to Becker's breakthrough work on the body's electromagnetic fields beginning in the late 1950s. While it may seem incredible that this was not followed up on at the time, it so happened that very shortly after the 1909 study results were published, electromedicine would be officially on its way out in the United States.

During the time of Frazee's experiments, the Carnegie Endowment for the Advancement of Teaching funded a study by the American Medical Association to look into electromedicine to see if there was anything to it. The committee appointed to do this study delivered its report the year following Frazee's findings and said there was no scientific basis for the use of electricity in medicine.[11]

In large part, that was due to the lack of sensitivity of then available electrical and electromagnetic measuring devices. Electrotherapists could point to therapeutic results but had no way to show how the applied electricity could possibly effect changes in the body. Unfortunately, it also allowed genuine frauds to be perpetrated by those so inclined, since no one could prove that they could not cure every disease they named, without expending more time and effort than most self appointed watchdogs wanted to apply to the task.

Not so the Flexner Committee. They did what such committees do by definition: If something could not be proved it could not be said to exist, so they dismissed electromedicine, as, then, did the American Medical Association.

Interestingly, just five years prior to that, the Chinese Emperor, embarrassed by the primitiveness of medical practice in his country, prohibited the further use of acupuncture in Chinese medicine, requiring physicians in his country to take up the more advanced, Western medicine in their practices instead.[12]

General Douglas MacArthur, similarly, forbade the "primitive" Japanese practice of shiatsu in medicine when U.S. forces occupied Japan in 1945. Fortunately the order was overturned by President Truman, and at the turn of the 21st century we find many practitioners of shiatsu therapy in the U.S. and around the world.[13]

So in the first ten years of the 20th century everyone everywhere wanted to update medicine and make it modern. Among the first steps taken was to get rid of electromedicine and acupuncture.

Modernizing medicine was no easier then than it is now, as it happened, and acupuncturists continued to practice in China, albeit quietly for a while. The communist regime both resurrected and formalized the practice of acupuncture when they came in. As a bonus, they forced China's last emperor to learn and practice acupuncture and moxibustion while he was imprisoned by them in the 1950s.[14] Its practice had been mainstreamed again by the time President Nixon's group visited there in 1971 and exposed its obvious usefulness. Members of his team essentially brought it home to America over a half century after it had been banned in its homeland. Meanwhile, Hitler chose as his personal physician, Theo Morell, a doctor with a thriving business in Berlin who was still using electrical stimulation to treat prostatitis and impotence in his private practice at the time.[15]

If so-called useless medicine has been hard to stamp out, however, it has always been just as hard to get something new started in medical practice. For example, scurvy, which had forever been a grave problem for seafaring nations, took the lives of three-fourths of Lord Anson's crew on his trip around the world as late as 1740-44, and the Channel Fleet had 2,400 cases of scurvy after just ten weeks at sea in 1778. But the latter losses occurred 25 years following the publication of Lind's *Treatise of the Scurvy* in which, following his experiments, he reported limes or lemons to be the prevention and the cure.[16] Eventually, it was to take the British Admiralty 40 years and thousands upon thousands of lost lives to get limes aboard its sailing vessels following Lind's discovery. Of course it was true that the ships' stores were already laden with other things, and no one wanted to replace a few rum barrels with limes.

Similarly, more British soldiers (8,000) died of typhoid fever in the Boer war in Africa than were killed in action, even though a professor of pathology at Britain's Netley Military Hospital had perfected a vaccine made of dead typhoid bacteria and recommended its use by the army. A successful trial of the vaccine in the Indian Army had proved its safety and effectiveness, the report appearing the same year the Boer War began.[17]

Becker reports the serendipitous finding in Sheffield Children's Hospital in England in the early 1970s that children up to eleven years of age who lose the tip of a finger, up to the first major crease behind the nail, will totally regenerate the finger tip including muscles, nerves, nail, and skin, provided it is a clean cut and no one attempts to treat it. Any attempt to suture the missing part back on, or close the wound by suturing a protective skin flap over it, etc., will result in a deformed or missing finger tip.

Surgeon Cynthia Illingworth, who discovered this phenomenon, began treating other children who had lost a fingertip by simply cleaning the wound and loosely bandaging it to keep the dirt out. Within four years she had documented several hundred regrown fingertips, and other clinical studies confirmed it. That was in 1974, and it was well publicized, yet 25 years later, doctors throughout the world are still maiming children's hands by diligently providing medical treatment for children with missing fingertips.[18]

Now that it had been purged of electrical charlatanism, medical practice in the U.S. continued as a proud melange of herbs, mustard packs, blood letting, mercury shots, cathartics, purges and the like. Since the use of safe intravenous drips would not be discovered until World War II was underway, many medications of the day, including not a few very elaborate food supplement preparations, were simply injected into the person via the sigmoid colon.[19]

Surgery was still a recognized field of medicine, of course. Among the more common surgical procedures in the early 20th century was cutting patients open and tying down their floating kidneys, thus curing backache. In that same era some surgeons decided that the colon was not only useless but also a deterrent to good health, so they had begun removing that also.[20]

By 1936, physicians still recognized that bad eyesight was often caused by "autointoxication due to imperfect elimination" and though no longer doing colonectomies, for better eyesight recommended a good cleansing of the colon whose poisons were still widely known to pollute the body and to be responsible for all sorts of ailments, including bad vision.[21]

Just prior to and during World War II we entered the magic bullet period in medicine, first with antibiotics, then with other medications, notably the psychoactive drugs. Western medicine quickly began to lose interest in purges, herbal remedies, any placebo effect from a warm bedside manner, and so forth, and entered its current drug-dominant phase. Pharmaceutical companies vied with one another to produce and market the next powerful, wide spectrum antibiotic and the next psychopharmacologic wonder. Their sales reps became the new postgraduate medical educators to the medical profession.

The transition, as usual, was not as fast as we sometimes think. The antibiotic sulfonamide had been used as a skin antiseptic as early as 1913, and the ability of sulphanilamide to kill streptococci, the agent then killing patients with septicemia was known as early as 1932, when I.G. Farben successfully researched, then patented it. The first report on penicillin had been published back in 1929.[22] Luckily, World War II was on, and there was an emergency need to do something about thousands upon thousands of wounded and dying out on the battlefield. Antibiotics were then rushed into medical practice.[23]

Interestingly, it was not penicillin that began the medical revolution as many people now think, but the use of the various new sulfa powders following the bombing of Pearl Harbor, that began the new antibiotic phase of medicine.[24] Slaughter, in 1946, furnished a vivid reminder of those heady days as the transition in medicine was still in progress. He breathlessly reported, "New methods of preparing the drug (penicillin) hold promise that soon it may be given by one or at most two injections (in patients suffering from gonorrhea), and probably will not even require hospitalization."[25]

It is interesting to speculate how much longer it would have taken antibiotics to enter medical practice if the war had not been on. Certainly the medical conservatives would have demanded years of research on the possible harmful effects of injecting the products of fungi directly into the human body. Many years of animal research would have been demanded therefore, and finally small initial trials on human volunteers, probably prisoners serving life sentences, would gradually be made. It is conceivable that wide spread use of antibiotics may have entered mainstream medicine no earlier than the 1960s had it not been for the terrifying war that was in progress.

The origins of today's cranial electrotherapy stimulation (CES)

In the late 1960s the *Dallas Morning News* carried a small filler about a portable electrical device that was being used to relax the engineers who drove the bullet train in Japan. It said that they would drive the train from Tokyo to Kyoto, then lie in a darkened room on a cot for a few minutes with this device connected to their head via electrodes. It was said to relax them prior to their return trip north. An enterprising engineering firm from Garland, Texas, whose business it was to research new products, sent a small delegation to Japan to check out the device. They returned to Dallas with the Russian Electosone device, which pulsed 100 times per second with a sinusoidal waveform. Its output was limited to 1.5 milliamperes (mA), and there were four electrodes, two to be placed over the eyelids and two to be placed at the base of the head in back. The device was about the size of a businessman's brief case, though much heavier due to its internal rechargeable batteries.

One of the engineers, Ray Gillmer, left the parent organization with this new idea and began NeuroSystems, Inc., in Garland Texas. He began to manufacture his Neurotone 101 that had treatment settings of either 50 Hz or 100 Hz, stimulated sinusoidally, on an 80% duty cycle, with stimulus intensity limited to 1.5 mA. Because of the uncomfortable pressure and visual effects when the frontal electrodes were placed over the eyes, he early on decided to place them just above the eyebrows on the forehead.

Later he added to his armamentarium transcutaneous electrical nerve stimulation (TENS) devices, galvanic skin response (GSR) biofeedback devices, and a device that did both CES and GSR biofeedback. He was making nationwide sales efforts by the early 1970s.[26]

Meanwhile, an early researcher in the U.S.A., Saul Rosenthal, M.D., led a group of scientists at the University of Texas Medical School at San Antonio in their study of the Russian Electrosone unit, which was called an electrosleep device, and later the Neurotone 101. In fact, during the 1960s and early 1970s CES in the U.S.A., like CES in most of the world, was called "electrosleep." Rosenthal and other researchers who followed were to expend much research time and effort using the device in an attempt to put people to sleep. It did not do so reliably, but it did seem to relax them and eliminate much stress in the process.

Consequently, beginning in the early 1970s sleep studies became increasingly rare apart from some that did achieve notable improvement of sleep when the subjects went to sleep at some later time, sometimes several hours after treatment. Serendipitously, it was discovered that CES reduced stress states, which included anxiety and depression. Research then began focusing on the treatment's ability to effectively treat depression and anxiety, such as that found in persons withdrawing from addictive substances, along with cognitive deficits that presumably sprang from the depression and anxiety states.

The Neurotone 101 was called before the FDA's Neurology Panel in 1978 after new laws required the assessment of the safety and effectiveness of devices then on the market. They suggested to Gilmer that the name "electrosleep" might be a misnomer. Gilmer suggested that they call it "cranial electrotherapy". The FDA wasn't willing to commit to the "therapy" part, and they settled on "cranial electrotherapy stimulation." The FDA decided that any small electric current that went across the head, from any medical device used in the U.S.A., was to be called cranial electrotherapy stimulation. Thus even TENS units, when they placed electrodes so that current flowed across the head would now be CES devices.

Electrosleep circles at that time spread throughout the world, but most notably in the Eastern European nations, plus several countries in Western Europe such as Austria, where an international electrosleep conference was held every three years. As a group these clinicians theoretically thought of CES as just another electrical stimulation whose intensity was reduced down from a stimulation continuum that began at its most intense with electroshock, then was reduced down in intensity to electroanesthesia, which in turn could be reduced down to electrosleep levels. In their thinking it had nothing to do with acupuncture points, meridian therapy, the yin and yang and such. It was, effectively, mini electroshock treatment, without the negative side effects of its cousins that stimulated at higher intensity.

Soon to come from a quite different theoretical perspective in Hong Kong, however, was Margaret Patterson. M.D. She was a British surgeon working in a hospital that used acupuncture for anesthesia during surgery. To avoid the concentrated staff effort involved in twirling inserted needles, plus the additional physiological insult to the patient from inserted needles, they developed the habit of applying small amounts of electrical stimulation to the acupuncture points instead. They were using a bipolar spike wave, AC current, pulse width of 0.6 milliseconds (mS) and a frequency of 111 Hz. After one such surgical procedure, the patient seemed amazed. He had not told them that he was a heroin addict beforehand, and yet later admitted to the staff that he was having no withdrawal symptoms even several days following the procedure.

This profoundly impressed Patterson and she assisted as her colleagues began trying this stimulation out on known addicts who were being withdrawn from various drugs or alcohol.[27] To her amazement, the treatment aborted the withdrawal syndrome in her patients, and a new therapy was born. She named it "neuroelectric therapy (NET)." She went on to discover (or decide, it was never clear) which pulse rates were best for which condition treated, and began to proselytize heavily for NET, both back in England and later in the U.S.A. She added disorder-specific electrical stimulus rates to NET's armamentarium, and thus moved away from the pure theoretical concepts of acupuncture, but not into the mini electroshock school.[28]

Both she, and now NeuroSystems were utilizing two electrodes instead of four, placed just behind the ears for the treatment. This new placement was well researched by both, and found to effect the same cures that had been obtained by either the frontal/occipital placement in the Neurotone treated patient, or the auricular (heart-lung) acupuncture points formerly used in NET.

By the late 1970s and early 1980s, both Margaret Patterson and Ray Gilmer were marketing a small, pocket size unit. The difference was that Gilmer's "Relaxpak" was limited to 100 Hz and 800 microamperes, now pulsing with a modified square wave. Dr. Patterson's had different frequency (Hz) capabilities, 10 Hz for serotonin production and turnover (from rat studies), below 75 Hz for barbiturate addictions, 75 Hz - 300 Hz for narcotics, 2000 Hz for cocaine, etc. The pulse was a bilateral, modified square wave of unstated intensity. She liked to keep her pulse widths between 0.1 and 1.5 mS. By 1986, she was on the eighth version of her device. A lot of secrecy was still being maintained surrounding its stimulus characteristics. Its stimulus intensity was not published, but she stated that available frequency rates should range from 1 Hz to 2000 Hz, so her newest device probably did.

At about that same time Dr. Daniel L. Kirsch was inventing microcurrent stimulators for pain treatment. He had begun his studies of electrical stimulation parameters as early as 1972, working with physician-acupuncturists. Like Patterson, his later work took him far afield from acupuncture. His present Alpha-Stim technology takes into account the pulse wave harmonics available in the specialized basic pulse characteristics of the stimulators he now has developed. In his pain treatment device he designed a technology that did not require numerous separate pulses per second, as in Patterson's device, since they are all readily available in the harmonics. These would later be made a part of his CES technology also.

The mini electroshock vs. acupuncture theories died down or became less important as other device manufactures attempted to enter the U.S. market. The FDA made it very difficult for all of them, even though the FDA had permitted entrance into the American market of TENS stimulators for pain control, electrical biofeedback monitors, cardiac pacemakers, and electromagnetic bone healing devices, among others, well after CES had been in medical use in the U.S. Unlike CES, these were for real medical problems, not mere psychiatric complaints. For more than 20 years and counting, the FDA has created two major blocks to the success of CES in the U.S. marketplace.

To comprehend this, it helps to know that the Device Amendment Act of 1976 required the FDA to call in for review and classification all medical devices on the market at the time the law was passed. Since they could not get to all of them right away, these devices were retained on the market in a so-called grandfathered open market status. In something of a semantic quirk, all devices were classified as either Class I, for devices that met all safety and effectiveness standards, and in addition had developed precise good manufacturing practice (GMP) guidelines, Class II, for devices that met safety and effectiveness standards but lacked the GMP guidelines, and Class III for those that were still undergoing basic research and had shown neither safety nor effectiveness. The latter were not allowed to be marketed in the U.S. The catch was that the FDA also had another Classification III, in which were put all grandfathered devices that they had not yet reclassified, but which legally remained on the market.

Like all electrical stimulators in the U.S.A., CES had earlier been declared a prescription only device, so it was not available over the counter in the U.S., and third party payers were usually billed for the treatment. When CES marketers attempted to make sales to medical professionals for the use of CES in treating their patients, third party payers invariably called the FDA regarding CES, and were invariably simply told that it was a Class III device. No additional explanation was given. The third party payer would hang up the telephone and refuse to pay for treatment with what they assumed was a research device. Medical insurers do not knowingly pay for research, of course. They presumably would have paid for grandfathered Class III devices, however, had they known or been told. An exception to FDA's practice in this regard occurred when a senator called the FDA at the request of a CES company in his home state and asked the status of CES. An FDA lawyer wrote him a fine letter explaining in detail the actual situation of CES being a grandfathered Class III device with legal access to the open market. This indicated that FDA personnel knew the difference in the two Class III categories, they just were not telling.[29]

The second thing of note that FDA did, to all appearances, was to make an in-house decision in the early to mid 1990s to get rid of CES once and for all. They published a call-up for CES in the *Federal Register*, and companies then on the market were required to submit all their scientific evidence for CES's safety and effectiveness. FDA's Neurology Panel was to go over all of this data and make its classification recommendation to the Commissioner. If no CES company complied, CES would automatically fall out of its grandfathered open marketing status and be taken off the market. Several companies sent in all of their data, however, including some that had legally come onto the market tied to the apron strings of the original grandfathered device. Only Electromedical Products International, Inc., submitted a full-blown Premarket Approval Application (PMA), the medical device equivalent of a new drug application.

FDA knew not to trust its Neurology Panel too far, since its earlier panel, convened in 1978, had recommended the approval of CES for the treatment of addictions. So FDA now inserted into the middle of this process one of its staff members who had a masters degree in mechanical engineering. Her task was to review all of the scientific studies, published in peer reviewed medical journals, plus several masters theses and doctoral dissertations, completed under supposedly competent university faculty. Every study, without exception, she discounted as not being science, for reasons she determined on a case by case basis as she read them. To say it another way, this rather low ranking staff member did something she presumably would not have had the political intestinal fortitude to do unless she was under a direct order from higher in the organization. She single handedly dismissed over 100 clinical and scientific studies, 90% of which were behavioral science studies, a subject not taught in schools of mechanical engineering, and then stated that there was nothing to present to the Neurology Panel which therefore would not be convened to review CES. Based on her analysis and recommendation, the Commissioner supposedly had no choice but to pull CES off the U.S. market once and for all, sending it back to square one as a research device. FDA's permission (its Investigational Device Exemption - IDE) would then be required prior to the initiation of any proposed research project with CES in the future. Simply by choosing to withhold the IDE, no future research studies would have been possible, and CES would have been dead once and for all in the U.S.A.

Luckily, Electromedical Products International, Inc., one of the few CES companies remaining, if not the only one, had in the interim accumulated enough earnings (and potential earnings, as it ultimately required) to file a law suit against the government, the result of which was that the FDA backed down. As of this writing CES remains in the grandfathered Class III category, and therefore legally still on the open market, but a reclassification petition with supporting documentation is on the FDA Commissioner's desk for his consideration in down classifying it to Class II. As luck would have it, that is one of the few procedures one can initiate with the FDA for which the FDA has no legally mandated response time limit. At this writing, the application has been on the Commissioner's desk for more than four years, and counting.

The major explanatory systems

When marketers go into the medical market place with a new treatment, physicians typically want to know how it does what it is said to do. While physicians used aspirin for over a hundred years before they knew about prostaglandins, they were not to be that easily persuaded to put electricity into a patient's head, unless of course it was the more acceptable electric shock (still in FDA's grandfathered Class III status as of this writing, and very much in active use). So it seemed necessary and advisable to discover CES's treatment mechanism, and that presented its own problems.

An interesting phenomenon that occurs when scientists around the world get together to discuss medical treatment, "electrosleep," in this instance, especially when it involves the head, is that there are in existence completely different theoretical medical explanatory systems. When these are translated into English, Americans find that although all the words are in their English vocabulary, they have no clue as to what the other person is saying. Or as one American researcher succinctly stated the problem following a paper read by a Yugoslavian researcher at an international CES conference in Bulgaria which had been simultaneously translated into English over our headphones, "What the hell?!"

The Russians have a theoretical science built on the great Pavlov's research and concomitant theoretical constructs. They conceptualize most neural conditions and events in terms of inhibition, disinhibition, neural excitation, conditioning and the like. Thus, in a paper given at an international congress on CES, one researcher reported, "According to current concepts (Land, Myasnikov), hypertension is a neurosis of the higher regions of the central nervous system which involves the appearance of stagnant foci of excitation in the cerebral cortex and adjacent subcortical structures. As a result, various autonomic-humoral disturbances develop, including increased arterial pressure."[30] He had researched the successful use of CES in patients with high blood pressure.

Another East Block researcher stated, "positive therapeutic effect(s) occur more frequently in patients showing signs of protective inhibition in the cerebral cortex," adding, "Patients with the best therapeutic results of electrosleep were distinguished by the extraordinary instability and speedy wearing off of their conditioned responses and by the presence of a well marked external and after-inhibition." It was concluded that the predominant defect in this group of patients was weakness of the excitation process, accompanied by a tendency towards the development of protective inhibition in the cortex.[31] In any event, CES successfully treated the condition.

Thus, a great number of positive findings by former East Block researchers are still lost to the American scientist and clinician because of our theoretical differences and, consequently, our ways of understanding and stating study findings.

In the West, we tend to conceptualize brain activity in terms of neurochemical reactions at the presynaptic/postsynaptic neural membrane juncture. Thus, Pozos and his group at the University of Tennessee Medical Center studied the cholinergic/adrenergic system in several experiments with dogs. They injected their subjects with reserpine, a dopamine reuptake blocker, then applied electric current to engender increased dopamine release into the synapse and consequent depletion when this was broken down by monoamine oxidase (MAO). This gave the dogs Parkinson-like symptoms. Then, while the reserpine was still blocking the dopamine reuptake, atropine was injected to act as a blocker to the postsynaptic uptake of acetylcholine, thereby preventing or reducing acetylcholine's effect on the postsynaptic membrane. Now the dogs' Parkinson-like symptoms disappeared, the dogs returning to normal behavior. To further check their theoretical system, the researchers removed the atropine and added physostigmine to the still reserpinized dogs. The physostigmine was intended to block the MAO breakdown of intrasynaptic acetylcholine, making more of it available. The dogs responded with their most profound Parkinson-like symptoms. Finally, the researchers removed all drugs from the dogs' bloodstream and found that dogs allowed to go about their normal activities recovered in three to seven days, while a similar group given CES stimulation recovered in two to eight hours.[32]

Similarly, Mark Gold and his group did a double-blind study in which medical inpatients who were addicted to narcotics were withdrawn using either alpha methyl dopa as an α-blocker at norepinephrine's postsynaptic receptor in the locus ceruleus (to make up for the relative lack of available β-endorphins to balance norepinephrine's stimulation effect), or CES. The CES group received no medication, but received stimulation for one hour per day during the withdrawal period, which lasted a minimum of three days. The physicians who evaluated the patients on a daily basis during their withdrawal could not tell which patients were on which treatment, until the α-blocker was removed from that group and they responded with rebound depression, presumably due to the newly MAO depleted levels of norepinephrine which had been built up in the intrasynaptic space. The CES patients, who were theoretically stimulated by CES to increase their β-endorphin production up to a prior homeostatic level, did not show rebound depression following the cessation of CES therapy.[33]

To restate, in the West we tend to theorize in terms of neurochemicals balancing each other in a homeostatic relationship in the brain. As a result, in medical practice we add additional chemicals to an unbalanced system, dopamine in Parkinson patients, for example, α-blockers (*e.g.,* clonodine in withdrawing alcoholics), β-blockers (*e.g.,* sometimes used in heart dysrhythmias), or MAO blockers to increase the effective amount of a given neurochemical being ejected from the presynaptic vesicles.

Where does the need for all of this intervention come from? Hans Selye, M.D., warned us some time ago that persons who experience continuing environmental stress will readjust their ongoing homeostasis to the stress response and experience recurring physiological problems as a result of our sympathetic neurohormonal system constantly being poised for the fight or flight reaction. If this continues, after a short time the entire immune system begins to break down.[34] That we as a people frequently shift into abnormal neuroelectrical states should not be surprising.

Our brain presumably evolved as we ambled over an open plain with a couple of goats, a cow and a few chickens to keep us company. Now we speed along the highway to work and back from 30 to 70 miles per hour, often work in high rise buildings where we can look out a window and see the ground some 15 floors or more below, then come home to our house, in a crowded neighborhood full of people we have never met.

For restful entertainment after dinner, we glue ourselves to the television and watch bodies blown apart with submachine guns, thrown out of the windows of skyscrapers or burned to death in spectacular conflagrations. In addition, we easily forget that there is a Central or a South America right on our doorstep until something really bad goes wrong down there and we get to see the resulting starving, bleeding, drowned, or mangled bodies in our living room on the six o'clock news. Ditto Afganistan, Africa, Bangladesh, etc.

For health reasons, it would obviously be best if we could get back to our brain's more normal homeostasis, but when we medicate the brain in an effort to force it back, we encroach upon the brain's natural mechanisms and it can never return to normal while the drug is present. Often the drug becomes essentially addictive in that it can not then be removed without sending the patient through the dreaded withdrawal syndrome complete with its intense depression, anxiety and sleeplessness, if not seizures.

CES on the other hand is intended to gently prod the various neurohormonal systems back into their pre stress homeostatic relationships. Once it has done that, CES ceases to have an effect, and no patient to date has shown habituation, much less an addiction to CES upon clinical follow-up of from one to two years post prescription.

A third major theoretical system, held in China and much of the Far East, theorizes in terms of man existing in a unified nature, the Tao, which contains and consists of polar and complementary aspects, the Yin and Yang. Nature is in constant motion, and when the Yin and Yang forces are in balance, life is harmonious and flourishes. Not so when the forces are out of balance. Man is seen as a microcosm of Nature. Chi is the life force in the body. Organ networks communicate with each other via an invisible web of channels transporting Chi.

These pathways are called meridian pathways. There are twelve paired meridians, half on the right side of the body and half on the left, plus two midline meridians. Dr. Robert T. Story gives an excellent summary of recent research in which these channels have been delineated with radioactive tracings, and gives some basic ideas of how these interact with the neuronal system in the body.[35] The Chi courses through the body in perpetual motion in channels that empty into one another, intersect, and have inner body as well as surface streams, connecting the interior with the exterior of the body. In a healthy person, Chi moves freely throughout the body. In the ill person, Chi is heavy, oppressive, constrictive and congestive. It is no longer moving freely.

Acupuncture is a process of stirring up the Chi so that stasis is overcome, thereby restoring circulation. The system then returns to normal. By eliminating congestion and activating circulation of Chi, then, acupuncture interrupts and disorganizes patterns of illness.[36]

The theoretical action of CES in this system would be to electrically stimulate the Chi when in stasis and encourage its free movement throughout the body once again.

New theoretical models

There is every evidence that we are on the threshold of moving on to new theoretical explanatory models in the West as of this writing. In the forefront of these theories are those regarding biologically closed electric circuits, put forth by Björn Nordenström, M.D.,[37] and the extraneuronal semiconducting ion flow network theory of Robert O. Becker, M.D.[38] Both men have spent their careers as research scientists, their work cutting across lines of established scientific and professional specialties.

Both systems recognize the current of injury in which the polarity at the site of an injury in the body turns positive almost immediately, then gradually back to negative as healing begins and continues. Both recognize that there is an electromagnetic energy field surrounding the electron flow channel, and that this can interact with electromagnetic pressure impinging on it from the outside to change the ion potential and ion flow characteristics inside the closed channel.

In more than 20 years of research, Becker elaborated the direct current system that flows not thorough the nerves, but through the ubiquitous nerve support cells, the glial, ependymal, and Schwann cells. These, he found, act as semiconductors, passing slow speed analogue DC current from the central to the peripheral body areas along the motor nerve support cells, and from the periphery toward the central body axes via the sensory nerve support cells. He speculated that the system interlocks physically with the nervous system and is most likely its precursor.

Once he had found the current of injury, Becker devoted a great deal of his career to studying these energy relationships as body parts repaired or regenerated in various lower animals, most notably the salamander. As a result of his work the FDA authorized the marketing of an electromagnetic device to treat nonunion bone fractures in 1979. By 1986, over 15,000 fractures had been treated with these devices. In 1984, the queen of England had a painfully strained shoulder successfully treated with two, 90-minute treatments with a pulsed electro-magnetic field device.[39]

Once Björn Nordenström had discovered biologically closed electrical circuits, his research led him into the bloodstream to discover what drew white blood cells and other disease fighting organisms to the wound site, followed by other blood components that nourished and supplied the wound as healing took place. He discovered that it was the electrical changes in the wound site and within the vascular system itself that was working the changes at the wound area. He went on to discover that the vascular system functions as a closed electrical system, whose blood elements serve as ion conductors while the vascular walls act as insulators. The arteries, the veins and the capillaries all have distinct and separate functions in this organic system. He concluded that the release of energy by injured and dying cells could be the driving force - the battery - of the intravascular electric circuits.

Both researchers, working separately, concluded that since these DC currents are electrical, and have electromagnetic fields, many, if not all of them can be measured with the extremely sensitive instruments now available. These fields are also sensitive to impinging electromagnetic fields from inside and outside the body.

Becker found that an external electromagnetic field imposed on the body's electro-magnetic field could reverse ion flow and change ordinary positive areas in the body, to negative and vice versa. By imposing a magnetic field around the normally negatively charged part of the head of a salamander he could force the charge into positive such as it was when the animal was under anesthesia. Immediately, whole body anesthesia resulted. Similarly, the human head records negative in front and positive in back, and both poles rotate positions when the person is asleep or is under general anesthesia.

In following up on his earlier findings, Becker worked with a hypnotist and discovered that under hypnosis the front of the person's head changed from its normal negative potential, dropping down toward zero as the hypnotic trance deepened. That is, the potential changed just as it would have in anesthesia, just not as far. Also, following a post hypnotic suggestion that a subject's arm would not feel pain, the arm potential went from negative to positive, just as it did when procaine was injected.

Meanwhile, Nordenström's research centered on cancer and he began to use electrodes inserted into cancers and nearby areas in the lung to test his theories. With his techniques, he reliably reduced or totally eliminated cancers up to four millimeters in diameter. In the process, he found the vascular-interstitial closed electric circuit, which represented energy pathways available in vascularized tissues. Its function is for blood vessels to serve as electrical conducting "cables" which are capable of connecting different regions of tissue over conducting interstitial fluid.

Interestingly, both Nordenström and Becker recognized acupuncture points as active areas for energy input into the body, and Becker went so far as to measure the unique electrical potential around each of the 50% of the points he found electrically active, a subject that others had also been investigating.[40] In systems described by both researchers there are theoretical mechanisms in which ions moving through the acupuncture meridians could enter the otherwise closed circuits. In Becker's system, the *Nodes of Ranvier* appearing as microscopic gaps between the Schwann cells lining the neural axon would be among several such sites where externally impinging ions could change the physical characteristics of the electrical impulse as it moves down the axon toward the dendrites. This would, in turn, effect a quantitative change in either the activating or inhibiting outcome of the neuron's fire. In Nordenström's system, charged membranes of the cells of the capillary walls admit impinging ions via gates and vesicles. When electrons cross an enzyme bridge through the capillary wall it closes this local, capillary circuit and forces ionic flow through the longer distance circuit of the arteries and veins. Also, in the presence of injury, the venous walls do not close, and ions from the blood interact quite readily with those in the immediate environment, such as any that might be coming in via the meridians.

Both researchers showed intense interest in and not a little fear from the high levels of electromagnetic pollution present in the modern world, saying unequivocally that these were surely having large, unknown, and most likely negative effects on the body's electrical and electromagnetic control functions.

Both systems, then, add new and additional concepts to our present theories about the body and its inner workings. Nordenström's words were, "[this] means that we must revise extensively our present concepts of conversion of energy in biochemical reactions."[41]

Among Becker's comments were, "I predict that research on this system will eventually let us learn to control pain, healing, and growth with our minds alone, substantially reducing the need for physicians. …A combination of biofeedback, recording electrodes, and the Super Quantum Interference Device, an ultrasensitive magnetometer, would seem to be the ideal setup for the next level of inquiry into the mind's healing powers."[42]

Other medical models are also taking shape at the turn of the 21st century. Many researchers and clinicians in the steadily growing neurofeedback field have a theory that a disregulation of the brain's firing patterns is responsible for most of the behavioral pathologies that we see in modern American medicine, including the depression, anxiety and insomnia that CES is condoned to treat. This theory holds that the thalamus is the command center in the brain that directs traffic flow to and from the body to the cortex and back again. Its firing pattern determines whether alpha, beta, theta or delta waves will be predominant in a given part of the brain at any given time, and in what combinations. These patterns, in turn, determine much of our behavior. Normal thalamic function can be altered by any number of things from psychological trauma to various kinds of physical trauma, and the thalamus will begin sending somewhat deranged firing orders into various parts of the brain causing depression, anxiety, insomnia, attention deficit disorder, eating disorders, addictions, and even uncontrollable criminal behavior by some individuals, to list a few. "Nearly all health problems, this model holds, flow from overarousal, underarousal, or instability in the central nervous system."[43] In this theoretical system, while neurotherapy acts to retrain specific, unwanted brain wave patterns in various parts of the brain, CES would be thought of as normalizing the overall firing pattern to bring it back into its pretrauma homeostasis.

Also having an increasingly important effect on present medical thinking is Candace P. Pert's report of the finding that all white blood cells throughout the body manufacture all of the so-called neurotransmitters, and that the brain reacts not only to neurotransmitters but even has insulin receptors, among others previously unexpected. White blood cell activities can be changed by emotional experiences, and these experiences can, in turn, change the way white blood cells behave. The relationship between the two have a memory effect, so that white blood cell changes that take place when an individual is depressed, can then cause depression when that pattern of white blood cell activity occurs again at some future time.[44] This has meant a basic reorientation in the way we think about the mind-body relationship in immune system functioning, as an example. It has changed the way researchers approach anti-aging research and cancer research, among many others. The effect on American medicine will surely grow at an ever quickening pace as more information regarding the "mind-body" system becomes available.

Another major player in our medical concepts will be the important new findings in neural regeneration. Until recently we have been taught that neurons develop in the infant, and once formed no more neurons are produced, and if any are lost for any reason in the adult, no more can be formed. Research is showing that not only are new connections between existing neurons constantly being formed and lost, but new neurons also grow to replace those that are lost in persons of any age.[45] This kind of finding will have a major impact on future directions of CES research. For example it has been found that the hypothalamus has been damaged, with fewer viable neurons present, in depressed people, but tends to recover when the depression is eliminated. CES will take a major stride in coming out of the closet in American medicine if it is found that CES stimulates neural regeneration in previously traumatized areas of the brain, in the process of its well documented ability to cure depression.

In the near future, it is more than likely that these theoretical systems will be further developed and will be seen as the major players in much of the neurochemical related changes that are so central to the present medical theories in the West. Dr. Daniel L. Kirsch has been an early theoretician heralding this new age.[46,47] New theories will give great importance to the fact that the major cellular functions of our bodies appear to be controlled by the body's own DC electrical field. The new theories will give us for the first time a way of conceptualizing the forces that can guide the development of the human body from the first divisions of the egg in the womb to the incredible multitudes of cell differentiations that result in the finished body, and how these are maintained in wellness or interrupted in illness.

The people who are already out there well ahead of these theories that are likely to be next molded into being, will continue to be pelted with stones by otherwise respectable people until sometime in the future when even these pioneers may be brought into the fold of scientific respectability. I refer to those persons who say they are passing energy into other persons by the laying on of hands, those who are sure that stones pass healing energy via their innate semiconducting properties, and those who focus their energies in prayer onto the diseased or disabled, among many others.[48]

Unlike these, CES fortunately has already found respectability within the old neuro-chemical explanatory system, but it can be expected that CES will also find a strong position in the newly developing theories in which incoming pulsed electrical stimulation will be seen to provide a helpful and perhaps even necessary push to the stalled flow of Chi in the body, or of some intransigent positive electrical potential remaining where a negative potential is wanted, either along the extraneuronal semiconducting analog pathways, or in the biologically closed electric circuits within the vascular system.

Meanwhile, CES has gone beyond its earlier uses in the drug free treatment of anxiety, depression and insomnia, and has recently been found to be highly effective in the treatment of fibromyalgia, multiple sclerosis, and other difficult pain conditions, among other things.[49,50]

As of this writing, CES has now completed its 40 year apprenticeship in American medicine and, like limes on British ships, is in the process of entering into its legitimate place in mainstream medical practice. That has begun to happen even as you read this.

The following chapters in this book will indicate what is known about CES to date.

Ray B. Smith, Ph.D., M.P.A.
Mineral Wells, Texas

References

[1] Gordon, Richard. The alarming history of medicine. New York: St. Martin's Press, 1993. P. 49.

[2] Electromedical Products International, Inc. Owner's manual: Alpha-Stim 100 microcurrent stimulator. EPII, Mineral Wells, Texas, 2002.

[3] Editors of Time-Life Books. Mysteries of the unknown; Powers of healing. Time-Life Books: Alexandria, Virginia, 1997. P. 88.

[4] Melzack, Ronald, & Wall, Patrick. Pain mechanisms: a new theory. *Science*, 150: 971-979, 1965.

[5] Editors of Time-Life Books, Ibid, P. 88.

[6] Berlioz, Louis, Memoires sur les maladie chronique, les evacuations sanguines et l'acupuncture. Paris: Croullebois, 1816.

[7] Sarlandiere, Jean Baptiste, Memoires sur l'ectro-puncture, considere`e comme moyen nouveau de traiter efficiacement la goute, les rhumatismes et les affectiones verveuses. Paris, 1825.

[8] Cohen, L.H. Galvanopuncture; with a successful case of operation by electrolysis in a glandular tumor. *New York Medical Journal*, 223:380-387, 1875.

[9] Becker, Robert O. & Selden, Gary, The body electric; electromagnetism and the foundation of life. William Morrow, N.Y., 1985. P. 172.

[10] Becker, R. Ibid. Pp. 74-75.

[11] Kirsch, Daniel L. & Lerner, Fred N., Electromedicine: the other side of physiology. In Weiner, Richard S. (Ed.) Pain Management; A practical guide for clinicians. St Lucie Press, Boca Raton, Florida, 1998, P. 830.

[12] Cameron, Meribeth E. The reform movement in China, 1898-1912. Standford University Press, Stanford, CA, 1931.

[13] Editors of Time-Life Books. Ibid. P. 55.

[14] Brackman, Arnold C. The last emperor. Carroll & Graf; N.Y., 1975, Pp. 322-323.

[15] Gordon, R. Ibid. P. 229.

[16] Gordon, R. Ibid. P. 60.

[17] Richardson, Robert G. Surgery: Old and new frontiers, N.Y.: Charles Scribner's Sons, 1968, P. 169.

[18] Becker, R. Ibid. P. 155-156..

[19] Gordon, R. Ibid. P. 162.

[20] Gordon, R. Ibid. Chapter 8.

[21] Peppard, Harold M. Sight without glasses, Doubleday, Garden City, N.Y., 1936. P. 25.

[22] Fleming, A. On the antibacterial action of cultures of a penicillin with special reference to their use in the isolation of B. influenzae. *British Journal of Experimental Pathology*, 10:226, 1929.

[23] Gordon, R. Ibid. Pp. 69-73.

[24] Slaughter, Frank G., The new science of surgery. Julien Messner; N.Y., 1946. Chapter 4, *God's Powders*.

[25] Slaughter, F. Ibid. P. 47.

[26] Personal communication from Ray Gilmer, 1980.

[27] Wen, H.L. & Cheung, S.Y. Treatment of drug addiction by acupuncture and electrical stimulation. *Asian Journal of Medicine*, 9:138-41, 1973.

[28] Patterson, Meg. Hooked? NET: the new approach to drug cure. Faber and Faber, London, 1986. Chapter 3.

[29] Personal communication with Larry Paros, 1992.

[30] Kostyukhina, N.A. Comparative evaluation of capillarographic data of hypertensives during treatment with pulse currents (electrosleep, interference currents, and thythmic galvanic collar). In Wageneder, F.M. & St. Schuy (Eds.), Electrotherapeutic Sleep and Electroanesthesia. Vol. II, Amsterdam, Excerpta Medica, 1970.

[31] Titaeva, M.A. Changes in the functional state of the central nervous system under the influence of a pulse current as used in electrosleep. In Wageneder, F.M. & St. Shuy (Eds.) Electrotherapeutic sleep and electroanaesthesia. International Congress Series, No. 136. Excerpta Medica Foundation, Amsterdam, 1967.

[32] Pozos, Robert S., Strack, L.F., White, R.K. & Richardson, Alfred W. Electrosleep versus electroconvulsive therapy. In Reynolds, David V. & Anita Sjoberg, (Eds.), Neuroelectric Research. Charles Thomas: Springfield, 23:221-225, 1971.

[33] Gold, M.S., Pottash, A.L.C., Sternbach, H., Barbaban, J. & Aunitto, W. Antiwithdrawal effect of alpha methyl dopa and cranial electrotherapy. Paper presented at Society for Neuroscience, 12th annual meeting, October, 1982.

[34] Selye, Hans, The stress concept: past, present and future. In Stress Research, Cary L. Cooper (Ed.) 1983, John Wiley and Sons, N.Y., Pp. 4-6.

[35] Story, Robert T. Comprehensive meridian therapy. New York Chiropractic College, Seneca Falls, N.Y., 1995.

[36] Beinfield, Harriet & Korngold, Efrem, Between heaven and earth; A guide to Chinese medicine. Ballantine Books: N.Y., 1991.

[37] Nordenström, Björn E.W., Biologically closed electric circuits; clinical, experimental and theoretical evidence for an additional circulatory system. Nordic Medical Publications: Stockholm, Sweden, 1983.

[38] Becker, R.O., The basic biological data transmission and control system influenced by electrical forces. *Ann NY Acad Sci*. 238:236-41, 1974.

[39] London Times, The. Rubbing shoulders, *The times*, London, 1984; Sept. 5:12(Col 1).

[40] Bergsman, O. & Wooley-Hart, A. Differences in electrical skin conductivity between acupuncture points and adjacent skin areas. *Am. J. Acupuncture*. 1:27-32, 1973.

[41] Nordenström, Björn E.W., Ibid. P. 319.

[42] Becker, Robert, Ibid. Pp. 239, 242.

[43] Robbins, Jim, A symphony in the brain. Grove Press: N.Y., 2000, pp 200-202.

[44] Pert, Candace B. Molecules of emotion; the science behind mind-body medicine. Simon & Schuster: N.Y., 1999, P. 182.

[45] Underwood, Anne. Searching for a new and improved Prozac. *Newsweek*, December 31, 2001.

[46] Kirsch, Daniel L. Electromedicine: the other side of physiology. In Weiner, Richard S. (Ed.) Pain management: A practical guide for clinicians, 6th ed., Chapter 60, CRC Press: Boca Raton, 2002.

[47] Kirsch, Daniel L. A practical protocol for electromedical treatment of pain. In Weiner, Richard S. (Ed.) Pain management: A practical guide for clinicians, 6th ed., Chapter 61, CRC Press: Boca Raton, 2002.

[48] Gerber, Richard, Vibrational medicine for the 21st century. Harper Collins: N.Y., 2000.

[49] Lichtbroun, Alan S., Raicer, Mei-Ming C., Smith, Ray B. The treatment of fibromyalgia with cranial electrotherapy stimulation. *Journal of Clinical Rheumatology*, 7(2), 2001 Pp. 72-78.

[50] Smith, Ray B. The use of cranial electrotherapy stimulation in the treatment of multiple sclerosis. In process, *The International Journal of Multiple Sclerosis Care*, 2002.

3

86 PIVOTAL SCIENTIFIC STUDIES OF CES

Cranial Electrotherapy Stimulation (CES) arrived in the United States from the former USSR, Europe, and Japan, where it was originally called electrosleep. It has also been called transcranial electrotherapy (TCET), neuroelectric therapy (NET), neurotransmitter modulation, and other names. CES is the designated term the United States Food and Drug Administration uses for this treatment in the USA. Whatever terminology the authors used was changed to CES in the abstracts to maintain consistency for the reader. The titles were not changed. The early literature of the 1960s and 1970s is often confusing because when it was called electrosleep, it was thought that CES could actually induce sleep. We now know it controls anxiety, thus enabling one to sleep better, and inducing sleep is not required for CES to achieve its effect.

Overall, based on the authors' conclusions of the outcomes of their studies, 91% (78) of the pivotal scientific studies had positive outcomes.

INDEX TO PIVOTAL SCIENTIFIC STUDIES

Note: numbers reference studies, not pages.

A. DISORDERS STUDIED:

Alcohol: 1, 2, 30, 41, 47, 48, 58, 59, 64, 65, 66, 68, 71, 83

Anesthesia: 6, 43, 74, 75

Anxiety: 1, 3, 13, 14, 16, 17, 19, 20, 21, 22, 27, 28, 30, 31, 34, 36, 40, 41, 42, 45, 46, 47, 48, 49, 51, 53, 54, 55, 56, 57, 59, 67, 68, 69, 70, 71, 78, 80, 81, 82, 83, 86

Attention Deficit Disorder: 22, 67, 85

Bronchial Asthma: 14, 36

Cerebral Palsy: 33, 38, 44

Cigarette Withdrawal: 48

Closed Head Injuries: 70, 75

Cocaine: 5, 48, 71

Cognitive Dysfunction: 25, 35, 58, 64, 66, 67, 70, 73, 85

Dental: 8, 24, 86

Depression: 1, 3, 9, 13, 14, 16, 20, 28, 30, 31, 34, 36, 39, 40, 41, 42, 47, 49, 51, 53, 54 61, 67, 68, 70, 71

Fibromyalgia: 32, 50

Gastric Acidity: 29

Headaches: 4, 12, 28, 50, 72

Heroin: 19, 48

Labor: 6

Learning: 35, 73, 85

Marijuana: 46, 48

Methadone: 18, 19, 48

Muscle Tone/Movement/Tremor: 15, 28, 33, 37, 38, 44, 53, 65

Opiate: 18, 46, 48

Pain: 8, 22, 23, 24, 28, 32, 43, 55, 61, 72, 75, 79, 85

Phobia: 69

Polysubstance Abuse: 1, 2, 36, 41, 48, 49, 58, 59, 71

Reaction Time, Vigilance: 26, 35, 38

Rehabilitation: 15

Sex Offenders: 81, 82

Sleep (Induction of, and Insomnia): 9, 11, 13, 14, 15, 16, 19, 20, 25, 26, 28, 31, 32, 34, 36, 37, 42, 48, 49, 51, 53, 54, 56, 63, 76, 77, 84

Stress: 21, 28, 40, 46, 59, 60, 65, 67, 78, 83

Suggestibility: 9, 55, 57

Withdrawal: 1, 5, 18, 19, 46, 48, 49, 65

B. MEASURING STRATEGIES - PHYSIOLOGICAL

Electrocardiogram (EKG): 33

Electroencephalogram (EEG): 2, 9, 11, 14, 16, 22, 23, 25, 26, 30, 34, 36, 37, 60, 63, 77, 84

Electromyogram (EMG): 4, 15, 17, 21, 34, 37, 45, 46, 81, 82, 83

Intracerebral Current: 10

Skin Conductance or Capacitance: 21, 34, 45

Blood Pressure, Pulse, Respiration, and/or Heart Rate: 14, 21, 33, 37, 75, 78

Body Chemistry:

Basal Acid Secretion:	29
β-Endorphins:	30, 61, 62
Catecholamine:	3
Cholinesterase:	61
Dopamine:	30
GABA:	30
Histamine Stimulated Gastric Output:	29
17-hydroxycorticosteroid:	16
Ketosteroids:	3
MAO-B:	29, 30
Melatonin:	62
Norepinephrine:	61, 62
Serotonin:	30, 61, 62
Serum thyroxine:	52
Tri-iodothyronin resin uptake:	52

Fantanyl Requirements During Anesthesia: 43, 74

Nitrous Oxide Requirements During Anesthesia: 75

Peripheral Temperature/Peripheral Vascular Tension: 4, 21, 45, 78, 81

C. MEASURING STRATEGIES - PSYCHOLOGICAL

Beck's Anxiety and/or Depression Inventory: 1, 41, 42

Benton Visual Retention Test: 66

Beta Nonverbal IQ Test: 66

Eysenck Personality Inventory: 42, 80

Global Evaluations - Subject: 8, 12, 20, 45, 48, 50, 51, 69, 72, 76, 86

Global Evaluations - Researcher: 14, 20, 48, 51, 53, 54, 56, 57, 72, 75, 76, 78, 80, 86

Hamilton Anxiety Scale (HAS): 1, 19, 27, 57

Hamilton Depression Scale: 1

Harvard Scale of Hypnotic Susceptibility: 55

Himmelsbach Scale: 1, 48

Institute for Personality and Ability Testing (IPAT) - Anxiety Scale: 59

Institute for Personality and Ability Testing (IPAT) - Depression Scale: 67

Izard's Differential Emotion Scale: 39

Minnesota Multiphasic Personality Inventory (MMPI): 30, 65, 84

Montgomery and Asberg Depression Rating Scale (MADRS): 49

Multiple Affect Adjective Check List (MAACL): 41, 47

NIMH Self Rating Symptom Scale (SRSS): 20

16-Personality Factors (16-PF): 46

Profile of Mood States (POMS): 32, 40, 59, 68, 70, 71, 83, 85

Rancho Los Amigos Scale: 7

Revised Beta Examination I.Q. Test: 58, 64, 66

Sexual Inventory: 82

State/Trait Anxiety Inventory (STAI): 17, 30, 40, 47, 55, 56, 59, 67, 78, 80, 81, 82

Taylor Manifest Anxiety Scale (TMAS): 16, 19, 30, 31, 42, 57

Visual Analogue Scale (VAS): 49, 86

WAIS (WISC) OBS Scales: 58, 67

Zung Depression Scale: 13, 14, 16, 30, 31, 51, 53, 54, 61

D. DEVICES USED IN THE PIVOTAL SCIENTIFIC STUDIES OF CES:

Alpha-Stim 2000, 350, CS, and 100: 4, 5, 17, 21, 22, 23, 28, 32, 35, 41, 45, 46, 60, 67, 69, 79, 81, 82, 86

Anesthelec: 6

CES Labs: 67, 70

Diastim: 49

Dormed: 31

Electrodorn: 29, 84

Electrosone 50: 13, 14, 16, 26, 34, 53, 54

Electrosom: 76

Grass S88 & Grass S1U5: 10

HealthPax: 2

Hess 100: 25

LB 2000: 1

Liss Stimulator: 23, 61, 62, 67, 73

LRDE model HB-1705: 63

Neurometer: 78

Neurotone 101: 9, 12, 20, 27, 42, 47, 55, 56, 58, 59, 64, 65, 66, 68, 80, 83

Neurotransmitter Modulator: 24, 38, 44

Pain Supressor: 33, 50, 72

RelaxPak: 40, 85

Somlec: 11, 57

Not specified: 3, 7, 8, 15, 18, 19, 30, 36, 37, 39, 43, 48, 51, 52, 71, 74, 75, 77

Although several studies did not specify the device used by name, some of those did specify the electrical characteristics. In some studies, the researchers made their own device.

E. RESEARCH METHODOLOGY:

Double-Blind, Placebo-Controlled: 1, 4, 6, 8, 12, 13, 18, 20, 21, 22, 23, 25, 27, 30, 31, 32, 35, 43, 47, 49, 51, 55, 58, 59, 60, 64, 70, 72, 75, 78, 79, 80, 81, 84, 86

Single-blind: 17, 19, 39, 54, 68, 74, 76, 77, 83

Controlled Study: 2, 3, 5, 14, 34, 40, 46, 57, 61, 66, 71, 73, 79, 82, 85

Crossover: 16, 26, 38, 42, 43, 80

Open Clinical Trial: 11, 15, 24, 29, 33, 36, 37, 41, 44, 48, 50, 52, 53, 54, 56, 62, 63, 65, 67, 69, 79, 82

Retrospective Study: 28, 45

Single Case Experimental Design or Case Study: 6, 9, 10

Follow-up: 5, 14, 15, 20, 21, 22, 36, 40, 42, 45, 48, 67, 84

1. Bianco Jr., Faust. The efficacy of cranial electrotherapy stimulation (CES) for the relief of anxiety and depression among polysubstance abusers in chemical dependency treatment. Ph.D. dissertation, The University of Tulsa Graduate School, Pp. 1-224, 1994.

Device: LB 2000, 100 Hz, 2mS, <1.5 mA, electrodes behind the ears at the mastoid process

After achieving Institutional Review Board (IRB) approval and informed consent, 65 polysubstance abusers with no history of psychosis were recruited from the Oklahoma Department of Human Services and split into 3 groups for this double-blind study using blinding boxes. Patients were at a lock-in unit at the Chemical Dependency Unit. 36 subjects (18 CES, 16 controls, and 5 sham CES) left against medical advice. 20 males and 9 females from 20 to 49 years old (mean of 31.3) completed the full course of 45 minutes daily for 6 - 14 days. 9 patients in group 1 (31%) were non-CES controls receiving standard treatment, 9 patients (31%) in group 2 received simulated CES plus standard treatment, 11 patients (38%) received active CES plus standard treatment. The revised Beck Anxiety and Depression Inventories, and the Symptom Check List of the Himmelsbach Scale were administered, along with an attention placebo control interview, and observer-rated measures employed by 2 researchers: the Structured Interview Guide for the Hamilton Anxiety and Depression Scales. In order to achieve a power of .8 (beta = .2), alpha was calculated at .05, effect size at .60, and N at 30 (10 per group). Scheffe tests were performed to determine the significance between the means of each of the 3 groups. There was no significant difference between variables at pre-test. However, analysis of variance (ANOVA) revealed significant post-test group differences.

Hamilton Anxiety means for CES pre-test was 24.44 ± 9.22 to a post-test of 7.09 ± 3.21, for sham CES pre-test was 22.56 ± 9.95 and post-test was 15.67 ± 7.92, and for controls pre-test was 20.56 ± 6.21 and post-test was 16.89 ± 9.06. Scheffe post hoc tests for Hamilton was significant between the CES and controls (P<.05) and between the CES and sham (P<.05), but not the sham and controls (P>.05) as measured by the observer ratings. Beck Anxiety post-test means were not significant, means for CES pre-test was 22.91 ± 10.99 to a post-test of 5.27 ± 5.23, for sham CES pre-test was 28.78 ± 15.21 and post-test was 9.33 ± 7.97, and for controls pre-test was 21.44 ± 9.89 and post-test was 9.78 ± 12.17. Although the self-reports showed no statistical differences between groups, there was a trend towards significance.

Hamilton Depression means for CES pre-test was 24.91 ± 6.67 to a post-test of 5.46 ± 2.91, for sham CES pre-test was 22.33 ± 10.14 and post-test was 14.56 ± 9.08, and for controls pre-test was 20.33 ± 6.56 and post-test was 17.44 ± 6.97. Scheffe post hoc tests for Hamilton was significant between the CES and controls (P<.05) and between the CES and sham (P<.05), but not the sham and controls (P>.05) as measured by the observer ratings. Beck Depression means were not significant, means for CES pre-test was 29.27 ± 10.25 to a post-test of 6.91 ± 4.46, for sham CES pre-test was 25.11 ± 10.86 and post-test was 11.22 ± 11.16, and for controls pre-test was 27.56 ± 9.74 and post-test was 12.11 ± 6.15.

The study did not control for medications. The author concluded that the active CES, when combined with the normal treatment regimen given at the treatment facilities was more effective in reducing anxiety and depression than the normal treatment regimen alone and the sham CES plus normal treatment regimen. Thus, the anticipated results regarding CES was supported, while the anticipated results regarding placebo effect was not supported. No side effects were reported.

2. Braverman, Eric, Smith, Ray B., Smayda, Richard, & Blum, Kenneth. Modification of P300 amplitude and other electrophysiological parameters of drug abuse by cranial electrical stimulation. *Current Therapeutic Research*. 48(4):586-596, 1990.

Device: HealthPax, 100 Hz, 20% duty cycle, 1.0 mA, no dc bias, square waves, electrodes at left wrist and forehead

Electrophysiological abnormalities are said to be hallmarks of the high risk individual for drug abuse and the drug abuser. P300 waves occur 300 mS after a cognitive auditory potential and have been shown to have a reduced amplitude in many alcoholics, which does not revert to normal even after continued abstinence. Earlier research has concluded that the need to modify these electrophysiological parameters could be of critical importance in the treatment and possibly the prevention of drug abuse. In this study 13 alcohol and/or drug abusers (9 - 81 years old, mean of 43.44) and 2 staff controls were selected as they entered the clinic for brain electrical activity mapping (BEAM, a computerized EEG). After providing informed consent, all were given 40 minutes of CES between pre- and post-CES BEAM scans. There were no significant changes in the controls. Following CES the patient's P300 amplitude increased significantly (P<.05) as analyzed by Fisher t-tests which compared the differences between the means and variances. The time went from a pretreatment of 308 ± 24 to 317 ± 26 msec post-treatment. The amplitude (dV) went from pretreatment of 7.0 ± 4.1 to 9.9 ± 6.0 post-treatment. Also, there were significant positive shifts in alpha, delta, theta and beta spectra in patients who were abnormal in one or more of these areas prior to CES treatment.

It was concluded that CES might be a significant non-drug treatment for the underlying electrophysiological disorder of the drug abuser, because the normalization of these electrophysiological parameters are characteristic of pharmaceutical treatment. The authors concluded that they believe the future is bright for prescriptive electricity, and that the electrophysiological changes that occur as a result of CES have the greatest implication for America's #1 health problem, drug abuse. No side effects were reported.

3. Briones, David F. & Rosenthal, Saul H. Changes in urinary free catecholamine and 17-ketosteroids with cerebral electrotherapy (electrosleep). *Diseases of the Nervous System*. 34:57-58, 1973.

Device: 100 Hz, 1 mS, positive pulses, cathodes over orbits, anodes over mastoids

7 male patients from 22 to 37 years old were given 30 minutes of CES for 5 days. 4 were "normal" volunteers and 3 were hospitalized psychiatric patients with neurotic anxiety and depression. Total free catecholamines were measured by bio-rad column (normal is 0 - 115 microgram per 24 hours) prior to and after 5 CES treatments. Pre- and post-testing means revealed a 23.9 to 47.4 microgram increase in 24 hour urinary free catecholamine across all patients, with the greatest rise in 2 anxiety patients and 1 volunteer who was slightly symptomatic. The average gain in 24 hour urinary 17 ketosteroids was 6.9 mgs, pretreatment mean was 18.5 and post-treatment was 25.4 (normal is 10 to 24 mgs per 24 hours). 2 patients had insignificantly reduced levels. The authors suggested that these findings probably reflected change at the hypothalamic or pituitary level in the brain. No side effects were reported.

4. Brotman, Philip. Low-intensity transcranial electrostimulation improves the efficacy of thermal biofeedback and quieting reflex training in the treatment of classical migraine

headache. *American Journal of Electromedicine.* **6(5):120-123, 1989. Also Ph.D. dissertation, City University Los Angeles, Pp. 1-117, 1986.**

Device: Alpha-Stim 2000GL, 0.5 Hz, 50% duty cycle, <500 µA, biphasic asymmetrical rectangular waves, ear clip electrodes

In this double-blind study, 36 females, ages 18 - 40, suffering from classical migraine headaches (ICD-9 346.0), completed informed consent and were randomly assigned to Quieting Reflex Training (QR) and placebo CES (N = 12), QR plus actual Alpha-Stim CES (N = 12), or CES only groups (N = 12). All groups were measured for temperature changes using thermal biofeedback (TB) via finger monitors on the dominant hand, and temporalis muscle electromyogram (EMG). All received 8 treatments, plus 1, 2, and 3 month follow-up sessions. Medication levels dropped dramatically from the initial session to the eighth session. Fischer t-tests were employed separately for investigation of CES and QR. Results were calculated using the formula of frequency x intensity of headaches. The findings were that groups receiving TB and QR, either with CES (pretreatment mean of 14.42 ± 6.26, post treatment of 4.50 ± 5.30) or with placebo CES (pretreatment mean of 15.33 ± 6.62, post treatment of 4.33 ± 4.46), responded significantly better than did the TB CES group alone (pretreatment mean of 14.00 ± 4.56, post treatment of 6.33 ± 4.38), but that the group receiving TB, QR, and CES responded significantly better (mean of .08 ± 0.28) than the TB, QR and placebo CES group (mean of .58 ± 1.19) or the TB and CES group (mean of 8.67 ± 6.60) at the 3 month follow-up period. Only the CES group showed significant carry over effects in finger temperature. EMG findings of the CES groups showed a recovery to normal 15 minutes after treatment. Those groups that did not receive the CES treatment were subsequently treated with CES and they achieved headache reductions comparable to those obtained in the TB, QR, and CES group.

Observations during the study suggested that CES may contribute to both a rapid rise of finger temperature during each session and to a homeostatic rise in finger temperature over time. It was suggested that this was possibly due to a hypothalamic mechanism. No subjects in CES or placebo CES groups reported side effects.

5. Brovar, Alan. Cocaine Detoxification with cranial electrotherapy stimulation (CES): A preliminary appraisal. *International Electromedicine Institute Newsletter.* **1(4):1-4, 1984.**

Device: Alpha-Stim 350, 0.5 Hz, 50% duty cycle, <500 µA, biphasic asymmetrical rectangular waves, ear clip electrodes

25 consecutive admissions to a drug abuse treatment hospital that qualified for DSM III diagnosis of cocaine abuse were included in the study. Patients were alternately assigned to a control group (N = 12), and Alpha-Stim CES treatment (N = 13), of which only 5 accepted while 8 refused. CES was given for 20 minutes twice a day for the 5 day inpatient treatment program. All 5 (100%) of the CES patients completed detoxification, compared with 75% of the other 20. All 5 (100%) of the CES patients completed the treatment program, compared with 63% of the CES refusers and 67% of the other 12 controls. A follow-up of the 3 groups from 6 to 8 months later showed that no CES patients had returned for treatment, while 50% of the CES refusers and 39% of the controls had recidivated. One of the latter had died of overdose.

The role of CES in the treatment of chemical dependency is of great interest since anxiety and insomnia are frequently present in the early stages of recovery and are a common precursor to relapse. The authors concluded that CES facilitated patient retention in a hospital detoxification and rehabilitation program for cocaine dependent persons. No side effects were reported.

6. Champagne, C., Papiernik, E., Thierry, J.P. & Noviant, Y. Transcutaneous cerebral electric stimulation by Limoge current during labor. *Ann Fr Anesth Reanim*. 3:405-13, 1984. (France)

Device: Anesthelec, 166 kHz, intermittent - 100 Hz, 3 electrodes: a negative electrode placed between the eyebrows and positive electrodes located in the retro-mastoid regions

In order to test the analgesic efficacy of CES during labor and delivery, a double-blind study was performed in 20 cases for whom analgesia was necessary. In 10 cases CES was used with the current on and in 10 cases as a sham. Labor and delivery were carried out by a medical team different from those who set up the CES. The results showed that this method, with or without nitrous oxide inhalation, decreased by 80% the number of epidural and general anesthesia that would otherwise have been unavoidable. To define the effects of this new method, maternal and fetal parameters of 50 deliveries carried out under CES were compared with 50 deliveries carried out under epidural analgesia. CES was used only if analgesia was required. This study was a retrospective comparison between two similar non-paired series. Despite the fact that analgesia obtained with CES was less powerful than with epidural analgesia, this method showed many advantages: total safety for the child and the mother, easy utilization, shorter labor time, decreased number of instrumental extractions and potentially reduced costs. Good acceptance and satisfaction for the mother should allow a rapid evolution of this new method.

7. Childs, Allen. Droperidol and CES in Organic Agitation, *Clinical Newsletter*, Austin Rehabilitation Hospital, 1995.

Device:100 Hz, electrodes below the mastoids

Confused and agitated post-head injury (or post-anoxic or post-stroke) patients, often referred to as "Rancho Level IV" from the Rancho Los Amigo I-VIII Scale, is described as, "The patient is in a heightened state of activity with severely decreased ability to process information. He is detached from the present and responds primarily to his own internal confusion. Behavior is frequently bizarre and non-purposeful relative to his immediate environment. He may cry out or scream out of proportion to stimulus even after removal. He may show aggressive behavior and attempt to remove restraints or tubes."

This is a case report of a 33 year old male Rancho IV patient given p.r.n. droperidol along with CES. The patient developed meningitis at age 14 which left him with a generalized tonic-clonic seizure disorder, but seizures were controlled until 2 years later when he suffered a significant concussion playing high school football. At that time he experienced up to 7 generalized tonic-clonic seizures a day, uncontrollable by medication. In 1989 he underwent a right temporal lobectomy which resulted in a disappearance of the seizures for 2 years. In 1991 he experienced the acute onset of status epilepticus and then prolonged coma. He was diagnosed with viral encephalitis. On awakening, his behavior deteriorated into confusion, sexual inappropriateness, and dangerous aggression. MRI showed left temporal ishemia and atrophy with enlargement of the left temporal horn and atrium of the left temporal ventricle. Topographical EEG showed increased right temporal and frontal slowing. Brain stem auditory, middle latency, and 40 hertz evoked potentials were all abnormal. Haldol, Norpramin, Verapamil, lithium, sodium amytal, and lorazepam were all ineffective.

In the first 7 months of his inpatient stay, he was physically aggressive 247 times, door rattling 1,983 times, exhibited 58 verbal threats, refused tasks 453 times, and attempted to elope 200 times. On introduction of droperidol, the assaultive episodes decreased from an average of 8 to 4 per week, with substantially diminished duration.

5 weeks after beginning p.r.n. droperidol, 30 minutes twice daily CES was added. There was an immediate lessening of tension in the first 3 weeks of treatment, and the violent assaults ceased. In addition to extinguishing the physical aggression, the p.r.n. droperidol-CES treatment was successful in decreasing the other 4 behaviors: door rattling down 76%, verbal threats down 100% (to zero), task refusal down 29%, and elopement attempts down 33%. Because of these dramatic changes in behavior, the patient no longer required continuous one-to-one supervision, and p.r.n. injections for explosive behavior became infrequent, then unneeded. Although the patient was still confused and required a closed treatment setting, he was no longer aggressive, which clearly had been his most problematic and dangerous behavior. No side effects were reported.

8. Clark, Morris S., Silverstone, Leon M., Lindenmuth, James, Hicks, M. John, Averbach, Robert E. & Kleier, Donald J. An evaluation of the clinical analgesia/anesthesia efficacy on acute pain using the high frequency neural modulator in various dental settings. *Oral Surgery, Oral Medicine, Oral Pathology.* **63(4):501-505, 1987.**

Device: high frequency neural modulator, 15 Hz, 4 mA, temporal electrodes, and intraoral to hand electrodes

50 healthy, nonpregnant dental patients from 16 to 60 years old were separated into an experimental group (N = 30), and placebo group (N = 20) in this double-blind study to evaluate the effectiveness of CES and peripheral stimulation as a substitute for local anesthesia in various dental procedures. The procedures included oral surgery, restorations, tooth extractions, root planing, pulp extirpation, and temporomandibular joint therapy. The degree of patient comfort and satisfaction, their request for local anesthetics, as well as manageability of pain control by the dentist was evaluated. In the treatment group, favorable responses ranged from 0.0% to 92.8%, depending on the procedures. 24 of 30 (80%) CES patients were able to undergo dental procedures without anesthesia. 15 of 20 (75%) of the placebo group required anesthesia. In the operative group, 13 of 14 patients were treated successfully with CES (P<.05), whereas only 3 of 7 placebo CES patients did well. All 3 of the CES patients and all 3 placebo CES patients required anesthesia for endodontic procedures. The treatment group gave an overall favorable rating of 71.8%, whereas the placebo group gave an overall favorable rating of only 8.5%. CES patients provided favorable comments about the procedure and all stated that CES would be their first choice in future visits. No side effects were reported.

9. Cox, Aris & Heath, Robert G. Neurotone therapy: A preliminary report of its effect on electrical activity of forebrain structures. *Diseases of the Nervous System.* **36(5):245-247, 1975.**

Device: Neurotone, 100 Hz, 2 mS, 500 µA

A 41 year old female patient with a history of severe depressive disorder was prepared with deep and surface electrodes for long-term brain study. She was given 2, 30 minute CES sessions with a crossover treatment/simulated treatment design, followed by pre-post EEG readings. After actual but not simulated treatment, the patient reported feeling drowsy and relaxed, and she remained in this relaxed state for about 30 minutes, after which she went to sleep for an hour. This was unusual for her. After the patient awakened, her relaxed state lasted 3 hours. There was also a well-developed alpha rhythm in the occipital cortex following actual but not simulated treatment, also unusual for her. Since she was not considered suggestible (several attempts at hypnotism to relieve her symptoms had been unsuccessful), the authors concluded that CES has a demonstrable physiologic effect in contrast to some published reports that it is only suggestive. No side effects were reported.

10. Dymond, A.M., Coger, R.W. & Serafetinides, E.A. Intracerebral current levels in man during electrosleep therapy. *Biological Psychiatry.* **10(1):101-104, 1975.**

Device: Grass S88 stimulator coupled with a Grass SIU5 stimulus isolation unit, 100 Hz, 0.1 - 1.5 mA, square waves stereotaxically placed electrodes implanted bilaterally in various temporal lobe structures

In the early days of CES research, the question often arose whether or not the electrical current from CES goes into the brain or simply scatters around the head via the skin or bones. This study measured current in a patient with temporal lobe epilepsy across chronically implanted electrodes in the anterior and posterior hippocampus and hippocampal gyrus. The electrodes were placed 1.1 cm apart. CES caused voltage drops between the electrodes from 0.1 to 1.5 mA. This was considered sufficient to elicit physiological response in brain tissue. No side effects were reported.

11. Empson, J.A.C. Does electrosleep induce natural sleep? *Electroencephalography and Clinical Neurophysiology.* **35(6):663-664, 1973.**

Device: Somlec 3, 20 Hz, 250 µS, DC pulses

This study was completed in the era when CES was called "electrosleep" and when it was thought that it had no effect other than putting people to sleep. In this study 8 student volunteers spent an acclimation night and two experimental nights in a sleep laboratory with CES and EEG monitoring. One went to sleep, the other 7 were made more alert on the EEG, but described it as an interesting, restful experience. CES was only given for 5 minutes although the author states that it is recommended that treatments last 1.5 - 2 hours. The authors concluded that while it did not make these (non-insomniac) subjects sleep, it is possible that CES may alter the mood of tense, anxious people so that they are more likely to get to sleep when they go to bed. No side effects were reported.

12. England, Ronald R. Treatment of migraine headache utilizing cerebral electrostimulation. Master of Science Thesis, North Texas State University, Denton, Texas, Pp. 1-38, 1976.

Device: Neurotone 101, 100 Hz, 2 mS., electrodes behind each ear

18 migraine patients, 6 males and 12 females ranging from 21 to 62 years old (mean of 37.9) were solicited by newspaper ads. After giving informed consent, 3 groups of 6 patients each were matched on the basis of headache intensity during a 2 week baseline period and divided into CES treatment, simulated treatment, and waiting list control groups. CES was given 45 minutes per day for 15 days, Monday through Friday. A Wilcoxon matched-pairs, signed-ranks test was calculated for the difference in scores for each of the variables of headache frequency, intensity, and duration. The frequency of headaches had not changed significantly by the end of the study. There was no significant difference in intensity of headaches after the second week of treatment. When both baseline periods were compared to the results of the third week of treatment, the CES group was

found to have significantly (P<.025) lower headache intensity ratings than the placebo group.

There was also a significant (P<.05) reduction in duration of headaches among CES patients over placebo after the second week. The waiting list control group reported improvement also, but they were asked to recall their week's experience over the telephone on Friday only, while the treatment and placebo groups were asked to keep a written record on a daily basis.

It was noted that the recordings may not have been comparable and that the variable of medication usage tended to confound the results. The frequency, intensity, and duration of pain did not change in the placebo patients during or following the study. The author concluded that CES does consistently better than placebo. No side effects from CES were reported.

13. Feighner, John P., Brown, Stuart L. & Olivier, J. Edward. Electrosleep therapy: A controlled double-blind study. *Journal of Nervous and Mental Disease.* **157(2):121-128, 1973.**

Device: Electrosone 50, 100 Hz, 1 mS, 100 - 250 μA, cathodes over orbits, anodes over mastoids

23 long term psychiatric patients who had been ill a minimum of 2 years with prominent anxiety, depression, and insomnia, and who did not respond to psychotherapy, psychopharmacology, and ECT in 4 cases, were given 2 weeks of CES and 2 weeks of sham CES in a double-blind crossover design. Treatments were for 30 minutes daily, Monday through Friday. Analyses were done by the 2-tailed Mann-Whitney U test. Scores on the Zung self rating depression scale improved significantly in both groups, but only after 10 days of active treatment, and never during the sham phase of treatment. Actively treated patients also improved significantly on other target symptoms, particularly anxiety and insomnia.

The CES/sham group means based on global ratings of anxiety was 4.5 on day 1, 2.5 on day 15 (P<.02), and 3.1 on day 26 (P<.10), and the sham/CES group was 4.4 on day 1, 4.0 on day 15 (P>.05), and 3.2 on day 26 (P<.05).

The CES/sham group means based on global ratings of depression was 4.0 on day 1, 2.8 on day 15 (P<.05), and 3.8 on day 26 (P>.05), and the sham/CES group was 3.8 on day 1, 3.9 on day 15 (P>.05), and 3.1 on day 26 (P>.05).

The CES/sham group means based on global ratings of insomnia was 4.6 on day 1, 1.9 on day 15 (P<.002), and 3.4 on day 26 (P<.05), and the sham/CES group was 4.0 on day 1, 4.4 on day 15 (P>.05), and 3.1 on day 26 (P<.02).

7 of 8 patients who exhibited significant improvement relapsed within the first month after treatment. 4 of 6 long term depressed patients were dropped from the study because of massive worsening of depressive symptoms, 2 of whom exhibited suicidal ideation. The remaining 2 depressed patients had an unremarkable course, but remained in the study. 3 patients benefited more from this therapy than any previous extensive psychiatric care.

14. Flemenbaum, A. Cerebral Electrotherapy (Electrosleep): An open clinical study with a six month follow-up. *Psychosomatics.* **15(1):20-24, 1974.**

Device: Electrosone 50, 100 Hz, 1 mS, cathodes over orbits, anodes over mastoids

28 anxiety, depression, and insomnia outpatients who had been symptomatic for at least 3 - 4 years and unresponsive to extensive previous treatments were divided into 3

groups and given 5, 30 minute CES treatments. 3 patients left the study, 1 due to complaints of worsening of her nervousness after 3 treatments, 1 left after 4 treatments and could not be located, another died of an overdose 3 months after the treatments, but before the researchers could determine why he left the study. Group I patients (N = 14) had no other serious complicating psychiatric disorders, Group II (N = 7) was comprised of patients whose target symptoms were secondary to physical, somatic difficulties, and group III (N = 4) had a history of psychotic episodes. All patients were on psychotropic drugs. Only historical controls were employed in this study. The Zung depression scale and clinical global impressions (1 - 7 scale) were employed pretreatment, and for follow-up at weeks 6, 16, and 24. By the 6th week the pathology for the 3 groups seemed to be reduced to approximately equal levels. An insignificant trend towards worsening was seen by the 24th week. Comparison of the final results with the pretreatment ratings shows statistically significant improvement (P<.01).

The author noted that at the end of the study 12 of the 25 patients were much, or very much improved, 8 had shown some effect, though minimal, and 5 were not improved or had become worse. Some of these chronic patients were practically asymptomatic, other psychophysiological symptoms like asthma and blood pressure had become controllable by regular medical treatment, and/or their target symptoms showed complete or nearly complete remission. Most remarkable of all, these changes occurred in patients who previously had not responded to extensive treatment. Although about 50% of the patients showed minimal improvement, or none at all, those who had beneficial results maintained them throughout the 6 month follow-up. The author added that side effects are virtually nonexistent. It was concluded that this treatment seems to be an excellent modality for patients. Its safety and economy recommend its freer trial.

15. Forster, Sigmund, Post, Bernard S. & Benton, Joseph G. Preliminary observations on electrosleep. *Archives of Physical Medicine and Rehabilitation.* 44:481-489, 1963.

Device: A device was fabricated, 20 Hz, 0.2 - 0.3 mS, 0.5 - 5 mA, rectangular pulses

This study was designed to test the effects of CES for inducing sleep, and as usual, had variable results. They did find that whether or not patients went to sleep, there is a clinically noticeable effect of CES upon muscle spasticity in patients with hemiplegia and paraplegia and upon muscle spasm in traumatic injuries such as low back syndromes. These results were confirmed with EMG readings in their 6 normal and 17 clinical patients. There were no controls so the effects of lying supine during an average of 3.56 sessions were not screened out. Although as amplitude was increased to 20 volts a feeling of slight dizziness approaching a headache was noted, the authors concluded that the technique appears to be entirely safe.

Follow-up of patients up to 1 year after treatment did not reveal any harmful effects. The authors suggested that CES may be a potentially valuable technique in the management of certain patients undergoing rehabilitation.

16. Frankel, Bernard L., Buchbinder, Rona & Snyder, Frederick. Ineffectiveness of electrosleep in chronic primary insomnia. *Archives of General Psychiatry.* 29:563-568, 1973.

Device: Electrosone 50, 100 or 15 Hz, 1 mS, 100 - 700 µA, square waves, cathodes over orbits, anodes over mastoids

17 insomniacs referred from local physicians with an average duration of symptoms for almost 20 years were given 15, 45 minute CES treatments Monday through Friday at

100 or 15 Hz, a week off, then 15 more treatments at 15 or 100 Hz in a cross-over design with each group split in half. Both the 100 Hz and 15 Hz groups appeared to be combined for the 3rd week and 7th week measurements. There were no changes in the EEG, sleep onset time, sleep efficiency, total number and duration of awakenings, etc. The Taylor Manifest Anxiety Scale did not change (pretreatment means of 21.0 ± 9.3, after 15 treatments: 19.9 ± 10.1, after 30 treatments: 19.2 ± 10.1, at 1 month follow-up 20.5 ± 9.6) nor did the Zung depression scale. 17-hydroxycorticosteroid levels did not change. All of these changes have been found in other controlled studies, so Frankel's findings stand virtually alone in the literature.

Note: From the write up, it is possible that the authors combined the two frequency groups for the final statistical analysis, even though Frankel noted in his introduction the comment made by Obrosov in the European literature that hertz of different levels should not be mixed when treating the same patient, as was done in this study, since beneficial effects can be eliminated or canceled out. We also now know that beneficial gains from CES treatment tend to increase following the initial treatment. Such effect, when present, would nullify the expected effect in cross-over designs involving placebo or other treatment.

A commonly reported innocuous side effect was mild blurring of vision lasting 15 to 30 minutes which resulted from the sustained mechanical pressure of the electrodes on the eyes.

17. Gibson, Thomas H. & O'Hair, Donald E. Cranial application of low level transcranial electrotherapy vs. relaxation instruction in anxious patients. *American Journal of Electromedicine.* **4(1):18-21, 1987. Also Ph.D. dissertation (THG), California School of Professional Psychology, Pp. 1-150, 1983.**

Device: Alpha-Stim 350, 0.5 Hz, 50% duty cycle, 50 µA, biphasic asymmetrical rectangular waves, ear clip electrodes

In this single-blind study, 64 volunteer subjects responded to newspaper advertisements, 32 males and 32 females, ranging in age from 22 to 55 years old (mean = 36.64), who scored 50 or above on the State Trait Anxiety Inventory (STAI), completed informed consent and were randomly assigned to 20 minutes relaxation training (RT) on audio tape only, Alpha-Stim CES only, RT plus CES, or to a control group which listened to a neutral audio tape and received sham CES. There were 8 males plus 8 females in each group. 9 of the original 73 subjects were dropped from the study due to failure to meet the study criteria or failure to show up. Treatment time was 1, 20 minute session. Relaxation was measured by frontalis muscle electromyogram (EMG) and a post treatment STAI. Subjects responded on the STAI significantly (P<.001) better than controls and equally to either RT alone with a means of 52.88 pretest to 32.19 post, CES alone: 52.31 pre to 30.06 post, or both RT and CES together: 53.69 pre to 30.44 post. The control group only dropped from 53.25 to 51.94. The EMG trend paralleled the STAI with means of 15.64 to 11.10 µV posttest in the RT alone, 17.12 to 11.17 µV in the CES alone, 17.41 to 9.77 µV in the combined group, and 14.14 to 14.47 µV in the control group. Analysis of variance for EMG scores showed highly significant F-ratios for the time variance term and the group X time interaction term. Results were further verified by Tukey tests for pair-wise comparisons.

The authors concluded that the results of this study indicate that Alpha-Stim CES may be a useful adjunctive therapy for short term treatment of symptoms of anxiety. The treatment appears to have about the same efficacy as the same amount of time of relaxation instructions, but is easier to administer. No side effects were reported.

18. Gold, M.S., Pottash, A.L.C., Sternbach, H., Barbaban, J. & Annitto, W. Anti-withdrawal effects of alpha methyl dopa and cranial electrotherapy. *Society for Neuroscience 12th Annual Meeting Abstracts.* **October, 1982.**

Device not specified.

Chronic opiate user inpatients were randomized for this double-blind study and given either alpha methyl dopa (Aldomet) or placebo 48 hours after abruptly removing methadone, or CES, or placebo CES. Aldomet and CES were both effective in controlling the effects of acute withdrawal. CES was also effective in controlling the effects of protracted withdrawal. No placebo condition was effective. The authors theorized that CES was effective by stimulating β-endorphin, which inhibited the noradrenaline activity at the locus ceruleus. No side effects were reported.

19. Gomez, Evaristo & Mikhail, Adib R. Treatment of methadone withdrawal with cerebral electrotherapy (electrosleep). *British Journal of Psychiatry.* **134:111-113, 1978. Also in Gomez, Evaristo & Mikhail, Adib R. Treatment of methadone withdrawal with cerebral electrotherapy (electrosleep). Presented at the annual meeting of the American Psychiatric Association, Detroit, 1974.**

Device: 100 Hz, 2 mS, 0.4 - 1.3 mA, electrodes from the forehead to mastoids

For this single-blind study, 28 male heroin addicts undergoing methadone detoxification, between 18 and 60 years old, were selected on the basis of having severe anxiety as measured by the Hamilton Anxiety Scale (HAS) and Taylor Manifest Anxiety Scale (TMAS), difficulties in sleeping, willingness to participate in the study for at least 2 weeks in a locked ward, and agreement not to take any tranquilizers or hypnotics while in the study. This was a self medicated withdrawal study in which methadone was given as requested by the patients as needed to control their withdrawal symptoms. The patients were then randomly divided into a CES treatment group (N = 14) who were taking 20 - 60 mg of methadone/day, a placebo group (N = 7) taking 30 to 40 mg/day, and a waiting in line control group (N = 7) taking 25 - 40 mg/day. CES or sham CES was given for 10 days, Monday through Friday, 30 minutes per day. After 6 - 8 CES treatments, methadone intake was 0 in 9 patients, with another 1 at 0 after 10 treatments. 3 were taking 10 - 15 mg after the 10 treatments. The other active patient dropped out of the study after the first treatment. The patients reported feeling restful and having a general feeling of well-being, their sleep was good and undisturbed after 3 treatments. The TMAS scores also came down significantly in the CES group with 7 patients dropping from a mean of 31 before CES to 20 after 10 days (normal is 8 - 18), while the others showed a 25 - 50% reduction. Sham CES patients showed an insignificant change in the mean TMAS scores from 29 to 27. The methadone intake did not change in 4 sham CES patients, and only dropped 5 - 10 mg in the other 3. These patients were anxious and depressed, and complained of difficulty sleeping and somatic problems. The 7 controls also did not do well, TMAS scores increased in 2 cases, was the same in 1, and only decreased 1 - 2 points after 10 days in the remainder. The methadone intake was the same in 3 controls, and decreased in the other 4 after 10 days. These patients were anxious and had difficulty sleeping. HAS scores were also diminished in the CES group but not the placebo or controls.

It was noted that with a higher current, the patient felt uncomfortable, but there were no skin burns.

20. Hearst, Earl D., Cloninger, C. Robert, Crews, Eugene L. & Cadoret, Remi J. Electrosleep therapy: A double-blind trial. *Archives of General Psychiatry.* **30(4):463-66, 1974.**

Device, Neurotone 101, 100 Hz, 2 mS, alternating and direct current, forehead to mastoid electrodes

28 psychiatric outpatients on medication and undergoing psychotherapy were divided into 4 groups, 22 received CES treatments or sham treatments using alternating current, and 6 more were divided into an alternating or direct current, or sham treatment group. A total of 14 received actual CES. All had 5, 30 minute treatments or sham treatments. Assessment was by the National Institute of Mental Health self rating scale (SRSS) and by physician and patient global ratings for sleep, anxiety, depression, and overall status. The groups did not differ substantially in the number of days they were symptomatic following treatment. However, the patients receiving active treatment were confirmed by Fisher's exact test for 2 x 2 contingency tables to be significantly ($P<.05$) less depressed than the sham group (79% vs. 21%). Other positive findings showed a trend ($P<.10$) towards improvements in the CES group over the sham in feeling lonely (64% vs. 21%), having feelings easily hurt (64% vs. 21%), and difficulty falling or staying asleep (71% vs. 29%). Physicians' and patients' global ratings showed an insignificant tendency towards improvement on the last day of treatment.

There was no significant differences between the groups 2 weeks post-treatment, and only 2 patients continued improvement, 1 relapsed after 1 month, while another relapsed in 2 months. A third patient showed marked improvement for 1 week, relapsed for 3 weeks, then responded again to biweekly treatments for 2 months. All 3 patients with sustained improvement had active treatment. Self rating scales did not indicate a significant improvement for anxiety, insomnia, or somatic complaints. No patient with primary affective disorder was adversely affected by CES.

The authors concluded that either CES may transiently increase the patients tolerance of their depressive symptoms without significantly altering symptom frequency, or that it has a transient mild effect on both symptom frequency and intensity without any appreciable change on the natural course of the illness. There was no report of side effects.

21. Heffernan, Michael. The effect of a single cranial electrotherapy stimulation on multiple stress measures. *The Townsend Letter for Doctors and Patients.* **147:60-64, 1995. Presented at the Eighth International Montreux Congress on Stress, Montreux Switzerland, February 1996.**

Device: Alpha-Stim 100, 0.5 Hz, 50% duty cycle, 100 µA, biphasic asymmetrical rectangular wave, ear clip electrodes

20 subjects complaining of generalized stress symptoms for at least 1 year, all of whom failed to respond to medication, were selected from the author's private practice and divided into real Alpha-Stim CES (N = 10) and placebo treatment (N = 10) in this double-blind study using double-blinding boxes. None of the treatment or placebo subjects perceived any sensation. Measurements of finger temperature, heart rate (HR), trapezius electromyogram (EMG), and brain capacitance were tested before, after, and 1 week following a single 100 µA, 20 minute treatment session at 0.5 Hz. Analysis was performed on each of the dependent variables using the paired t-test. All subjects in the CES treatment

group showed immediate declines in EMG and heart rates with simultaneous increases in finger temperature and capacitance. These changes were all significant at the P<.05 level of confidence with confirmation of the experimental hypothesis that CES would reduce stress related physiological measures. The results with CES on EMG, HR, and finger temperature were significant at the P<.025 level. The placebo group showed small insignificant fluctuations up and down in all dependent measures.

One week follow-up measures in the CES group showed carryover effects in EMG and HR, but were not significant at the .05 level for finger temperature or capacitance. The author concluded that the psychophysiological reduction in stress response found in this study may be the probable correlate and necessary preconditions for the anxiety reduction frequently found in the CES literature. No side effects were reported.

22. Heffernan, M. Comparative effects of microcurrent stimulation on EEG spectrum and correlation dimension. *Integrative Physiological and Behavioral Science.* **31(3):202-209, 1996.**

Device: Alpha-Stim 100, 0.5 Hz, 50% duty cycle, <500 µA, biphasic asymmetrical rectangular waves, ear clip electrodes, and silver 1½ inch self-adhesive electrodes

Two mathematical derivatives of electroencephalogram (EEG), fast fourier transform (FFT), and non-linear, system dynamic measures of correlation dimension from chaos analysis were used to assess the objective effects of Alpha-Stim earlobe (CES) versus Alpha-Stim mid-trapezius muscle stimulation on brain EEG. These measures were considered to be clinically relevant since low points in the FFT have been associated with attention deficit disorder (ADD), and declining correlation dimension has been associated with onset of epilepsy.

30 subjects from the author's practice who completed informed consent were randomly assigned to 1 of 3 treatment groups: earlobe, trapezius, and a double-blind placebo control. 18 female and 12 male subjects between 40 and 70 years old (mean of 65) participated. Typical symptoms included head, neck, and shoulder pain of several years' duration, with 75% having been diagnosed with some level of auto-immune disease, primarily of a rheumatoid type. All subjects also displayed symptoms of slow wound healing, fatigue, and periodic flare-ups of joint inflammation. After an initial 5 minute rest period, 10 minutes of Alpha-Stim treatment of 100 µA at 0.5 Hz, or placebo, was given between 2, 2 minute EEG recordings. 4,000 data points were generated for each subject representing successive EEG amplitudes in the 2 minute EEG records. Results showed that trapezius stimulation proved more effective in producing significant declines in FFT spectral smoothing, with an average standard deviation (SD) in the FFT of 1.1, as compared to the CES group showing a SD of 2.9. Correlation dimension of both trapezius and CES groups increased significantly (P<.001) as compared to placebo, with the correlation dimension measures for earlobe being 5.7, trapezius 5.6, and placebo 3.7.

The author discusses the significance of using stimulation of body sites for promoting clinically beneficial effects in brain electrophysiology as evidenced by improved FFT and correlation dimension. Significant changes in FFT, represented as spectral smoothing, followed trapezius microcurrent stimulation, suggesting a clinical application to treat low amplitude FFT bands associated with anxiety disorders (5 - 12 Hz), and ADD (12 - 14 Hz). As correlation dimension increases in EEG data, the eigenvectors transverse many more paths, avoiding a collapse into fixed point attractors and resultant pathologic brain electrical patterns. This study's effects on raising return plot complexity and correlation dimension may only apply to microcurrent devices that have complex or chaotic waveforms, such as the Alpha-Stim. Not all commercially available stimulators have such parameters. No side effects were reported.

23. Heffernan, Michael. The effect of variable microcurrents on EEG spectrum and pain control. *Canadian Journal of Clinical Medicine.* 4(10):4-11, 1997.

Devices: Alpha-Stim 100, 0.5 Hz, 50% duty cycle, 500 μA, biphasic asymmetrical rectangular wave; Liss Stimulator, 15 Hz, 500 Hz, and 15,000 Hz, 50% duty cycle, 500 μA; BK Instruments control device, 0.5 Hz constant square wave, 500 μA, all using silver electrodes bilaterally on the wrists

50 subjects were evaluated in this two part double-blind study in which the researcher proposed a model of spectral smoothing using EEG (API Neurodata system) as a measure of regeneration and pain reduction. In phase 1, 2 minute spectral averages of root mean square EEG amplitude versus frequency were compared between 2 groups: a normal group of pain free persons (N = 10), and an age (40 - 65 years old, mean of 60), sex matched group of pain patients (N = 10) with degenerative joint disease (DJD). The pain patients had at least 8 hours of pain per day for at least 2 years, and the pain-free subjects had no pain for 2 years. Pain-free subjects produced smooth declining spectral curves (mean deviation in RMS = 0.2, P>0.1), whereas the pain group showed many irregularities, and significant "unevenness" in EEG spectral arrays (mean deviation in RMS = 2.4, P<.01). On the basis of these findings and prior research the researcher proposed using spectral smoothing as a model to evaluate the effectiveness of differing microcurrent stimulators in safely treating pain patients.

In phase 2, 30 pain patients, half males, half females, 30-65 years old, with at least 2 years of DJD of hip, shoulder, knee, or back, confirmed by X-ray, and unresponsive to medication, completed informed consent and were randomly assigned to 1 of 3 groups. Double-blinding was achieved by placing the stimulators out of sight of both the investigator and subjects. They were each given a 5 minute test dose of stimulation from 3 differing stimulators, a 15 Hz, 500 Hz, and 15,000 Hz device (Liss Stimulator); a 0.5 Hz, random, biphasic asymmetrical device (Alpha-Stim); and a continuous 0.5 Hz non-CES device for control (BK Instruments). Using current limited, 500 μA stimulation bilaterally to the wrists, post stimulation spectral smoothing and pain control was found to be superior with the Alpha-Stim (deviation from normal FFT 3.1 pre to 0.4 post (P<.01). Although all 3 stimulators produced approximately a tenfold increase in RMS amplitude, the control 0.5 Hz device (deviation from normal FFT 2.7 pre to 2.6 post, P>0.1) and the Liss Stimulator (deviation from normal FFT 2.8 pre to 3.0 post, P>0.1) both produced considerable distortion from the EEG spectrum of normal, pain free subjects. Ordinal 5-point pain scales before and after stimulation showed that only the Alpha-Stim produced significant pain control with the 5 minute test dose 4.5 to 2.1, (P<.01), versus 4.3 to 4.5 (P>0.1) with the Liss Stimulator, and 4.6 to 4.8 (P>0.1) with the control device.

The researcher discusses these findings by proposing a theory of rapid pain control from regenerative restoration of normal cellular electrical fields. This theory of rapid pain reduction by electric field restoration is then contrasted with pain control by stress induction and increased production of endorphins. Finally the researcher discusses implications of using the spectral smoothing of both EEG and body fields as a model of reversing the negative, carcinogenic effects of externally applied extremely low frequency

(ELF) when used therapeutically or delivered inadvertently from human electrical power usage. No side effects were reported.

24. Hochman, Richard. Neurotransmitter modulation (TENS) for control of dental operative pain. *Journal of the American Dental Association.* 116(2):208-212, 1988.

Device: Neurotransmitter Modulator, electrodes across temples

This is a study of 600 dental procedures over a 1 year period. Although the author refers to the device as a TENS, electrodes were placed across the temples for 10 minutes prior to each procedure which makes the treatment CES by definition. The procedures ranged from vigorous subgingival scaling to endodontic. Results were evaluated for pain control related to procedure type, and the patients' skepticism about the procedure. Results were considered positive if the patient reported greater than 90% reduction in pain and did not request the additional administration of local anesthetic. More than 76% of the patients in all procedures reported 90% or greater success using CES for dental analgesia. For the 71 scaling and prophylactic procedures, more than 83% reported successful pain reduction, and for the 473 restorative procedures, more than 76% reported pain reduction success. For 29 crown preparations, 55% reported success. The majority of patients were skeptical about the procedure but after experiencing CES they were more comfortable with CES than they were with previous dental experiences.

The author concluded that from the results obtained during 1 year of treating a variety of patients requiring a broad scope of dental treatments, CES was found to provide a safe, noninvasive, readily acceptable, adjunctive analgesic modality to maintain patient comfort through the majority of dental procedures for most patients. Additional, unexpected positive results were found when the patients reported "feeling more relaxed than usual." No side effects were reported.

25. Hozumi, S., Hori, H., Okawa, M., Hishikawa, Y. & Sato, K. Favorable effect of transcranial electrostimulation on behavior disorders in elderly patients with dementia: a double-blind study. *International Journal of Neuroscience.* 88:1-10, 1996.

Device: HESS-100, 6 to 80 Hz, 256-530 µA, repetitive rectangular electric pulses, 6-8 V, 0.2 mS

The efficacy of CES for sleep-wake and behavior disorders in elderly patients with dementia was tested in a double-blind study. The subjects were 27 inpatients with multi-infarct dementia (12 males and 15 females, aged 58-86). They were randomly divided into two groups: active treatment (N = 14) and placebo treatment (N = 13). CES was performed for 20 minutes from 10:00 AM every morning. The active or placebo treatment was performed for 2 weeks in each group. CES was significantly effective in behavior disorders such as wandering or nocturnal delirium, and decreased motivation during the daytime. It was also effective in improving night sleep. Electroencephalograms confirmed increased vigilance levels in the daytime both during and after the treatment.

26. Itil, T., Gannon P., Akpinar, S. & Hsu, W. Quantitative EEG analysis of electrosleep using frequency analyzer and digital computer methods. *Electroencephalography and Clinical Neurophysiology.* 31:294, 1971.

Device: Electrosone 50

10 male volunteers received EEG recordings with 2 days of CES and 2 days of sham CES in a cross-over design. Patients who exhibited no decrease of vigilance when CES

was off also showed no significant changes when CES was on. Those showing a slight-to-moderate drowsiness during the off recording did show a slight-to-moderate sleep pattern when the CES was on. There was no significant EEG difference between the on and off sessions recorded during resting time. However, during reaction time measurements there was an increase in 5-10 Hz activity and a decrease in fast alpha and beta activity when CES was on as compared with the recordings taken with CES off. No side effects were reported.

27. Jemelka, Ron. Cerebral electrotherapy and anxiety reduction. Master's thesis, Stephen F. Austin State University. May 1975.

Device: Neurotone 101, 100 Hz, 2 mS, <1.5 mA, anodes on forehead, cathodes on mastoids

28 pychiatric inpatients on the psychiatric ward in a Texas state prison were given 7, 30 minute CES treatments or sham treatments in a double-blind protocol. Active devices were preset to 100 Hz at 100 µA. Anxiety was measured by the Hamilton Anxiety Scale, and a student derived anxiety index. CES patients improved significantly on both anxiety measures, while the sham treated controls did not. No significant negative responses to the treatment were found.

The author concluded, "Results of this study indicate that CES effectively and efficiently reduces anxiety. The dramatic changes in... measures of anxiety were obtained in a short period of time (7 days). Since treatments can be administered by a trained assistant or nurse, there is little demand on the professional's time." Abstract courtesy of Ray B. Smith, Ph.D., M.P.A.

28. Kirsch, Daniel L. Postmarketing survey of Alpha-Stim CES patients.

Device: Alpha-Stim 100, 0.5 Hz, 50% duty cycle, <600 µA, biphasic asymmetrical rectangular waves, ear clip electrodes

A postmarketing survey was originally conducted during October, 1995 of all known health care practitioners using Alpha-Stim CES technology. A total of 313 individual patient report forms were received. Another survey was conducted in 1998 ending in April 1998 when 187 more forms were received providing combined data on a total of 500 patients reported by 47 physicians. 172 males, and 326 females were identified, ranging from 5 to 92 years old. 21 of the forms were completed on inpatients, the balance on outpatients. 41% of the patients were reported to have completed CES treatment, and 43% were still receiving treatment at the time of the survey. 10 patients discontinued treatment because it was not efficacious, 3 discontinued due to undesirable side effects, 13 because their insurance ran out, and 20 for other reasons.

Most of the reports included multiple symptoms. A degree of improvement of 25% or greater was considered to be clinically significant. The data is summarized below and analyzed in greater detail in Chapter 13.

There were 349 reports of using the Alpha-Stim for anxiety. 327 of 349 patients (93.70%) reported significant improvement in their anxiety. No patient's anxiety was made worse by the treatment, 8 (2.29%) reported no change, 14 (4.01%) reported a slight improvement up to 24%, 39 (11.17%) reported a fair improvement of 25 - 49%, 89 (25.50%) reported a moderate improvement of 50 - 74%, 181 (51.86%) reported a marked improvement of 75 - 99%, and 18 (5.16%) reported a complete (100%) recovery from their anxiety.

241 of 259 patients (93.05%) reported significant improvement in their stress. No patient's stress was made worse by Alpha-Stim CES treatment, 6 (2.32%) reported no change, 12 (4.63%) reported a slight improvement, 37 (14.29%) reported a fair improvement, 70 (27.03%) reported a moderate improvement, 124 (47.88%) reported a marked improvement, and 10 (3.86%) reported a complete recovery from their stress.

165 of 184 (89.67%) reported significant improvement in their depression. No patient's depression was made worse by Alpha-Stim CES treatment, 8 (4.35%) reported no change, 11 (5.98%) reported a slight improvement, 31 (16.85%) reported a fair improvement, 38 (20.65%) reported a moderate improvement, 82 (44.57%) reported a marked improvement, and 14 (7.61%) reported a complete recovery from their depression.

107 out of 135 (89.26%) reported significant improvement in their insomnia. No patient's insomnia was made worse by the treatment, 16 (11.85%) reported no change, 12 (8.89%) reported a slight improvement, 17 (12.59%) reported a fair improvement, 34 (25.19%) reported a moderate improvement, 45 (33.33%) reported a marked improvement, and 11 (8.15%) reported a complete recovery from their insomnia.

In addition, significant results of 25% or greater was reported in 260 out of 286 (90.91%) for pain relief, in 136 out of 151 (90.07%) for headache, and 245 out of 259 (94.59%) for muscle tension.

Side effects were all mild and self-limiting: 472 (94.4%) reported none. 6 (1.2%) reported dizziness as a side effect, and 2 (0.4%) reported nausea, both of which normally occur when the current is set too high or in patients with a history of vertigo, 3 (0.6%) reported skin irritation, 1 each (0.2%) reported, anger, a metallic taste, a heavy feeling, or intensified tinnitus.

29. Kotter, Gary S., Henschel, Ernest O., Hogan, Walter J. & Kalbfleisch, John H. Inhibition of gastric acid secretion in man by the transcranial application of low intensity pulsed current. *Gastroenterology.* 69(2):359-363, 1975.

Device: Electrodorn 1, 100 Hz, 1 mS, 0.1 - 1.5 mA, rectangular wave, cathodes frontal, anodes occipital

Following up on an earlier positive study in primates, 5 hospitalized adult male volunteers from 28 to 58 years old completed informed consent and had their basal acid secretion rate in their stomachs measured by intragastric titration utilizing a pH-sensitive telemetry capsule that was swallowed while held on a tether outside the subject's body. On a randomized basis, no current was passed through the electrodes during one of the tests, whereas a mean of 1 mA was applied during the other. Acid secretion was halted during or after CES. In a second study, 12 subjects had histamine-stimulated maximal acid output (MAO) reduced by an average of 30% with CES, with individual reductions ranging from 5.7% to 53.2%. There was no acid reduction during simulated CES treatments. A third study showed histamine-stimulated acid output decreased by 6.3 - 46.5%, with an average of 27.3% below control values in 6 volunteers. Acid secretion gradually began again when CES was terminated. The results of all 3 studies (N = 23) indicate that CES can cause a highly significant reduction in both basal and histamine stimulated gastric acid output. No side effects were reported.

30. Krupitsky, E.M., Burakov, A.M., Karandashova, G.F., Katsnelson, J., Lebedev, V.P., Grinenko, A.J. & Borodkin, J.S. The administration of transcranial electric treatment for

affective disturbances therapy in alcoholic patients. *Drug and Alcohol Dependence.* **27:1-6, 1991.**

Device: 70 - 80 Hz, 4 - 7 mA, square waves, cathodes on forehead, anodes behind ears

20 alcoholic patients with affective disorders who volunteered were equally divided by chance into 2 groups for this double-blind, placebo controlled study. All patients were abstinent for at least 3 weeks, so their affective disturbances were not alcohol withdrawal syndrome (AWS) symptoms. They were all weakly or moderately depressed, and exhibited a high level of reactive and personal anxiety. The CES group (N = 10) had 20 treatments over a 4 week period, and the placebo group (N = 10) were given a weak current, but otherwise the same conditions. There was considerable improvement in the CES group on the MMPI depression scale and Zung's test. Reactive anxiety of the active CES group by STAI (pre-test mean of 51.7 ± 3.14 to post-test 30.6 ± 2.15, P<.05), Personal anxiety by STAI (pre-test mean of 51.4 ± 3.09 to post-test 13.8 ± 5.15, P<.05), and anxiety by Taylor's scale (pre-test mean of 26.6 ± 1.79 to post-test 14.0 ± 3.63, P<.01) were all reliably diminished. The placebo group demonstrated a tendency toward a definite aggravation of the state and some increase of affective disturbance on all tests: STAI reactive anxiety (pre-test mean of 51.7 ± 2.81 to post-test 63.0 ± 3.44, P<.05), personal anxiety (pre-test mean of 66.9 ± 2.71 to post-test 51.2 ± 4.93), Taylor anxiety (pre-test mean of 20.5 ± 1.99 to post-test 28.0 ± 3.21).

The activity of MAO-B in blood platelets and GABA concentration in blood were increased in the CES group after 20 treatments. The concentration of serotonin, dopamine, and β-endorphin in blood were not substantially changed. The changes of biochemical indices were not registered in the control group where the tendency towards decreased MAO-B and GABA level in blood corresponded with a definite increase of affective disturbances at the end of the course. EEG analysis showed that the latency of α-rhythm appearance in occipital leads after eye closing was decreased after CES, whereas in the control group it was practically not changed and considerably exceeded the indices of the CES group. The CES patients became more tranquil, well-balanced, active, and their mood was improved.

The authors concluded that CES is an effective non-pharmacological method to treat affective disturbances (*e.g.,* anxiety, depression) in alcoholic patients in remission. They also stated that CES was not accompanied by side effects or complications and was well tolerated by the patients, and that CES tends to avoid side effects and complications sometimes observed in pharmaceutical antidepressant therapy and tranquilizers.

31. Levitt, Eugene A., James, Norman McI. & Flavell, Philippa. A clinical trial of electro-sleep therapy with a psychiatric inpatient sample. *Australian and New Zealand Journal of Psychiatry.* **9(4):287-290, 1975.**

Device: Dormed, 100 Hz, 50 - 200 µA, square pulses, cathodes over orbits, anodes over mastoids

This is a double-blind study of 13 chronically distressed patients, 6 male and 7 female, 23 - 63 years old, in an inpatient psychiatric hospital (length of stay, 2 months to 16 years). All were on anti-depressant and/or tranquilizing medication, with 9 on sleep medication. They were diagnosed with schizophrenia (N = 4), alcoholism (N = 2), psychotic depression (N = 2), and mixed neurosis and disorders of personality (N = 5). 5 received CES treatment and 6 received simulated treatment for 10 sessions over 2 weeks, 30 minutes per session. Instrument malfunction made it impossible to complete the treatment program with 2 active CES patients. There were no significant changes between groups on the Taylor Manifest Anxiety Scale or the Zung Self-Rating Depression Scale. Clinician ratings of anxiety and insomnia were found to agree to an extremely limited extent with results on the anxiety and depression scales. 4 of 5 of the active CES patients showed a decrease on Taylor, while the 5th remained constant, for an average drop of 4.4. 5 patients improved with placebo while the remaining 1 got worse, an average drop of 3.2. Therapist ratings of anxiety showed 2 patients to be improved, 2 unchanged, and 1 worse following active CES. Of those receiving sham treatment, 1 was rated improved, 2 unchanged, and 3 more anxious. The Zung depression scores for 2 CES patients showed improvement while the other 3 showed an increase. 5 of 6 sham patients showed a decrease in depression, and 1 was more depressed. Clinician ratings of depression noted improvement in 3, no change in 1, and increased depression in 1 receiving active CES, while 3 sham CES patients improved, and 3 were unchanged.

The authors noted that since nightly sedatives were administered the fact of a nonsignificant increase in sleep was hardly surprising. Subjects in both groups reported slight blurring of vision lasting 30 to 45 minutes following treatments. This supports the findings of other researchers that the blurred vision effect was mechanically caused by pressure from eye electrodes, and not electrical current.

32. Lichtbroun, Alan S., Raicer, Mei-Ming C., and Smith, Ray B. The treatment of fibromyalgia with cranial electrotherapy stimulation. *Journal of Clinical Rheumatology*. 7(2):72-78, 2001. Presented at the Fifteenth Annual International Symposium on Acupuncture and Electro-Therapeutics, Columbia University, New York, October 1999.

Device: Alpha-Stim 100, 0.5 Hz, 50% duty cycle, <600 μA, biphasic asymmetrical rectangular waves, ear clip electrodes

After successful clinical use of Alpha-Stim cranial electrotherapy stimulation (CES) in the first author's rheumatology practice, and IRB approval from Robert Wood Johnson Medical School, a double-blind, placebo-controlled study was undertaken in which 60 randomly assigned patients who completed informed consent were given either 3 weeks of subsensation (100 μA) CES treatment at 0.5 Hz for one hour daily (N = 20), sham treatment (N = 20), or served as controls for any placebo effect in the sham treated patients (N = 20). All patients met the diagnostic criteria of the American College of Rheumatology. The age range was from 23 to 82 years old (mean of 50). There were 2 men and 58 women suffering from fibromyalgia from 1 to 40 years, (mean of 11 years).

Treated patients showed a significant improvement in tender point scores (p<.01), and a significant improvement in self-rated scores of general pain level (p<.002). The number of subjects rating their quality of sleep as poor dropped from 60% at the beginning of the study to 5% (p<.02). In addition, there were significant gains in the self-rated feeling of well-being (p<.05), and quality-of-life (p<.03), plus fairly dramatic gains in 6 stress related psychological test measures of the Profile of Mood States. No placebo effect was found among the sham treated patients.

After the double-blind study, 23 of the 40 control patients opted for actual CES in an open clinical trial where they could increase the current in accordance with the standard clinical protocols for Alpha-Stim CES. They also showed a significant improvement in tender point scores (p<.001), and in self-rated pain (p<.005), quality of sleep (p<.001), feeling of well-being (p<.001), and quality-of-life (p<.001). Overall there was a 27%

reduction in self-rated pain, and a 28% decrease in the tender point scores of the treated group.

According to a review of 34 studies of prescription drug treatment for fibromyalgia, adverse effects from drugs are seen in 20% of fibromyalgia patients who use them, and improvement from drugs was reported as 28% at best. In addition, unlike with the use of medication, there is no ongoing cost to the patient after purchase of the CES device. Accordingly, the authors concluded that Alpha-Stim CES is as effective as the best drug therapies, with no negative side effects, and deserves further consideration as an additional agent for the treatment of fibromyalgia.

33. Logan, Michael P. Improved mechanical efficiency in cerebral palsy patients treated with cranial electrotherapy stimulator (CES), 1988.

Device: Pain Suppressor, 15,000 Hz, 50mS, 500 - 700 µA, electrodes placed above ears

36 spastic type cerebral palsy patients completed informed consent and were divided into 18 CES and 12 placebo CES in this double-blind study. Both groups performed a graded exercise test on a Tunturi bicycle ergometer. Pedaling speed was recorded in revolutions per minute (RPM), and the resistance to pedaling in Newtons (N). The workload was started at 0 and increased by 2 N every 2 minutes based on heart rate (HR), blood pressure (BP), and ability to maintain pedal velocity. An EKG measured HR every minute. Expired gases were measured every minute, and BP every 2 minutes. 6 patients were dropped from the study because 3 were not able to maintain pedaling motion, while another 3 voluntarily withdrew. The absolute test value differences were subjected to a 2 factor analysis of covariance. The mean poststimulation mechanical efficiency (ME) in the CES group increased by 19.1% (from 50.3 to 59.9), while the placebo group dropped by 9.1% (53.3 to 48.4). Workloads of treated patients improved by an average of 43% (mean of 65.9 to 94.3). This is a remarkable increase, especially when one considers that the placebo retest scores declined by 5.5% (mean of 75 to 70.9). The F statistics for the unit factors in ME was significant at the .0003 level.

The authors concluded that the results indicate that CES does, in fact, improve the work performance of cerebral palsy patients and that the most likely explanation is that spasticity was reduced in the actively treated patients. There was no report of side effects.

Dr. Logan received the Richmond Award from the American Academy for Cerebral Palsy and Developmental Medicine for this study.

34. McKenzie, Richard E., Rosenthal, Saul H. & Driessner, Jerry S. Some psycho-physiologic effects of electrical transcranial stimulation (electrosleep). American Psychiatric Association, *Scientific Proceedings Summary*. 1971. Also in *The Nervous System and Electric Currents*, Wulfsohn, N.L. & Sances, A. (Eds.) Plenum: New York, Pp. 163-167, 1976.

Device: Electrosone 50, 100 Hz, 1mS, 0.1 - 1.9 mA, cathodes over orbits, anodes over mastoids

8 psychiatric patients with a clinical history of chronic anxiety with depression and insomnia, and 4 normal staff "controls" were given 1, 30 minute CES treatment a day for 5 days. Psycho-physiological measurements were made on day 1 and day 5. All patients had slower EEG frequencies with increased amplitude in the fronto-temporal areas following CES. 7 patients showed increased quality and quantity of alpha with increased amplitude in the occipital-parietal leads. The submental EMG showed increased relaxation but was too

variable to be a reliable measure. The skin potential recordings (SPR) revealed a definite overall state of relaxation as the treatments progressed from an average of 24.55 millivolts to an average level of 12.75. Normal controls were comparable with the patients exhibiting a drop in SPR's of 25.29 to 5.76. The subjective reports of the normal subjects were unexpected. Only a mild sedative effect was expected. However, 3 of the 4 normals reported an activation or alerting effect. One of these reported hyperalertness with hyperirritability. A second experienced a helpful increase in energy and another a feeling of alertness. 2 normal subjects experienced feelings of euphoria with periods of silliness or giddiness, along with this they felt a lack of worry about real situational problems. In fact, they were worried over not being able to worry. All of these effects dissipated rather rapidly in 24 - 48 hours.

The authors noted that blurring of vision due to eye electrode pressure was fairly uniform over the small control sample and was not especially uncomfortable.

35. Madden, Richard & Kirsch, Daniel L. Low-intensity electrostimulation improves human learning. *American Journal of Electromedicine*. 4(2):41-45, 1987. Also Ph.D. dissertation (RM), City University Los Angeles, Pp. 1-95, 1987.

Device: Alpha-Stim 350, 0.5 Hz, 50% duty cycle, 200 µA, biphasic asymmetrical rectangular waves, ear clip electrodes

103 normal, healthy volunteer subjects without typing skills responded to recruitment efforts. 21 failed to satisfy the inclusion criteria or declined to participate. Of the remaining 82, 4 did not show up. 78 (29 males and 49 females) completed this double-blind study. They were randomly assigned to receive either 1, 20 minute Alpha-Stim CES treatment session (N = 39), or sham treatment (N = 39). The performance measuring device was a computer game called MasterType designed to teach typing skills, while measuring speed and accuracy. A baseline trial was conducted without stimulation. Immediately following the first trial, the subjects received real or sham CES and began the second trial. All subjects completed a total of 4 trials. Performance products (PP's) were obtained by multiplying rate per minute and accuracy scores following the completion of each trial. Prestimulation means of the first 2 trials were calculated as PPt1 (performance product for the first trial). PPt2 represented poststimulation or sham stimulation. The dependent variable was the performance gain score (PG) computed by taking the difference between t1 and 12 performance products represented as PG = PPt2 - PPt1. All t-tests were employed at the 0.01 confidence level. CES subjects improved significantly on the computer task involving psychomotor cognitive skills, with a PP4 - PP2 PG mean of 5.6 ± 2.2. Unexpectedly, 12 (30.8%) of the sham patients actually experienced a decrement in performance, and none improved significantly: PP4 - PP2 PG mean of 0.7 ± 2.3.

The authors concluded that this study demonstrates the efficacy of CES in improving human learning and performance. Normal or learning disabled children might also be taught more efficiently under the immediate or residual effects of CES in classroom settings. Others seeking increased alertness, concentration, and performance may also benefit, such as police officers, automobile drivers, air traffic controllers, surgeons, pilots, and athletes. No side effects were reported.

36. Magora, F., Beller, A., Assael, M.I. & Askenazi, A. Some aspects of electrical sleep and its therapeutic value. In Wageneder, F.M. and St. Schuy (Eds). *Electrotherapeutic Sleep and*

Electroanaesthesia. Excerpta Medica Foundation, International Congress Series No. 136. Amsterdam, Pp. 129-135, 1967.

Device: 30 - 40 Hz, 2 mS, 2 mA, forehead to occipital fossa electrodes

20 hospitalized patients suffering from long-lasting insomnia with anxiety, obsessive and compulsive reactions, morphine and barbiturate addiction and involutional depression were given 2 - 4 CES treatments weekly for 2 - 3 hours a day for a total of 10 - 20 treatments. 5 of the 20 showed no improvement, 11 had sedative effects, and 4 had hypnotic effects. The 15 responders all had normal restoration of their sleep rhythm as measured by EEG. Parallel with the return to a normal sleep pattern, all the other psychiatric signs: anxiety, depression, agitation, delusions, abstinence syndrome, improved so that all these patients were able to leave the hospital. Follow-up for 8 - 12 months after treatment revealed no relapse.

Also 9 children (aged 5 - 15 years) suffering from severe, long-lasting bronchial asthma, resistant to conventional treatment, including steroids, were given 3 - 24 (mean of 15) CES treatments once a week for 1 - 2 hours. The asthmatic attacks stopped completely in 3 children and 4 months later the children felt well without taking any drugs. 2 children showed objective improvement, no wheezes were found on examination, and the frequency and severity of wheezing spells were diminished. One child showed slight improvement, 2 did not respond at all. None suffered an asthmatic attack for 24 hours following CES. Placebo conditions did not cause any improvement. The authors concluded that it appears that CES may be an adjunct to the treatment of asthma in children. Because of the selection for trial of the most severe cases available, resistant to any other known treatment, even slight results are encouraging.

It was also noted that no ill-effects were noted on prolonged and repeated observations in dogs and in humans.

37. Magora, Florella, Beller, A., Aladjemoff, L., Magora, A. & Tannenbaum, J. Observations on electrically induced sleep in man. *British Journal of Anesthesiology.* **37:480-491, 1965.**

Device: 100 Hz, 10 - 100 Hz, 1 - 10 mS, 0.4 - 5 mA, square pulses, cathodes over orbits or forehead, anodes over mastoids

The authors were studying CES to determine what it took to put a patient to sleep. They varied hertz, amplitude, pulse width and the like, performing 65 experiments. The subjects were healthy volunteers, 5 females and 10 males with ages ranging from 30 - 45 years, 2 patients with Parkinson's disease (a 62 year old female and a 82 year old male), and 1 male, 65 years old, with dystonia musculorum. All subjects were advised to refrain from taking any drugs 12 hours prior to the experiments. In a group of 7 healthy subjects, the 2 patients with Parkinson's, and the 1 with dystonia musculorum, sleep did occur in most of the experiments as measured by objective criteria (respiration, EEG, EMG).

An unexpected finding was that the involuntary movements in the patients with Parkinson's and dystonia musculorum were changed in character during the passage of current, and eventually completely eliminated, as evidenced by clinical and EMG observations. Sleep was not induced in a second group of 13 healthy individuals, although in 7 a definite change was obvious consisting of lack of blinking, preference for eyes closed, passiveness, and disruption of the idea pattern obvious in conversation. On questioning, after the current was discontinued, these subjects had no evaluation of the lapsed time and stressed that while the current was on they felt detached from their surroundings and had an agreeable feeling throughout the experiment. No ill effects were observed after repeated experiments in the same and different individuals.

38. Malden, Joan W. & Charash, Leon I. Transcranial stimulation for the inhibition of primitive reflexes in children with cerebral palsy. *Neurology Report.* **9(2):33-38, 1985.**

Device: Neurotransmitter Modulator

In this double-blind crossover study 20 children (2.5 months to 15 years old) with normal intelligence and mild to severe spastic cerebral palsy completed informed consent and were then divided into real and placebo CES groups, each having 6 weeks of 2, 10 minute daily treatments and then the groups were reversed. The results were evaluated using the Malden Gross Motor Rating Scales I, II, and III, and the Advanced Gross Motor Skills Scale, which together constitute a total gross motor picture. Group A (active/placebo) had an original assessment of 37.2 measured an average of 13.1 months prior to the study, 52.9 at the start of the study, 79.4 at crossover, and 81 at the end of the study. The mean improvement of 26.5 points for Group A with active treatments was significant compared to the mean value of 1.6 points during the placebo period. Group B (placebo/active) had an original assessment of 36.83 measured an average of 37.16 months prior to the study, 85.4 at the start of the study, 87.9 at crossover, and 102 at the end of the study. The mean of Group B during the placebo period of 2.5 points was not significant compared to the 14.1 gain during the active period.

The authors concluded that the results of this study are highly significant and would seem to indicate that the treatment of children with spastic cerebral palsy with CES in addition to physical therapy is superior to conventional treatment offered alone. Placebo treatments have little further effect beyond that of conventional treatment. No side effects were reported.

39. Marshall, Alan G. & Izard, Carrol E. Cerebral electrotherapeutic treatment of depressions. *Journal of Consulting and Clinical Psychology.* **42(1):93-97, 1974.**

Device: 100 Hz, 1 mS, 0.5 - 1.5 mA, cathodes over orbits, anodes over mastoids

40 depressive inpatient volunteers without a chronic psychotic history (30 females and 10 males, aged 25 - 70 years) in a state psychiatric hospital were given 30 minute CES treatments for 5 successive days while on the regular hospital regimen. All of the patients were taking medication, part of the effect of which was usually sedative. Both active CES (N = 20), and simulated CES controls (N = 20) improved significantly on the DES+D II modification of Izard's Differential Emotion Scale. Heart rate, blood pressure and sleep records were also maintained, but they were largely invalidated by sources of variability associated with hospital routine.

Note: The first author made the CES device used in this study and reports that although no patients were burned, he and 1 pilot subject suffered second-degree burns behind 1 ear at the point of electrode contact. The 2 burned controls took almost 3 times the amount of current as the patients (1.4 mA versus 0.5 mA average). Such burns are very rare when using commercially manufactured CES units using <1 mA.

40. Matteson, Michael T. & Ivancevich, John M. An exploratory investigation of CES as an employee stress management technique. *Journal of Health and Human Resource Administration.* **9:93-109, 1986.**

Device: RelaxPak, 100 Hz, 2 mS, <1 mA, electrodes behind ears

40 members of an executive MBA program at the University of Houston, employed in middle management positions in various sized corporations, volunteered as CES subjects. 22 similar subjects served as unmatched controls. 8 of the CES subjects were unable to complete the treatment including 4 who left the study early due to complaints of headache. The final number of active CES subjects was therefore 32. The subjects ranged in age from 28 - 48. CES was given 30 - 40 minutes per day for 14 days. Measures employed were a stress questionnaire developed by the U.H. faculty, the POMS, and the STAI. Significant differences (between P<.05 and P<.001, two-tailed test) were found on all the measures among the CES subjects whereas the control group of 22 showed no meaningful change (positive or negative) on any of the variables.

A follow-up measure 2 weeks post study found that 11 of the 13 variables were still significantly improved in the treatment group, only the Reeder stress measure and the vigor-activity scale of the POMS failed to maintain a significant difference 2 weeks after CES was discontinued. State anxiety went from a mean of 42.84 pre-test to 36.47 post-test (P<.001) to 39.28 on follow-up (P<.05). Trait anxiety went from a mean of 42.41 pre-test to 40.06 post-test (P<.01) to 40.38 on follow-up (P<.05). The POMS Tension-Anxiety scale went from a mean of 16.22 pre-test to 10.74 post-test (P<.001) to 10.59 on follow-up (P<.001), the Depression-Dejection scale went from a mean of 12.22 pre-test to 8.47 post-test (P<.001) to 8.06 on follow-up (P<.01), the Anger-Hostility scale went from a mean of 16.59 pre-test to 12.22 post-test to 11.41 on follow-up (P<.001), the Fatigue-Inertia scale went from a mean of 12.69 pre-test to 9.25 post-test (P<.001) to 9.34 on follow-up (P<.001), the Confusion-Bewilderment scale went from a mean of 8.84 pre-test to 6.97 post-test (P<.01) to 6.63 on follow-up (P<.01).

The authors concluded that CES users reported a fewer number of health complaints, which manifested themselves with less intensity, a lower degree of sleep problems, less stress, faster discharge of tension, depression, anger, fatigue, and confusion, a greater degree of vigor, and lower levels of both state and trait anxiety.

41. May, Brad & May, Carole. Pilot project using the Alpha-Stim 100 for drug and alcohol abuse. August, 1993.

Device: Alpha-Stim 100, 0.5 Hz, 50% duty cycle, biphasic asymmetrical rectangular wave, ear clip electrodes

14 male volunteers in 2 recovery homes for several days to 7 months received 25, 1 hour Alpha-Stim CES treatments. Multiple Affect Adjective Check List (MAACL) means showed a significant and dramatic decline in the anxiety scores by mid test dropping from 4.07 pretest to 1.00 mid test and maintaining 1.00 post-test. Depression (3.42 pretest to 0.79 mid and post-test) and hostility scores (2.43 pretest to 0.71 mid and post-test) were also reduced significantly, while significant increases were seen in self-worth, feeling expression, and capacity for intimate contact. The Beck Depression Inventory dropped from 14.50 pretest to 5.00 midtest to 3.50 post-test.

The investigators commented that verbal feedback was equally exciting. One participant said afterwards, "something inside me has shifted and I just know I'm never going to take another drink of alcohol again." Another said, "I've been sober for about 75 days, but it feels like I've been sober for years." No side effects were reported.

42. Moore, J.A., Mellor, C.S. Standage, K.F. & Strong, H. A double-blind study of electro-sleep for anxiety and insomnia. *Biological Psychiatry*. 10(1):59-63, 1975.

Device: Neurotone, 100 Hz, 2 mS, mean of 480 μA

17 persistent anxiety and insomnia patients (21 - 60 years old, mean of 37.7), without evidence of psychosis, were given 5, 30 minute CES treatments or simulated treatments in a cross-over design after providing informed consent. The patients were told not to make any changes in their medication. There was improvement in all measures but 1 during the first week, but no significant difference between groups on the Taylor Manifest Anxiety Scale, Beck's Depression Inventory, or Eysenck's Lie, Neuroticism, or Extraversion scales, except that improvement of subjective insomnia was noted during active treatment (P<.05). The mean change in ratings over the first week for clinical anxiety was 0.62 for active CES and 0.61 for sham, for subjective anxiety was 0.37 for active and 0.55 for sham, and on Taylor was -0.75 for active and 2.55 for sham. Over the second week the mean for clinical anxiety was 0.27 for active CES and 0.31 for sham, for subjective anxiety was 0.00 for active and 0.88 for sham, and on Taylor was 1.87 for active and 2.25 for sham.

The authors concluded that five, 30 minute sessions might not be sufficient to elicit the effects studied. Also the current was unusually low for the device used. Curiously, the authors noted up front, in the abstract, that despite largely negative findings, several subjects reported a remarkable improvement in their symptoms some 2 - 3 weeks after CES. Note: While this was called a double-blind study, only the patients, and not the therapist were blind to treatment conditions. No side effects were reported.

43. Naveau, S., Barritault, L., Zourabichvili, O., Champagne, C., Prieur, G., Limoge, A., Poynard, T. & Chaput, J.C. Analgesic effect of transcutaneous cranial electrostimulation in patients treated by Nd:YAG laser for cancer of the rectum. A double-blind randomized trial. *Gastroenterol Clin Biol.* **16:8-11, 1992. (France)**

Device: 166 kHz, intermittent - 100 Hz, three electrodes: a negative electrode placed between the eyebrows and positive electrodes located in the retro-mastoid region

The aim of this double-blind crossover randomized trial was to assess if CES could decrease the dose of fentanyl required in patients with rectal cancer treated by Nd:YAG laser. 50 patients, 29 women, 21 men, mean of 78 years old (range: 53 - 96 years), were treated by 2 laser sessions with an interval of 48 hours between each session. Active and sham CES were given in random order for the 2 laser sessions. The major end point was the quantity of fentanyl injected when the score of pain was greater than or equal to 5 according to a visual analogue scale. Age, sex, body weight, tumor location and length, tumor circumferential extent and luminal patency, duration of laser session, amount of energy delivered per session (watt-seconds), and number of patients with deep sedation did not differ between the 2 groups. There was no interaction between the order of treatments and the treatment effects. The mean quantity of fentanyl with CES was 29 micrograms and 42 micrograms when sham CES was given. There was a decrease of 31% in the quantity of fentanyl with active CES (P<.05). Results were not affected either by the treatment order nor by tumor location. There were no side effects in either group.

44. Okoye, Renee & Malden, Joan W. Use of neurotransmitter modulation to facilitate sensory integration. *Neurology Report.* **10(4):67-72, 1986.**

Device: Neurotransmitter Modulator

16 patients, from 5 - 25 year old, with neurological diagnoses ranging from minimal cerebral dysfunction to cerebral palsy and spastic quadriplegia having at least borderline intelligence were divided into 3 groups for this 12 week study. The CES groups were

treated twice daily. Assessments were made using the Southern California Sensory Integration Test, and the Jebsen hand function test. The design copying scores for patients who received CES without occupational therapy (OT) averaged 59%. Patients receiving OT without CES averaged 35%, and patients receiving both CES and OT averaged 88%. Motor accuracy showed a tremendous improvement in the 2 CES groups over the OT-only group, with the CES-only group changing 43% in their dominant hand, and 21% in their non-dominant hand, the OT-only group averaging 15% in their dominant hand, and 45% in their non-dominant hand, and the combined therapy group averaging 53% change in their dominant hand, and 68% in their non-dominant hand.

In conclusion, the authors stated that CES patients whose scores showed moderate impairment during pre-test trials improved to within normal limits in a 12 week period, and that these findings were remarkable. No side effects were reported.

45. Overcash, Stephen J. A retrospective study to determine the efficacy of cranial electrotherapy stimulation (CES) on patients suffering from anxiety disorders. *American Journal of Electromedicine*. 16(1):49-51, 1999.

Devices: Alpha-Stim 2000, 350, CS, and 100, 0.5 Hz, 50% duty cycle, <500 μA, biphasic asymmetrical rectangular waves, ear clip electrodes

197 patients diagnosed with anxiety disorders (DSM 300.02, 308.3, 300.00), referred by local physicians, and given an average of 8.9, 25 minute Alpha-Stim CES treatments at 0.5 Hz in conjunction with other treatments from 1989 to 1995 were evaluated. Over 80% of the patients were also provided with an Alpha-Stim on loan to take home and use daily or twice a day. 15 patients did not complete the program, primarily for financial reasons. Of the 182 who completed the prescribed course of therapy, 55 were male, 127 were female, with an average age of 35.6. 26% had unsuccessful treatment with anxiolytic medication. 16% had used antidepressant medications, alcohol, individual psychotherapy or behavior modification therapy. 58% had no previous therapy for their anxiety disorder. All patients were asked to rate their current anxiety on a 0 - 100 scale, with 100 being the highest amount of anxiety they could imagine. Post treatment assessments were made at the beginning of their last session. Pre and post treatment assessments were also made for some patients on 3 objective physiological measures, electromyogram (EMG), electrodermal response (EDR), and peripheral temperature (temp). 73 patients had EMG evaluations, and an average of 8.6 treatments. The EMG group dropped from a pretreatment mean of 15.8 μV to a post treatment of 4.5 μV. 83 patients had EDR evaluations, and an average of 7.4 treatments. The EDR group dropped from a pretreatment mean of 14.6 to a post treatment of 7.6. 26 patients had temp evaluations, and an average of 12.6 treatments. The temp group rose from a pretreatment means of 81.2° F to a post treatment of 92.1° F. The subjective 0 - 100 scale for all 182 patients dropped form 62.3 to 14.8. Individual (as opposed to average) results were subjected to paired t-tests. There were significant (P<.05) positive changes on all objective and subjective criteria. The mean differences were 9.10 ± 2.00 μV for the EMG analysis, 6.89 ± 1.08 for the EDR, $9.91°$ F ± 2.69 for the temp, and 27.46 ± 16.34 for the 0 - 100 scale. There was a significant correlation (86%) between the perceived anxiety ratings and the objective measures. No patients were on any anxiolytic or antidepressant medication when they left treatment successfully.

At 6 to 8 month follow-up 73% of the patients were "well satisfied" with their treatment and had no significant regression or other anxiety disorders, 18% were "satisfied" but had some problem with anxiety since they stopped the treatment, and 9% chose not to respond, had significant symptoms since they stopped the treatment, or in 1 case, "was not satisfied" with the treatment. There were no reported short or long term side effects. (Note: Follow-up is from original manuscript, it was omitted in publication).

In conclusion, the author noted that the results appear to be immediate in most cases, and that CES treatment seems to have long lasting results as long as the patient is given a minimum of 4 to 6 treatments.

46. Overcash, Stephen J. & Siebenthall, A. The effects of cranial electrotherapy stimulation and multisensory cognitive therapy on the personality and anxiety levels of substance abuse patients. *American Journal of Electromedicine.* 6(2):105-111, 1989.

Device: Alpha-Stim 2000, 0.5 Hz, 50% duty cycle, <500 µA, biphasic asymmetrical rectangular waves, ear clip electrodes

32 marijuana users with various psychophysiological stress disorders diagnosed with generalized anxiety disorder and substance abuse disorder were referred from family practitioners and randomly assigned to a control group (N = 16) in which they were treated with biofeedback electromyogram (EMG) training, Quieting Response (QR) relaxation tapes and psychotherapy, or a CES experimental group (N = 16) which was treated with biofeedback EMG training, QR, psychotherapy, plus multisensory emotional therapy using the Relax and Learn System and Alpha-Stim CES. There were significant differences in the outcomes of the two groups. Although little change was recorded in EMG readings through the second treatment, by the fifth treatment the improvement was remarkable. The experimental group was able to reduce their mean EMG from 38 to 3.2 µV. The control group also reduced their mean EMG from 41 to 9.6 µV. Analysis of variance (F = 5.43, P<.01) indicate significant differences between the groups. The experimental group averaged the same amount of relaxation at the end of 8 sessions that the control group reached in 10.

In the 16PF personality test, there were significant differences between groups in 4 areas. Nervous tension was reduced in both groups. The experimental group was significantly more planful (4.0 pretest to 7.2 post-test, P<.01) in the self sufficiency test, a good indicator of reduction in anxiety levels, whereas there was no change in the control group (4.6 to 4.6). In area of dominance, a measure of assertiveness, the experimental group had a significant gain from 3.2 to 7.1, while the control group had an insignificant gain of 4.0 to 4.3. Ego strength for the experimental group rose from 3.0 to 7.6 which represents a significant (F = 6.95, P<.01) increase in decision making skills, while the control group had an insignificant gain (F = .28, P>.75) from 2.8 to 3.0. The experimental group was also able to reduce their use of marijuana more quickly testing drug free in only 6 weeks, and sustained over a longer period of time than the control group which was drug free in 9 weeks. No side effects were reported.

47. Passini, Frank G., Watson, Charles G. & Herder, Joseph. The effects of cerebral electric therapy (electrosleep) on anxiety, depression, and hostility in psychiatric patients. *Journal of Nervous and Mental Disease.* 163(4):263-266, 1976.

Device: Neurotone 101, 100 Hz, 2 mS, cathodes over orbits, anodes over mastoids

60 inpatient volunteers (59 males, 1 female) in a V.A. hospital suffering from either anxiety or depression were randomly assigned to CES treatments or simulated treatments. The diagnoses included alcohol addiction, depressive neurosis, manic-depression, anxiety

neurosis, drug dependence, organic brain syndrome, schizophrenia, psychotic depressive reaction, hypochondriacal neurosis, hysterical neurosis, adult adjustment reaction, social maladjustment, acute alcohol intoxication, personality disorder, passive-aggressive personality, and situational disturbance. Both groups were given 10, 30 minute treatments. All subjects in both groups improved significantly (P<.001) on the Multiple Affect Adjective Check List (for anxiety, active CES means was 12.06 pre-test to 8.67 post-test, for placebo CES 11.47 to 7.90) and on both the State Scale of the STAI (active: 64.93 to 45.20, placebo: 52.17 to 44.10) and Trait Scale of the STAI (active: 52.10 to 46.67, placebo: 50.47 to 43.77).

The authors noted that no attempt was made to control the amount or type of psychotropic medication administered to the patients and most of the subjects in the study were on psychoactive drugs. No side effects were reported.

48. Patterson, Margaret A., Firth, Jean & Gardiner, Richard. Treatment of drug, alcohol and nicotine addiction by neuroelectric therapy: Analysis of results over 7 years. *Journal of Bioelectricity.* **3(1&2):193-221, 1984.**

Device: asymmetrical rectangular pulse, 0.22 mS, 1 - 2,000 Hz (depending on addiction), 1.5 - 3 mA, 1 cm diameter electrodes

186 drug and alcohol patients (114 male, 72 female) participated in this study between 1973 and 1980. All completed informed consent. 113 were treated as inpatients. The mean number of drugs used by these patients was 19.8 out of 41 drugs surveyed. Daily amounts used ranged from 300 mg prescribed heroin to 9 g of street heroin, 1/2 to 10 g of cocaine, 40 to 800 mg of methadone and up to 70 tablets daily of various narcotics and psychotropic drugs. An exclusion criterion was any patient suspected of having psychosis. Patients were treated continuously for the first 6 days, then for progressively shorter times during days 7 - 10, resulting in 6 hours of treatment on day 10. Nursing staff recorded detailed data for 1 year, and patients recorded self-ratings on quality of sleep and overall abstinence syndrome (AS). AS was recorded on a 0-4 Himmelsbach scale with 4 indicating the worst and 0 indicating the absence of each of 19 symptoms or signs with the maximum possible in each assessment being 76 points. Craving and anxiety were recorded separately. Records were also kept of the time taken to fall asleep, the number of hours of sleep, and the overall quality of sleep on a 4-point scale by both nurses and the patients.

Classical physiological signs of withdrawal did not occur. AS was analyzed for each different drug group. A Kruskall-Wallis test for K dependent groups determined that there was a significant difference between the rank sums of the various modes of use of the main drug (chi square = 18.23, df = 4, P<.05). The mean for intravenous use showed the highest AS. Patients treated a second time with CES experienced a considerable decrease in AS on the second treatment compared to the first. A difficult finding to explain was that the few who insisted they had no AS were those using excessively heavy amounts of drugs.

CES rapidly reduced both acute and chronic withdrawal symptoms of all chemical substances, without drugs and with no negative side effects. Of the 186 patients, 98.4% were successfully detoxified, with marked feeling of well-being. Anxiety is not normally diminished by drug substitution, including the use of clonidine-like drugs, and it is usually increased by gradual drug withdrawal, but in this study 95% were free of craving, and 75% were free of anxiety by the 10th day of CES. For 80% craving disappeared within 4 months of CES. Whereas normal sleep patterns normally take 2 months to return after withdrawal from heroin and amphetamines, up to 4 months after barbiturate withdrawal, and several weeks after stopping alcohol, the majority of the CES patients regained a normal, drug free sleep pattern between the third and ninth night on CES.

Out of 126 patients who took drugs with the potential for causing withdrawal convulsions, 60 (47.6%) took above maximum therapeutic doses. Seven (5.5%) had seizures. Only 1 patient, who had previously suffered multiple convulsions, had more than 1 brief seizure. He had been taking 1,000 mg pentobarbital, 1,000 mg chlormethiazole, and 60 mg flurazepam daily for 3 years, and was on phenytoin on admission. No patient except the 1 cited experienced delirium tremens and none had hallucinations or delusions.

There were 8 deaths over an 8 year period. All were drug addicts. The average time between CES and death was 22 months, with only 1 being less than 1 year. None of these deaths were associated with CES. This 6.1% death rate compares favorably with 12% reported in a representative sample of 128 patients of London Drug Dependence Clinics over 10 years, or 23% in New York City over 20 years.

The drop out rate over 7 years was only 1.6%, prompting the authors to suggest that this was one of the most significant indicators of patient acceptability and clinical effectiveness when compared to other programs cited with drop out rates of 71%, 45%, and 90%.

Of a 50% response to follow-up, 78.5% were addiction-free (80.3% of drug addicts) 1 to 8 years after CES, with an average time in rehabilitation of only 16 days. Alcohol, marijuana and cigarette use was decreased in 64%. Diminished drug use was reported in 76% of recidivists. 17% had 1 treatment after CES (another CES treatment or other hospital treatment), and 1% had 2 treatments. This compares favorably with a U.S. government survey showing that 26% to 43% had repeat treatments every year after the initial treatment, for up to 6 years. 23.5% of the CES patients used alcohol as a temporary substitute, compared to 60% in the U.S. government survey.

There was a consistent improvement in quality of life measures, relationships, and some reductions in alcohol, marijuana, and cigarette use. There was a 75% overall improvement in the health of these patients, with no long-term illnesses or negative physical effects on health which could have resulted from CES.

49. Philip, P., Demotes-Mainard, J., Bourgeois, M. & Vincent, J.D. Efficiency of transcranial electrostimulation on anxiety and insomnia symptoms during a washout period in depressed patients; a double-blind study. *Biological Psychiatry*. 29:451-456, 1991.

Device: Diastim, 350 Hz, 0.7 mS, 1 - 1.2 mA, rectangular monophasic pulses, cathodes over orbits, anodes over mastoids

21 psychiatric inpatients suffering major depressive disorders according to DSM III-R criteria were divided into 2 groups for this double-blind study. The active CES group (N = 10) had 3 males and 7 females (age 44.9 ± 10.3) with an average length of depressive illness of 56 months (1 - 156). The placebo group (N = 11) had 3 males and 8 females (age 36.4 ± 13.8) with an average length of depressive illness of 64 months (range of 5 - 222). All patients completed informed consent. The treatment withdrawn upon admission consisted of benzodiazepines (9 of 10 active and 8 of 11 placebo), barbiturates (1 of 10 active), antidepressant drugs (5 of 10 active and 8 of 11 placebo), and neuroleptics (1 of 10 active and 1 of 11 placebo). The study began on the first drug-free day. Depressive pathology was evaluated daily by the Montgomery and Asberg Depression Rating Scale (MADRS). Sleep was evaluated using a sleep diary and questionnaire. Visual analog scales evaluated anxiety, fatigue, arousal, and life events. Student's paired t-tests were used to

analyze the data. During the 5 day washout period, the natural development of symptoms consists of a rise in anxiety and an exacerbation of sleep disorders. In 2 cases, benzodiazepine withdrawal induced epileptic seizures in patients devoid of epileptic history. These seizures did not occur during CES sessions. The depressive criteria in the CES group paralleled that in the placebo group. Anxiety and sleep criteria showed divergent changes between groups. Anxiety on MADRS was exacerbated in the placebo group but reduced in the CES group (P<.01). The same was true of the ninth criteria of MADRS, pessimism about the future and feelings of guilt and failure. There were no other significant changes on MADRS in either group. Sleep duration improved in the CES treatment group, but was significantly worsened in the placebo group (P<.05). Feelings of fatigue and alertness revealed a positive change in the CES group (P<.05), but not in the placebo group.

The authors concluded that the effects of a drug washout period are markedly attenuated by CES, which is of interest in the management of psychotropic drug withdrawal. No side effects were reported.

50. Romano, Thomas. The usefulness of cranial electrotherapy in the treatment of headache in fibromyalgia patients. *American Journal of Pain Management.* 3(1):15-19, 1993.

Device: Pain Supressor, 12,000 to 20,000 Hz, 35μS, <4 mA, electrodes across temples

100 consecutive fibromyalgia syndrome (FS) patients (23 males ages 22 - 58, mean = 45, and 77 females ages 18 - 65, mean = 46) in a rheumatology practice with severe chronic headache unresponsive to outpatient treatments of medications (NSAIDS, beta blockers, tricyclics, and ergots), biofeedback, low tyramine diet, local injections, and physical therapy were given CES units and instructed to use them for 20 minutes, 4 times daily while continuing their medications. 75 completed the study. Dolimetry using a pressure algometer was performed at 6 active typical "tender" sites just before CES and 1 - 2 months after. Patients were also asked to rate their headache severity on a 1 - 10 scale (1 = no effect, 10 = totally effective in relieving headaches) before CES, at a subsequent visit, and at follow-up.

CES proved to be effective in FS-related headache patients. Approximately 50% of FS patients using CES regularly reported a significant decrease in the frequency and intensity of their headaches. The mean pretreatment headache intensity score was 8.1 (7.8 for males, 8.4 for females). After 1 - 2 months of CES treatment, the mean score was 4.7 (4.5 for males, 4.8 for females). The difference in the mean scores was 3.4 (3.3 for males, 3.6 for females) and there was definite subjective improvement. Dolimetric testing of 450 sites (6 per patient) revealed that 42% (189) were improved (values increased >1 kg/1.54 cm▣), 19% (86) were worse, and 39% (175) were unchanged. 8 patients reported absolutely no benefit, 6 stated they were entirely free of headaches, while 15 (20%) reported CES efficacy as a "7", indicating moderate improvement in both frequency and severity of headaches. 38 (51%) rated improvement as a "7" or greater.

The author concluded that CES is a helpful adjunct in the treatment of FS patients with headache previously unresponsive to more conventional techniques. No side effects were reported.

51. Rosenthal, Saul H. Electrosleep: A double-blind clinical study. *Biological Psychiatry.* 4(2):179-185, 1972

Device, 100 Hz, 1mS, 0.5 - 1.2 mA, orbit to mastoid electrodes

22 neurotic and personality disorder patients (including 2 inpatients) with anxiety, depression, and insomnia (20 females, 2 males 26 - 63 years old, mean = 43.1 years) were divided into active (N = 11), or sham groups (N = 11), each given 5, 30 minute treatments in a double-blind design. A psychiatrist used a 1 - 7 clinical rating scale before the first and after the final treatment for 3 areas of symptomatology: anxiety, sleep disturbance, and depression. The Zung depression scale was also employed at the same times. Patients receiving active treatment had a marked clinical improvement over patients receiving placebo treatment. Of the 11 CES patients, 8 showed a marked improvement, 2 showed a partial improvement, and 1 showed no improvement. Of the placebo group, 1 showed marked improvement, 2 showed partial improvement, and 8 showed no improvement. Average "total clinical ratings" on anxiety, sleep disturbance, and depression fell from 11.3 before CES treatment to 3.2 following treatment. The placebo group only fell from 12.2 to 9.5. In anxiety, the CES group fell from 4.3 to 1.4 while the placebo group only fell from 4.4 to 3.2. 8 of the patients who had sham treatments were then given real CES.

Patients receiving active treatment following inactive treatment responded better than patients receiving inactive treatment, but did not respond as well as those who received active treatment first. For example, the anxiety score fell from 4.0 to 2.5. At the end of the CES treatment, patients felt no confusion, memory loss, or disorientation. They usually reported a calm, relaxed sensation during the treatment, and a feeling of sedation with a desire to sleep following the treatment.

The author stated that he can not help being a little skeptical at his own results. He added that no treatment in common experience is as effective with this type of patient as these results indicate. No side effects were reported.

52. Rosenthal, Saul H. Alterations in serum thyroxine with cerebral electrotherapy (electrosleep). *Archives of General Psychiatry*. 28(1):28-29, 1973.

Device: 100 Hz, 1 mS

41 patients and non-patient subjects (20 males, and 21 females) were studied before and after 4, 30 minute CES treatments. The serum thyroxine level showed a consistent rise with an increase in 28 and a fall in 13 of 41 subjects (P<.05 by a 2 tailed t-test on the D scores). Increases ranged up to 2.5 µg/100ml with an average of 0.3 µg/100 ml. Among males, 10 of 20 showed substantial rises of 0.5 µg/100ml or more (P<.01), and no male subjects showed similar decreases. There was much more variability in the female population. Changes in tri-iodothyronine resin uptake were not significant.

The author hypothesized that these effects were due to direct hypothalamic stimulation, and not placebo effects. No side effects were reported.

53. Rosenthal, Saul H. & Wulfsohn, Norman L. Electrosleep: A preliminary communication. *Journal of Nervous and Mental Disease*. 151(2):146-151, 1970.

Device: Electrosone 50, 100 Hz, 1 mS, 0.5 - 1 mA, cathodes over orbits, anodes over mastoids

10 chronic anxiety, depression, and insomnia patients (25 - 65 years old) unresponsive to medication were selected from a psychiatric "medication clinic" and given from 7 to 10, 10 - 30 minute CES treatments. 6 completed the course of therapy, 4 dropped out because of inability to afford transportation to the clinic, medical illness, recovery after 1 treatment, or not liking the treatment. An additional 3 psychotically depressed inpatients were treated for a total N of 9. Of the 6 outpatients, 5 had relatively total remission, and 1 was a

treatment failure. Of the 3 inpatients, 2 were treatment failures and 1 had partial improvement. The average score overall for the 9 patients for sleep disturbance fell from 5.8 to 2.9, while the anxiety rating fell from 5.7 to 3.0. The clinical depression rating fell from 5.8 to 3.6 and the Zung Depression Scale scores fell from an average of 62.7 to 44.8. The 5 responders were all females with an average age of 47.6. Their sleep disturbances fell from 5.6 to 1.0 (no sleep disturbance), anxiety fell from 6.0 to 2.0, depression fell from 5.6 to 1.4 with Zung score falling from 60.4 to 29.2. 3 patients reported discontinuing sleeping pills that they had been taking for months or years.

There was no side effects reported in any of the patients other than a transient blurring of vision reported by several of the patients, probably associated with the forced closure of the eyes by the eyepads for 1 hour, which cleared within 15 - 30 minutes after treatment.

54. Rosenthal, Saul H. & Wulfsohn, Norman L. Studies of electrosleep with active and simulated treatment. *Current Therapeutic Research*. 12(3):126-130, 1970.

Device: Electrosone 50, 100 Hz, 1 mS, 100 - 250 µA, cathodes over orbits, anodes over mastoids

12 psychiatric outpatients, unresponsive to medications, were selected from an outpatient medication clinic. All were suffering from chronic anxiety, depression, and insomnia. They were given from 5 to 10 CES treatments. They were evaluated before treatment on a 1 - 7 (7 = severe) scale and Zung Self-Rating Scale and reevaluated after 5 sessions. 9 of the 12 patients had relatively total remission of their symptoms, 2 were treatment failures, and 1 was considered to show partial improvement. Overall, the average rating for sleep disturbance fell from 5.8 to 2.3, anxiety fell from 5.9 to 2.7, depression dropped from 5.2 to 2.3 and the average score on the Zung scale fell from 57.4 to 36.3.

Following the 5 treatments, 8 of 12 were completely asymptomatic with regard to insomnia. 6 patients selected in the same way were given simulated CES treatments on a single-blind basis. 2 of the 6 remained unchanged. 4 showed partial improvement. None showed the dramatic complete remission that was seen with active CES treatment. The average rating on the anxiety scale for the sham group fell from 4.7 to 4.3, sleep disturbance fell from 6.0 to 4.0, depression fell from 4.8 to 3.7 and the average rating on the Zung scale fell from 55.8 to 46.8.

The authors noted that the only side effect was a transient blurring of vision, reported by several of the patients, which cleared within 15 minutes after treatment. It was probably due to the forced closure of the eyes and the pressure of the eye pads. It was seen less often with later patients, and this may be due to less tight placement of the electrodes.

The authors concluded that somewhat to their surprise, 9 of 12 patients showed marked responses to treatment.

55. Ryan, Joseph J. & Souheaver, Gary T. Effects of transcerebral electrotherapy (electrosleep) on state anxiety according to suggestibility levels. *Biological Psychiatry*. 11(2):233-237, 1976.

Device: Neurotone 101, 100 Hz, 2 mS, electrodes on forehead and mastoids

42 psychiatric inpatients (41 males and 1 female) at a Veterans Administration hospital without psychosis or neurological impairment manifesting signs of anxiety either not on medication or not responding satisfactorily to medication who gave informed consent were selected for this double-blind study. They were rated as high suggestible (N = 12) or low suggestible (N = 12) as measured on the Harvard Scale of Hypnotic

Susceptibility. Half of each group were randomly assigned to active or simulated CES and given a pre-test STAI. This yielded 6 patients per cell for the 2 x 2 factorial design. The remaining patients were treated, but excluded from the study because they scored in the medium suggestibility range. Experimental subjects ranged in age from 21 to 59 years (mean = 38). Treatments were 5, 30 minute sessions on successive days. 6 - 9 days following the last treatment each subject again completed the STAI. The active CES patients mean pre-test to post-test state anxiety scores were reduced from 58.33 to 43.50 for the low suggestibility group, and from 57.66 to 50.66 for the high suggestibility group. The placebo patients pre-test to post-test state anxiety scores were only reduced from 57.33 to 57.16 for the low suggestibility group, and from 56.33 to 55.00 for the high suggestibility group. Subjects in the active CES group showed significantly greater anxiety reduction than did subjects in the placebo condition ($P<.01$, $F = 8.26$). There was no overall effect of suggestibility, nor was there a significant interaction between suggestibility and type of treatment. That is, CES was related to positive changes, and no placebo effect could be found as measured by the suggestibility level of patients.

The authors stated that the management of anxiety is a significant problem for medical and psychiatric practitioners. Chemotherapy, although highly effective in many cases, cannot be considered the final regime. Total reliance upon prescription medications predisposes the patient to possible untoward side effects, physiologic dependence, and overdose. The development of a safe, effective, and economical treatment for anxiety is worthy of serious investigation. They then concluded that this study demonstrated that active CES produced significantly greater reductions in anxiety than did a simulated treatment. No side effects were reported.

56. Ryan, Joseph J. & Souheaver, Gary T. The role of sleep in electrosleep therapy for anxiety. *Diseases of the Nervous System*. 38(7):515-517, 1977.

Device: Neurotone 101, 100 Hz, 2 mS, electrodes on forehead and mastoids

40 neurotic inpatients at a Veterans Administration hospital exhibiting significant symptoms of anxiety without psychosis or neurological impairment, either not on medication or not responding satisfactorily to psychotropic medication, who gave informed consent were given the A-State Scale of the STAI which measures various emotional reactions such as tension, worry, apprehension, and nervousness. Each patient underwent 5, 30 minute CES treatment sessions, with a therapist in the room to record clinical observations of sleep indicators (*e.g.,* snoring, shallow breathing, difficulty in arousal after treatment). 6 - 9 days after treatment the patients completed the A-State Scale again. 10 males (21 - 59 years old, mean = 34.10) were selected for which there existed a definite agreement between patient and therapist that sleep had occurred during 2 or more treatment sessions. Similarly, 10 no-sleep patients (9 males, 1 female, 26 - 57 year old, mean = 41.9) were also selected. Both groups improved significantly ($P<.001$) on the State Anxiety Scale of the STAI, with no significant differences in improvement in the sleep group when compared with the no-sleep group based on a 2 x 2 ANOVA with repeated measures on pre- and post-treatment scores. The sleep group went from a pretreatment mean anxiety score of 59.20 ± 12.72 to 49.00 ± 18.52 post-treatment. The no-sleep group means fell from 59.80 ± 9.89 to 41.90 ± 15.07.

It was concluded that sleep is not necessary for the effects of CES to occur. No side effects were reported.

57. Sausa, Alan D., & Choudhury, P.C. A psychometric evaluation of electrosleep. *Indian Journal of Psychiatry.* **17:133-137, 1975.**

Device: Somlec, 16 volts

160 anxiety patients were divided into 4 groups: group A, simulated CES; group B, auditory stimulus; group C, CES; group D, CES plus auditory stimulus. Patients were pre and post-tested on the Taylor Manifest Anxiety Scale (TMAS), the Hamilton Anxiety Scale (HAS), and by clinical evaluation. The patients had been given 30, 30 minute treatments on a 3 per week schedule. Statistics were not performed but percentages were computed. In the CES group C, there was a 35% improvement on the TMAS, 45% on the HAS, and 35% on clinical evaluations. In the simulated CES group A, there was a 0% improvement on the TMAS, 5% on the HAS, and 10% on clinical evaluations. In the auditory group B, there was a 20% improvement on the TMAS, 25% on the HAS, and 25% on clinical evaluations. In the combined group D, there was a 60% improvement on the TMAS, 80% on the HAS, and 75% on clinical evaluations.

The authors concluded that the results of this study indicate that the suggestibility and the process of transference produced an improvement rate of 10% clinically and 5% on the Hamilton Anxiety Scale, and CES is beyond doubt, a useful adjunct in the management of anxiety. No side effects were reported.

58. Schmitt, Richard, Capo, Thomas, Frazier, Hal & Boren, Darrell. Cranial electrotherapy stimulation treatment of cognitive brain dysfunction in chemical dependence. *Journal of Clinical Psychiatry.* **45(2):60-63, 1984.**

Device: Neurotone 101, 100 Hz, 2 mS, <1 mA, electrodes behind each ear

This double-blind study involved 60 alcohol and polydrug abuser inpatient volunteers with an average age of 33.9. Treatment effects were assessed pre and post-test on the Revised Beta Examination and 3 subscales of the WAIS that are clinical indicators of organic brain syndrome (digit span, digit symbol, and object-assembly). 88% of the patients were initially dysfunctional on 1 or more of the 3 WAIS scales, with 63% dysfunctional on 1 or more of the Beta subtests. 40 patients received CES or sham CES treatments, and a third, control group of 20 participated in the normal hospital program without access to CES devices. The study was completed by 87% of the CES treated patients (N = 26), 60% of the sham-treated patients (N = 6), and 85% of the controls (N = 17). It was noted that 80% of the sham-treated patients, but only 20% of the treated patients had complained about the ineffectiveness of CES treatment. Following the study, 2 of the complaining sham patients were given CES and they both said it was a highly effective treatment with WAIS testing supporting these claims. Using Fisher's t-tests, CES treated patients made significant (P<.01) gains on all measures of brain function over and above the 2 control groups. No placebo effects were found. Significant gains were also made on the Revised Beta Examination I.Q. test among CES patients but not by the controls.

The authors concluded by agreeing with Dr. Ray B. Smith's speculation that a treatment program in which patients are treated specifically for cognitive dysfunction is not only humane but can also add to the effectiveness of other treatments in a rehabilitation setting. No side effects were reported.

59. Schmitt, Richard, Capo, Thomas & Boyd, Elvin. Cranial electrotherapy stimulation as a treatment for anxiety in chemically dependent persons. *Alcoholism: Clinical and Experimental Research.* **10(2):158-160, 1986.**

Device: Neurotone 101, 100 Hz, 20% duty cycle, <1 mA, electrodes behind each ear

60 inpatient alcohol and/or polydrug abusers (mean age = 33.9) volunteered for this double-blind study. 30 were given CES, 10 sham CES, and 20 served as normal hospital routine controls. Dependent measures of anxiety were the Profile of Mood States, the IPAT Anxiety Scale, and the State Trait Anxiety Index. The CES and sham patients received 15 daily, 30 minute treatments. Based on Fisher t-tests of the means, CES treated patients showed significantly greater improvement on all anxiety measures than did either control group. There were no differences in response between older and younger patients, or between the primarily drug or alcohol abusers. No placebo effect was found on any of the measures.

The authors concluded that CES is rightfully gaining increasing use in American medicine as it gains increasing confirmation as a significant treatment adjunct for stress and cognitive dysfunction in chemical dependency treatment programs, regardless of the chemical of abuse or the age range of the patients treated. No side effects were reported.

60. Schroeder, Mark James. Acquisition and quantitative analyses of EEG during CES and concurrent use of CES and neurofeedback. Doctoral dissertation, The Graduate School of the University of Texas at Austin, Pp. 1 - 191, 1999.

Device: Alpha-Stim 100, 0.5 and 100 Hz, 50% duty cycle, 30 - 80 μA, biphasic asymmetrical rectangular waves, ear clip electrodes

This Institutional Review Board approved study describes the quantitative changes of the electroencephalogram (EEG) due to 30 - 80 μA of Alpha-Stim CES and the concurrent use of CES in 3 neurofeedback (NFB) sessions. 12 normal male subjects between the ages of 20 - 50 were tested. Subjects were right handed and right eye dominant. They had no previous head injury requiring medical attention, no history of epileptic seizures or convulsions, were never treated for insomnia or depression, and were not taking psychoactive prescription drugs.

Instrumentation methods to acquire artifact-free EEG during CES were developed and compared. A noise-cancellation technique was used to eliminate CES noise from the EEG. Each subject underwent a double-blind, crossover design under five treatment conditions: 1) Sham/Control (no treatment), 2) 0.5 Hz CES, 3) 100 Hz CES, 4) 0.5 Hz CES/NFB, 5) NFB. All treatments were administered to each subject for 20 minutes on different days. Occipital EEG data was acquired before, during, and after the treatment. From the processed EEG data, 22 different parameters were analyzed for changes due to the various treatment conditions. Among these parameters was a newly developed alpha modulation index. The alpha modulation index delineates the characteristic waxing and waning of the alpha rhythm from the more general case of alpha activity using a method based on complex demodulation. The index performed well when applied to simulated and physiological data. Thorough statistical analyses were applied to each experimental EEG parameter and treatment relative to the sham control. Each of the four types of treatment was compared with the controls on a paired t-test. A 2^2 ANOVA factorial design compared each of the 4 treatment conditions against each other. A time analysis of variance was also computed for each treatment against the controls to partial out any effects from the position in the study at which subjects received each treatment.

The principal experimental results indicate that both the 0.5 Hz and 100 Hz CES significantly shift the alpha band power distribution downward in frequency relative to control as shown by the alpha mean frequency variable in the EEG. 100 Hz CES also significantly reduces the relative amount of beta band power over time relative to control. NFB alone shifts the beta band power frequency significantly upward relative to control. There is a significant inverse interaction in the alpha index parameter during the combined CES/NFB treatment nullifying the increase in the parameter from each treatment alone, however the combined CES/NFB treatment may cause an increase in the physiological DC potential of the EEG. These findings suggest that Alpha-Stim CES elicits changes in the EEG that are quantifiable and beneficial to people with stress related disorders. The author concluded that the fact that both 0.5 Hz and 100 Hz CES, two completely different treatment parameters, showed significant changes from pre to post treatment for the same variable lends strong support to the claim that the effects seen are real.

No negative side effects were found during or following the study. No subject left the study early, nor did any complain about any study parameter during or following the study.

61. Shealy, C. Norman, Cady, Roger K., Wilkie, Robert G., Cox, Richard, Liss, Saul & Clossen, William. Depression: a diagnostic, neurochemical profile and therapy with cranial electrical stimulation (CES). *Journal of Neurological and Orthopaedic Medicine and Surgery.* **10(4):319-321, 1989.**

Device: Liss Pain Suppressor

14 non-smoking adults (6 males, 8 females, 22 - 72 years old) with no known illness served as Group 1 controls. Group 2 were 14 intractable chronic pain patients (5 males, 9 females, 30 - 68 years old). Group 3 were 9 chronic pain patients considered by themselves to be hopeless (3 males, 6 females, 32 - 60 years old). Group 4 were 11 patients with long-standing depression of more than 2 years unresponsive to 2 or more antidepressant drugs (3 males, 8 females, 30 - 67 years old). Fasting blood levels of serotonin, β-endorphin, norepinephrine, and cholinesterase were taken, along with the Zung test for depression, before and after 20 minutes of CES given daily for 2 weeks. In the depressed patients there was a significant elevation of serotonin (mean of 33.18 ± 9.33 pre-test to 44.64 ± 9.10 post-test P<.0089) and a significant decrease in cholinesterase (mean of 13.82 ± 2.86 pre-test to 10.45 ± 3.04 post-test P<.0067). There was a clinical lifting of depression in 60% of depressed patients and an improvement in pain complaints in 44% of the pain patients.

The authors concluded that CES may be of therapeutic value in depression and in chronic pain. No side effects were reported.

62. Shealy, C. Norman, Cady, Roger K., Culver-Veehoff, Diane, Cox, Richard & Liss, Saul. Cerebralspinal fluid and plasma neurochemicals: response to cranial electrical stimulation. *Journal of Neurological and Orthopaedic Medicine and Surgery.* **18(2):94-97, 1998.**

Device: Liss Stimulator, 15, 500 and 15,000 Hz, <4 mA, 50% duty cycle

5 asymptomatic volunteer nonsmokers (4 females) ranging in age from 23 to 60 years, provided informed consent for this study to ascertain whether or not levels of cerebral spinal fluid (CSF) neurochemicals can be correlated with serum plasma. Subjects had a blood sample taken while lying at rest prior to a spinal tap taken from the subarachnoid space. Subjects then underwent 20 minutes of CES. 10 minutes later blood and CSF samples were taken again. 5 additional subjects, all female, underwent the same procedure with blood tests alone. CSF responses to CES were most marked for serotonin and β-endorphin. Plasma responses to CES were greater for melatonin and slightly higher for norepinephrine. Plasma responses for β-endorphin exhibited an average increase of 50%

over baseline. Melatonin levels after CES rose <20% after CES in CSF, and 28 - 40% in plasma. Norepinephrine in CSF rose 3 - 15% following CES, whereas the plasma level increased 20 - 25%. CSF levels of β-endorphin increased up to 219%, whereas plasma levels increased up to 98%. Following CES the CSF levels of seratonin increased approximately one and one-half to twice baseline, whereas in the blood they increased only 15 - 40%. There was little change in the cholinesterase level in CSF after CES, and the plasma level varied between -6% and +15%. No statistical analyses was attempted. The authors concluded from this study that hypothalamic modulation may explain the reported antidepressant effect of CES. No side effects were reported.

63. Singh, Baldev, Chhina, G.S., Anand, B.K., Bopari, M.S. & Neki, J.S. Sleep and consciousness mechanisms with special reference to electrosleep. *Armed Forces Medical Journal India* **(New Delhi). 27(3):292-297, 1971 (also see animal studies of CES).**

Device: LRDE model HB-1705, 5 Hz to 30 KHz, 800 µA, square waves, cathodes over orbits or forehead, anodes at suboccipital region

4 normal human subjects showed increased alpha index on EEG immediately following CES (30 to 45 minutes), which culminated in spindle and slow sleep after a variable interval. In 6 patients suffering from subjective insomnia, CES resulted in increased alpha activity and a subjective feeling of well being but was not accompanied by either slow or paradoxical sleep. No side effects were reported.

64. Smith, Ray B. Confirming evidence of an effective treatment for brain dysfunction in alcoholic patients. *Journal of Nervous and Mental Disease.* **170(5):275-278, 1982.**

Device: Neurotone 101, 100 Hz, 2 mS, <1.5 mA, electrodes below each ear

100 male alcoholic inpatient volunteers (drinking for an average of 21 years with an average age of 42.2) were randomly assigned to either active or sham CES treatments for this double-blind study, 40 minutes per day, 5 days a week, for 3 weeks. Both groups had scored in the dysfunctional category on the Revised Beta Examination IQ tests before the study. 5 treatment and 10 controls left the study early and were not counted in the final tabulations. The treatment was given below sensation threshold. The CES group made significant gains on the Beta IQ test at or beyond the .05 level of confidence on subtest I (mazes) from a pretreatment mean for the active group of 8.53 to a post-treatment mean of 10.74, with the sham group testing at 8.48 pretreatment to 8.37 post, and on subtest IV (spatial relations) from a pretreatment mean for the active group of 7.18 to a post-treatment mean of 8.80, with the sham group testing at 7.21 pretreatment to 7.32 post-treatment. While the active group was completely back into the scoring pattern of published norms, the sham group did not improve.

The author concluded that in addition to the obvious considerations for the patient such treatment and recovery denotes, it also appears to be a thoughtful thing to do for those involved in other areas of the treatment effort, and whose efforts usually depend heavily on the cognitive functioning of the patient. It should aid treatment immeasurably, for example, if the patient can remember from one treatment session to the next what transpired in the session just preceding. No side effects were reported.

65. Smith, Ray B., Burgess, A.E., Guinee, V.J. & Reifsnider, L.C. A curvilinear relationship between alcohol withdrawal tremor and personality. *Journal of Clinical Psychology.* **35(1):199-203, 1979.**

Device: Neurotone 101, 100 Hz, 2 mS, <1.5 mA, electrodes below each ear

53 male alcoholic patients (mean of 44 years old) who were withdrawing from heavy drinking (mean = 9.57 years drinking) were monitored using the Lafayette Instrument Company's Steadiness Tester, hole type, Stop Clock, 1/100 second, and Tone Response hand tremor test along with the MMPI before and after 40 minutes of CES. All patients had been withdrawing for 96 hours or less, and were receiving Librium 25 mg t.i.d., and Dalmain 30 mg at bedtime. 5 patients whose tremor score did not vary more than ± 1 full second were discarded from the study because the reaction time of the experimenter who controlled the on/off switch on the tremor apparatus was found to vary within this limit. In keeping with an inverted U-curve theory of responsiveness to CES, high stress patients who tremored very little initially, tremored more following CES, while low stress patients who tremored more initially, tremored less following CES. This could be a major source of confusion in the typical linear statistical analysis involved in CES research.

The data fit the researchers' original hypothesis that withdrawing alcoholics would tremor less as their internal stress increased beyond a certain point, as indicated by MMPI score elevations. This may explain the somewhat disconcerting finding that sometimes as few as 80% of known alcoholics tremor during withdrawal, a response heretofore thought of as diagnostic of the addiction process by many researchers. Drug therapy alone did not alter the stress-tremor relationships found. No side effects were reported.

66. Smith, Ray B. & Day, Eleanor. The effects of cerebral electrotherapy on short-term memory impairment in alcoholic patients. *International Journal of the Addictions*. 12(4):575 -562, 1977.

Device: Neurotone 101, 100 Hz, 2 mS, 100 - 710 µA, electrodes below each ear

227 alcoholic patients (average age of 42) were given CES (N = 198) or served as time controls (N = 29). CES was given 40 minutes a day, Monday through Friday, for 3 weeks. CES significantly (P<.001) reduced brain dysfunction in all active treatment patients when compared with the controls on the Beta nonverbal I.Q. Test and the Benton Visual Retention Test of short term memory loss. The dysfunctional process continued to deteriorate in many of the controls, with a mean loss of 55% over an average 21 day period. The matched CES treatment patients improved an average of 84% during the same time period.

The authors concluded that they again found that the more serious disabled alcoholic patients tend to leave early while the less seriously involved stay on for treatment and that CES treatment halts or reverses this trend. This would be helpful if only because it holds the patients for other kinds of therapy offered. However, they also found no other treatment that alters the short-term memory impairment of their patients making CES a valued adjunct to other treatment approaches. No side effects were reported.

67. Smith, Ray B., Cranial electrotherapy stimulation in the treatment of stress related cognitive dysfunction, with an eighteen month follow up. *Journal of Cognitive Rehabilitation*. 17(6):14-18, 1999.

Devices: Alpha-Stim CS, CES Labs, and Liss Stimulator (randomly assigned)

This study compared the effects of 3 randomly assigned CES devices (Alpha-Stim, CES Labs, Liss Stimulator) in the treatment of stress related attention deficit disorder (ADD) in 23 children and adults, 9 males, 14 females, 9 - 56 years old (average 30.96) with an average education level of 10.56 years. All had been diagnosed as having generalized anxiety disorder (61%), and/or depression (45%), and/or dysthymia (17%), with difficulty in focusing when attempting cognitive tasks, difficulty in "connecting" when initially focused on a cognitive task, and once connected, having difficulty remaining on task or tracking it. CES treatments were given daily, 45 minutes per day for 3 weeks. All 3 CES devices were effective based on Duncan's Range test in significantly (P<.001) reducing depression as measured on the IPAT depression scale (mean of 19.38 ± 8.44 pretest to 13.19 ± 7.00 post test), state and trait anxiety scales of the State Trait Anxiety Inventory (mean state anxiety was reduced from 39.95 ± 11.78 pretest to 29.76 ± 6.99 post test, and the mean trait anxiety was reduced from 43.90 ± 11.31 pretest to 32.19 ± 7.50 post test), and in increasing the Verbal pretest (mean of 99.38 ± 13.20 to post test of 107.50 ± 14.13), Performance (mean of 107.4 ± 15.05 to 126.6 ± 14.2), and Full Scale I.Q. scores on the WISC-R or WAIS-R I.Q. tests (mean of 103.2 ± 13.7 to 117.6 ± 14.28). Overall, 18 (86%) of the subjects tested showed improvements in their depression, 18 (86%) in state anxiety, 18 (90%) in trait anxiety, and 100% had an increase in their Full Scale I.Q. scores, 22 (96%) in their Verbal I.Q. scores, and 100% improved their Performance I.Q. scores. Several of the adult subjects reported that they felt "mentally normal" for the first time in their lives.

An 18 month follow-up found 18 of the original 23 subjects available to return for testing. Overall, they performed as well or better than in the original study. None of the scoring changes in anxiety or depression between post study and follow-up testing were found to be significant. The initial Full Scale I.Q. increase held up over the 18 month period while there was a slight, but significant rise in the Verbal I.Q. score (t = 2.37, df = 17, P>.05) and a similar slight, but significant decrease in the Performance I.Q. (t = 3.75, df = 17, P>.01). The author concluded that this study gives strong support for the clinical use of treating stress related cognitive dysfunction in both children and adults.

68. Smith, Ray B. & O'Neill, Lois. Electrosleep in the management of alcoholism. *Biological Psychiatry.* **10(6):675-680, 1975.**

Device: Neurotone 101, 100 Hz, 2mS, <1.5 mA, frontal and occipital electrodes

72 male alcoholic inpatients (average age of 42.4, drinking for an average of 22 years with an average of 5 years of heavy drinking) were given either CES (N = 24 at end of study) or simulated CES (N = 23 at end of study), 40 minutes a day for 15 days. All patients were also receiving medication and psychotherapy. Norms were derived from 342 inpatient alcoholics. The CES group improved significantly (beyond the 0.001 level of confidence) on all 5 negative subscales of the Profile of Mood States while the control group improved on only 2 subscales: Tension-Anxiety and Depression-Dejection. The mean scores were: Tension-Anxiety (pre-test active CES mean of 12.61 ± 1.39 to 6.30 ± 0.79 post, control pre-test 12.22 ± 1.37 to 6.43 ± 0.95 post), Depression-Dejection (pre-test active CES mean of 12.32 ± 1.73 to 4.52 ± 0.87 post, control pre-test 12.80 ± 1.79 to 6.80 ± 1.56 post), Anger-Hostility (pre-test active CES mean of 6.75 ± 1.41 to 1.21 ± 0.42 post, control pre-test 6.63 ± 1.34 to 5.92 ± 1.50 post), Vigor-Activity, a positive score where higher numbers are better (pre-test active CES mean of 14.76 ± 1.21 to 15.08 ± 1.02 post, control pre-test 14.76 ± 1.25 to 13.00 ± 1.40 post), Fatigue-Inertia (pre-test active CES mean of 6.18 ± 1.12 to 1.91 ± 0.53 post, control pre-test 6.45 ± 1.29 to 4.05 ± 1.32 post), and Confusion-Bewilderment (pre-test active CES mean of 8.08 ± 0.99 to 3.92 ± 0.49 post, control pre-test 8.00 ± 0.96 to 6.08 ± 0.67 post). The CES group also improved significantly on Total Mood Disturbance while the controls did not (pre-test active CES

mean of 65.29 ± 6.62 to 40.33 ± 4.69 post, control pre-test 63.96 ± 6.56 to 47.29 ± 6.12 post).

The groups had to be matched following the study prior to statistical analysis, since a majority of the most seriously stressed controls (N = 13) had left the hospital against medical advice, along with 12 CES patients. No side effects were reported.

69. Smith, Ray B. & Shiromoto, Frank N. The use of cranial electrotherapy stimulation to block fear perception in phobic patients. *Current Therapeutic Research*. 51(2):249-253, 1992.

Device: Alpha-Stim CS, 0.5 Hz, 50% duty cycle, <600 μA, biphasic asymmetrical rectangular waves, ear clip electrodes

After gaining IRB approval, 31 persons responded to public media announcements requesting subjects who had been medically diagnosed as having 1 or more phobias. 25 were females (81%). All gave informed consent. The age ranged from 26 - 66 (average 48.69) with an average length of time since their phobia was diagnosed as 16.33 years (range 1 - 44 years). 65% (N = 20) were on medications, and of these, 60% (N = 12) were taking alprazolam. Each subject served as his/her own control. The subjects were asked to imagine themselves in their phobic stimulus situation and rate their fear on a 7 point scale. The authors cited an earlier study that reported internally elicited phobic thoughts produced as much and, at times, greater subjective anxiety, fear, and physiological activity than similar thoughts triggered externally by pictures or verbal statements about phobic objects.

Following 30 minutes of Alpha-Stim CES stimulation, and while the stimulation was still on, they were asked to frighten themselves as before. 1 subject left the study before the program began citing increased situational anxiety as the reason. 4 subjects, appearing to be elated, rated their end-of-study fear as 0, which was not on the scale. That left a useable N of 26. While 77% (N = 20) rated their fear as moderate to extreme going into the study, 85% (N = 22) rated their fear from very low to none following the CES stimulation (mean of 3.33 ± 1.22 pre-test to 1.96 ± 0.76 post-test). The results reached significance beyond a probability of .0001.

The authors concluded that, from their data, it appears that CES may be successfully instituted while patients are on medication. By the same measure, CES appears to be equally as effective without supportive medication and might be a useful tool with which to withdraw from such medication. Since CES devices are portable, its use by the patient in most phobic situations would appear feasible. No side effects were reported.

70. Smith, Ray B., Tiberi, Arleine & Marshall, John. The use of cranial electrotherapy stimulation in the treatment of closed-head-injured patients. *Brain Injury*, 8(4):357-361, 1994.

Device: CES Labs, 100 Hz, 20% duty cycle, <1.5 mA

21 closed head injured patients with an average age of 30, and time since injury ranging from 6 months to 32 years (mean = 11) completed informed consent. They were randomly assigned to CES treatment (N = 10), sham treatment (N = 5) or control "wait-in-line" (N = 6) groups. The statistician was also blinded, being given the data in 3 unidentified groups, making this a triple-blind study. The CES and sham groups had 12 treatments, daily over a period of 3 weeks. They were pre and post-tested on the Profile of Mood States (POMS). The CES treated subjects, but not the sham treated subjects or controls, improved significantly on every POMS subscale. Tension/anxiety was reduced

from a mean of 12.33 ± 7.36 to 8.78 ± 5.09 in the CES treated group, while it rose from 13.00 ± 6.21 pre-test to 14.36 ± 8.25 post-test in the sham group, and barely changed from 12.33 ± 8.07 to 12.50 ± 5.87 in the control group. Depression/dejection changed from 17.11 ± 12.35 to 12.06 ± 8.71 in the CES treated group, and from 20.91 ± 17.79 pre-test to 18.18 ± 12.47 post-test in the sham group, and from 20.00 ± 14.45 to 16.17 ± 9.48 in the control group. Anger/hostility changed from 13.67 ± 11.20 to 10.39 ± 7.49 in the CES treated group, and from 16.73 ± 8.27 pre-test to 17.55 ± 12.22 post-test in the sham group, and from 14.83 ± 11.50 to 14.83 ± 6.18 in the control group. Fatigue/inertia changed from 7.44 ± 6.75 to 5.33 ± 3.96 in the CES treated group, and from 9.46 ± 7.83 pre-test to 8.09 ± 6.63 post-test in the sham group, and from 8.17 ± 7.41 to 6.50 ± 5.82 in the control group. Confusion/bewilderment changed from 8.50 ± 6.75 to 6.22 ± 3.96 in the CES treated group, and from 10.55 ± 5.87 pre-test to 10.27 ± 5.10 post-test in the sham group, and from 9.67 ± 6.15 to 10.50 ± 5.01 in the control group. Total Mood Disturbance was reduced from a mean of 45.11 ± 41.95 to 31.89 ± 23.84 in the CES treated group, and from 52.73 ± 41.95 pre-test to 52.33 ± 36.64 post-test in the sham group, and from 47.83 ± 43.25 to 45.67 ± 24.16 in the control group. 1 patient on sham CES was seen to have a seizure. No negative effects from CES treatments were seen.

The authors concluded that physicians caring for closed head injury patients may well try adding CES therapy, a non-medication prescription, to the treatment of this heavily medicated patient population.

71. Smith, Ray B. & Tyson, Richard. The use of transcranial electrical stimulation in the treatment of cocaine and/or polysubstance abuse, In Process, 2002.

Device: No stimulation parameters of CES were given.

146 inpatients (31 males, 8 females, 14 - 46 years old plus 1, 69 year old, mean = 29.50) were selected in the order of their admission to the hospital. 25% were primary alcohol abusers, while 47% were abusing cocaine. 39 patients were given 45 minutes of CES treatments daily for 1 to 3 weeks. 107 patients served as controls (90 males, 27 females, 17 - 49 years old, mean = 29.20). All were pre and post-tested on the Profile of Mood States (POMS). Patients treated for 1 week with CES did not differ statistically from the controls on the six POMS subtests. Patients receiving CES for 7 days to 3 weeks improved significantly on all of the 6 POMS subscales. On the Tension-Anxiety subscale the CES group had a mean of 9.00 ± 5.05, while the controls mean was 10.94 ± 7.17 (P<.03). On the Depression-Dejection subscale, the CES group was 10.22 ± 5.48, while the control mean was 15.09 ± 12.28 (P<.0001). On the Anger-Hostility subscale, the CES group was 9.00 ± 5.05, while the control mean was 10.97 ± 7.17 (P<.03). On the Lack of Vigor subscale, the CES group was 13.48 ± 8.82, while the control mean was 14.77 ± 6.50 (P<.03). On the Fatigue-Inertia subscale, the CES group was 5.09 ± 3.91, while the control mean was 8.30 ± 9.25 (P<.0001). On the Confusion-Bewilderment subscale, the CES group was 6.39 ± 3.04, while the control mean was 8.84 ± 5.73 (P<.001).

When cocaine patients were analyzed separately, those receiving 7 days to 3 weeks of CES stimulation improved significantly on 4 of the 6 POMS subscales. When cocaine patients were compared with persons with other addictions, no differences in response to CES were found.

The authors concluded that CES, which had already been shown to be an effective treatment for alcoholic patients, is also effective for patients who have abused drugs in the cocaine family. It can be inferred that CES could function well as a core program element in addiction treatment programs. No side effects were reported.

72. Solomon, Seymour, Elkind, Arthur, Freitag, Fred, Gallagher, R. Michael, Moore, Kenneth, Swerdow, Bernard & Malkin, Stanley. Safety and effectiveness of cranial electrotherapy in the treatment of tension headache. *Headache*. 29:445-450, 1989.

Device: Pain Supressor, 12,000 to 20,000 Hz, 35µS, <4 mA, electrodes across temples

112 patients were enrolled in a multicenter double-blind study of tension headaches. Inclusion criteria were that patients had to have tension headaches requiring analgesic agents for at least 1 year, with at least 4 headaches per month. Patients were excluded with diagnosis of migraine, cluster, or medication-rebound headaches, pregnancy, major physical, mental, or neurological problems, recent history of drug dependency, or implanted electrical devices. Informed consent was obtained. Patients were instructed on the use of the CES device and to treat each headaches for 20 minutes, and if necessary, again for 20 minutes, 20 minutes after the first treatment. The study lasted up to 10 weeks, but terminated after 4 headaches. Patient and physician global evaluations were the primary efficacy variables. Following use of the active unit (N = 57), patients reported an average reduction in pain intensity of approximately 35%. Placebo patients (N = 55) reported a reduction of approximately 18%. The difference was statistically significant (P = 0.01). The active unit was rated as moderately or highly effective by 40% of physicians, and by 36% of patients. Both physicians and patients scored the placebo unit moderately or highly effective in 16% of the patients. The difference in order outcomes was statistically significant. Means of changes in headache severity of the 2 groups was 6.1 pre-test to 4.0 post-test for the active group (-34.4%, P<0.001), and 6.4 to 5.2 for the placebo group (-18.8%, P<0.001). 17 patients left the study early due to adverse events (2 active, 2 placebo), no effect (3 in each group), non-compliance (1 each), and 5 others reasons. 6 of 57 in the active group, and 7 of 55 in the placebo group had 1 or more adverse events. The incidence of adverse events was not significantly different between the active and the placebo groups for any of the reported symptoms.

The authors concluded that it appears that CES is safe, and should be considered in the management of tension headaches as an alternative to the chronic usage of analgesics.

73. Southworth, Susan. A. study of the effects of cranial electrical stimulation on attention and concentration. *Integrative Physiological and Behavioral Sciences*. 34(1):43-53, 1999.

Device: Liss Stimulator, 15, 500 and 15,000 Hz, <4 mA, 50% duty cycle

There have been several anecdotal accounts that CES enhances attention and the ability to learn new tasks in a normal population, but only one published investigation confirms that CES improves attention using the Alpha-Stim CES (Madden and Kirsch, 1987). The purpose of this study was to corroborate the findings of Madden and Kirsch, using more precise measures of attention, such as a Continuous Performance Test (CPT). A pretest and posttest CPT was given to 2 groups. The control group consisted of 21 subjects who received the placebo treatment. The experimental group of 31 subjects received 20 minutes of CES. 4 measures of the CPT showed significant gains in attention: Number of Hits, P=.010 Hit RT ISI Change, P=.016, Risk Taking, P=.055; and Attentiveness, P=.054. Based on subjects who demonstrated improvement by 1 standard deviation on 2 different measures of the CPT, 31% of the experimental group improved versus 4% of the control group. The author concluded that the use of CES as a method of increasing attention is a promising area that requires further investigation.

74. Stanley, Theodore H., Cazalaa, Jean A., Atinault, Alain, Coeytaux, Raymond, Limoge, Aimé & Louville, Yves. Transcutaneous cranial electrical stimulation decreases narcotic requirements during neurolept anesthesia and operation in man. *Anesthesia and Analgesia.* **61(10):863-866, 1982.**

Device: 3 mS on - 10 mS off sequence, 250 - 300 mA (average intensity was 0 mA) biphasic asymmetrical nonsquare wave, nasion to mastoid electrodes

IRB approved. The influence of CES on fentanyl requirements was evaluated in 50 patients undergoing urologic operations with pure neuroleptanesthesia (droperidol, diazepam, fentanyl, and air-oxygen) with simultaneous CES (group I) or without CES (group II). All patients had silver electrodes applied, but current was only delivered to group I. All patients had anesthesia induced with droperidol (0.20 mg/kg IV), diazepam (0.2 mg/kg IV), and pancuronium (0.8 mg/kg IV), and, after tracheal intubation, had anesthesia maintained with fentanyl in 100 μg intravenous increments every 3 minutes whenever and as long as systolic arterial blood pressure and/or heart rate were >20% of control (preanesthetic induction) values. Fantanyl requirements averaged 6.1 ± 0.5 and 7.9 ± 0.4 μg/kg/min for a mean total dosage of 9.0 ± 0.9 and 12.5 ± 0.8 μg/kg for the entire operation in groups I and II respectively. These differences between groups were statistically significant (P<.05).

This study demonstrates that CES augments the analgesic effects of fentanyl and thus reduces fentanyl requirements during urologic surgery with neuroleptanesthesia. The authors noted that analgesia with CES appears to be achieved without harmful effects to the patients and without increases in the duration of postoperative respiratory or central nervous system depression.

75. Stanley, Theodore H., Cazalaa, Jean A, Limoge, Aimé & Louville, Yves. Transcutaneous cranial electrical stimulation increases the potency of nitrous oxide in humans. *Anesthesiology.* **57:293-297, 1982.**

Device: 167 kHz, 250 - 300 mA (average intensity was 0 mA), 3 mS

IRB approved. 90 urological patients and 30 abdominal surgery patients (total N = 120, with a mean age of 47 ± 13 years) were randomly assigned to 1 of 3 active CES groups (1E, 2E, 3E), or 1 of 3 control groups (1, 2, or 3), with N = 30 per group. Groups 1 and 1E received 75% N_2O, groups 2 and 2E received 62.5% N_2O, groups 3 and 3E received 50% N_2O. After 20 minutes of N_2O or N_2O and CES, patients were given a painful stimuli of a Kocker clamp clamped to the second ratchet applied to their upper, inner thigh for 1 minute. An observer blind to the CES condition and the amount of N_2O recorded patient movement due to the painful stimulus. Additional recordings made by the blinded observer were systolic blood pressure (SBP), heart rate (HR), respiratory rate (f), and minute ventilation (V) measured before N_2O or N_2O plus CES, after 20 minutes, and following the 1 minute of painful stimulation. 20 minutes after all procedures, the patients were asked if they remembered any painful stimulus. Data was evaluated by chi-square test, analysis of variance, and Student's paired and unpaired t-tests. P<.05 was considered statistically significant. Breathing N_2O resulted in a significant, but similar small increase in SBP in all groups but no change in HR in any group. Breathing N_2O slightly increased f and V in groups 1 and 1E but produced no significant changes in f and V in any of the other groups. HR, SBP, f, and V were not significantly different in the 6 groups after 20 minutes of breathing N_2O. Painful stimulation did not significantly change HR, f, or V when compared to values obtained 1 minute prior to the stimulus in any group. SBP also was unchanged with painful stimulation in all groups except in control group 3 in which it became significantly increased. During painful stimulation, SBP was significantly higher in control group 3 than in all other groups. Movement with and memory of the Kocker clamp application, as well as the postanesthetic pain in the area of clamp application were significantly lower in the CES groups at all N_2O concentrations. As might be expected, positive responses increased in all groups as the N_2O concentrations decreased. A plot of percent of patients moving with painful stimulation during N_2O and N_2O plus CES versus concentration of N_2O indicates that CES increases the potency of N_2O approximately 37%, at least to this form of painful stimulation. The authors also concluded that CES prolongs the analgesia after recovery of consciousness, and that the data suggests that CES appears to be equivalent to 35 - 40% N_2O or between 0.3 and 0.4 MAC in analgesic potency when combined with N_2O.

Theoretically, it should be possible to use lower concentrations of inhalation anesthetics and lower doses of narcotics and other intravenous supplements when using CES. As a result, major organ system alterations in function should be less during anesthesia and postoperative recovery should be faster. In addition, the use of CES during operations may provide residual postoperative analgesia without chemical analgesic administration. These possible advantages of CES, if proven true in subsequent studies, could certainly alter both the research and clinical directions of anesthesiology. No side effects were reported.

76. Straus, Bernard, Elkind, Arthur & Bodian, Carol A. Electrical induction of sleep. *The American Journal of the Medical Sciences.* **248:514-520, 1964.**

Device: Electrosom (built for this study), 1.8 - 2.0 mS, 30 - 40 Hz, eye to mastoid electrodes

This was a very early study to see if CES could induce sleep. 34 hospitalized insomnia patients were given 6 - 12, 30 minute CES treatments, and simulated CES, and Phenobarbital on successive nights. Results were based on observations by nurses, and self-evaluations of the patients. There were more good nights' sleep from CES than placebo treatment according to both nurse's and patients' evaluations, and a corresponding difference of fewer poor nights' sleep (P<.05). Nurses evaluations of the CES and Phenobarbital was almost the same, although the patients indicated more good nights' sleep with Phenobarbital. No side effects were reported.

77. Taaks, H., and Kugler, J. Electrosleep and brain function. *Electroencephalograpy and Clinical Neurophysiology.* **24:62-94, 1968.**

Device: 100 Hz, 600 µA, cathodes on orbits and anodes on neck

In this early study attempting to put people to sleep, 7 female depressives (17 - 65 years old) were given CES for 20 minutes or a sham CES (actually 5 minutes of CES) for 20 minutes, 3 or 4 times on 7 successive days and measured for sleep or wakefulness with EEG, EOG, respiratory abdominal movements and body movements recorded for 20 minutes. The stages of sleep according to Loomis were determined visually for 40 second periods. Some slept under either condition, some did not. No side effects were reported.

78. Taylor, Douglas, N. Effects of cranial transcutaneous electrical nerve stimulation in normal subjects at rest and during stress. Ph.D. dissertation, Brooklyn College of the City University of New York, Pp. 1-88, 1991.

Device: Neurometer, sinusoidal waveform of 5, 100, or 2,000 Hz, 0 - 10 mA (mean of 260 µA was used), ear clip electrodes

This IRB approved dissertation is comprised of 3 studies evaluating the physiological and psychological effects of CES. All subjects signed informed consent forms. In a pilot study 30 normal, healthy subjects (13 males, 17 females, 18 - 33 years old) were divided into treatment-blind active and placebo CES, and no treatment groups. They were given 1, 30 minute 100 Hz CES treatment. One-way multivariate analysis of variance confirmed by Duncan's test revealed significant (P<.05) reductions in systolic (post-treatment mean of 90.29 ± 6.18 as a percentage of pre-treatment means in the active group, 97.01 ± 7.22 in the placebo, and 97.03 ± 7.38 in control) and diastolic blood pressure (post-treatment mean percentage of 91.07 ± 4.94 in the active group, 97.84 ± 3.48 in the placebo, and 98.82 ± 7.51 in control) and anxiety based on the State-Trait Anxiety Inventory (post-treatment mean percentage of 79.44 ± 14.44 in the active group, 94.6 ± 9.1 in the placebo, and 91.88 ± 9.3 in control), but was not significant in pulse rate, peripheral vascular tension, or skeletal muscle activity.

A second study, using double-blind procedures to test 5, 100, or 2,000 Hz on 90 healthy volunteers (20 males, 70 females, 18 - 25 years old), found significant reductions among the active 100 Hz CES group only in systolic blood pressure (post-treatment mean percentage of 96.4 ± 6.14 in the active 5 Hz group, 90.57 ± 7.58 in the active 100 Hz group, 100.05 ± 4.16 in the active 2,000 Hz group, 97.19 ± 4.26 in the placebo, and 98.53 ± 4.38 in control) and diastolic blood pressure (post-treatment mean percentage of 96.46 ± 6.91 in the active 5 Hz group, 90.40 ± 4.75 in the active 100 Hz group, 99.4 ± 5.67 in the active 2,000 Hz group, 99.06 ± 7.74 in the placebo, and 99.8 ± 4.75 in control), and pulse rate (post-treatment mean percentage of 97.3 ± 4.24 in the active 5 Hz group, 89.22 ± 6.13 in the active 100 Hz group, 97.88 ± 5.87 in the active 2,000 Hz group, 101.71 ± 7.92 in the placebo, and 99.07 ± 5.17 in control), but was not significant for peripheral vascular tension or anxiety, and not when using 5 Hz or 2,000 Hz sine-wave CES. In the second study, anxiety scores did change in the active groups, but it also changed in the placebo group (post-treatment mean percentage of 84.8 ± 18.49 in the active 5 Hz group, 79.18 ± 12.93 in the active 100 Hz group, 84.4 ± 11.11 in the active 2,000 Hz group, 89.54 ± 14.77 in the placebo, and 93.16 ± 20.28 in control).

A third double-blind study of 90 subjects (26 males, 64 females, 18 - 25 years old) was designed to answer the following questions: 1) Can CES attenuate the physiological and psychological response of normal subjects to 3 minutes of standardized stress (mental arithmetic)?, 2) Are the effects of CES immediate? 3) Do the effects of CES last after the current is turned off? 4 different CES groups were compared to a no treatment control group. Group 1 received an active 30 minute CES treatment, and another active treatment during a 3 minute stress phase immediately following, Group 2 received an active 30 minute CES treatment, and a placebo treatment during the 3 minute stress phase, Group 3 received placebo CES both times, and Group 4 received a placebo 30 minute CES treatment and an active CES treatment during stress. Significant effects were reductions in systolic blood pressure (post-treatment means as a percentage of pretreatment 93.33 ± 5.99 in Group 1, 90.83 ± 5.08 in group 2, 97.39 ± 6.32 in group 3, 96.06 ± 5.45 in Group 4, and 97.72 ± 4.03 in the control group), pulse rate (post-treatment means of 92.89 ± 8.72 in

Group 1, 92.83 ± 8.95 in group 2, 97.22 ± 13.23 in group 3, 97.89 ± 5.78 in Group 4, and 100.61 ± 5.78 in the control group), and anxiety (post-treatment of 80.28 ± 12.51 in Group 1, 84.11 ± 12.19 in group 2, 96.11 ± 8.74 in group 3, 94.72 ± 11.31 in Group 4, and 93.22 ± 8.27 in the control group), but not in diastolic blood pressure or peripheral vascular tension.

The author concluded that only the first question can be answered from this study. MANOVA revealed no significant group differences in physiological or psychological response to mental stress. The overall conclusion of the 3 studies was that CES can bring about reductions in anxiety, blood pressure, and pulse rates and that these effects are not due to placebo. No side effects were reported.

79. Tomaszek, David E. & Morehead, Kenneth. The use of CES in reducing pain in spinal pain patients. *In process,* 2002.

Device: Alpha-Stim SCS, 0.5 Hz, 50% duty cycle, <500 µA, biphasic asymmetrical rectangular waves, ear clip electrodes

38 patients in a neurosurgery practice who were waiting for surgical implantation of dorsal column stimulators for spinal pain reduction were treated with the Alpha-Stim SCS. 18 of these were in an open clinical trial where they used them 3 times a week in the physician's office, setting the intensity to the level they wished, These patients were asked to rate their pain on a 0 - 10 scale when it was at its least intensity (mean of 4.8 pre CES to 3.5 post), at its greatest intensity (8.9 pre to 7.4 post) and as it was generally (6.45 pre to 5.20 post).

The 20 other patients were provided CES devices to use at home, preset at 200 µA, as either active treatment (N = 10) or sham treatment (N = 10), 1 hour a day for 3 weeks. The CES treated group improved significantly while the sham group did not. Pain at its least intensity improved 17% in the CES treated group vs. a 23% worsening of pain in the sham treated group. Pain at its greatest intensity improved 19% from CES and 1% from sham treatment. General pain levels improved 26% from CES while the general pain levels in the sham treated group worsened by 11%. No side effects were reported.

80. Von Richthofen, C.L. & Mellor, C.S. Electrosleep therapy: a controlled study of its effects in anxiety neurosis. *Canadian Journal of Psychiatry.* 25(3):213-229, 1980.

Device: Neurotone 101, 100 Hz, 2 mS, <1.5 mA, anodes on forehead, cathodes on mastoid

10 patients with anxiety neurosis (6 males, 4 females, 17 - 52 years old) on medication, were given 5, 30 minute sessions of CES or simulated CES in a double-blind, cross-over design. Results were made by psychiatric clinical assessment using a 0 - 7 scale, Eysenck Personality Inventory, State-Trait Anxiety Inventory, and Complaint Checklist. Both groups improved significantly and were not different from each other either before or following the study.

It should be noted that the placebo group received actual current across their foreheads, which can be considered a form of CES that could have accounted for their results. No side effects were reported.

81. Voris, Marshall, D. An investigation of the effectiveness of cranial electrotherapy stimulation in the treatment of anxiety disorders among outpatient psychiatric patients,

impulse control parolees and pedophiles. Delos Mind/Body Institute, Dallas and Corpus Cristi, TX, Pp. 1-19, 1995.

Device: Alpha-Stim 100, 0.5 Hz, 50% duty cycle, 200 µA, biphasic asymmetrical rectangular wave, ear clip electrodes

After achieving IRB approval and informed consent, 105 parolees and psychiatric patients diagnosed with anxiety (STAI >40, EMG >6µV, Temp 75 - 95) were randomly assigned to either group A: Alpha-Stim CES (N = 40), group B: sham CES (N = 35), or group C, controls (N = 30) by assigning conditions to chairs, during group sessions conducted over a 10 day period, and allowing the subjects to sit wherever they would like in a group setting. The study was triple-blind which was accomplished by the use of identical double-blinding boxes, with either of 2 options selected, and by the statistician being blinded to all conditions for analyses. All subjects were tested on the State Trait Anxiety Inventory (STAI), electromyogram (EMG), and peripheral temperature (temp) before and after a single 20 minute application of CES treatment, except the control group, which sat in the same room but was not connected to any device. All CES subjects, but not placebo or controls had significant effects. STAI in the active CES group had a pretest median of 50 ± 8.12 to post-test median of 34 ± 7.39. STAI in the sham group had a pretest median of 51 ± 8.58 to post-test median of 50 ± 8.46. STAI in the control group had a pretest median of 48 ± 5.96 to post-test median of 48 ± 8.81. EMG in the active CES group had a pretest median of 10.40 ± 7.12 µV to post-test median of 3.80 ± 4.98 µV. EMG in the sham group had a pretest median of 12.55 ± 10.45 µV to post-test median of 12.95 ± 10.65 µV. EMG in the control group had a pretest median of 8.00 ± 9.11 µV to post-test median of 9.95 ± 9.69 µV. Temp in the active CES group had a pretest median of $90.0°$ F ± 5.63 to post-test median of $93.60°$ F ± 3.36. Temp in the sham group had a pretest median of $90.5°$ F ± 4.90 to post-test median of $91.65°$ F ± 4.81. Temp in the control group had a pretest median of $92.2°$ F ± 5.59 to post-test median of $92.45°$ F ± 5.89. The probability of achieving these results by chance on the STAI is $P<.0001$ for CES vs. sham or controls, and $P<.3902$ for sham vs. controls, on the EMG it is $P<.0001$ for CES vs. sham or controls, and $P<.6693$ for sham vs. controls, and on peripheral temperature it is $P<.0141$ for CES vs. sham, $P<.0011$ for CES vs. controls, and $P<.3109$ for sham vs. controls.

The author stated that when they began the research, several members of the team had significant doubts as to the effectiveness of this technology. In addition, the concerns of FDA caused further concern and suspicion regarding this technology. But after this project, they concluded that they are completely convinced as to the value of this treatment methodology for many of their patients. No side effects were reported.

Reviewer's Note: The FDA visited this researcher 4 times, but try as they might, they could find no problems with this research, concluding that, "Our review of the inspection report submitted by the district office revealed that there were no deviations from the regulations observed during the inspection." Signed by David R. Kalins, Chief, Program Enforcement Branch I, Division of Bioresearch Monitoring, Office of Compliance, Center for Devices and Radiological Health of the Food and Drug Administration.

82. Voris, Marshall D. & Good, Shirley. Treating sexual offenders using cranial electro-therapy stimulation. *Medical Scope Monthly.* **3(11):14-18, 1996.**

Device: Alpha-Stim 100, 0.5 Hz, 50% duty cycle, <500 µA, biphasic asymmetrical rectangular waves, ear clip electrodes

For a period of 6 weeks, 2 groups of convicted male pedophiles controlled by the Dallas Probation Department were treated using relaxation training and Alpha-Stim CES. Individuals were randomly assigned to treatment groups by numbers out of a hat. Group A consisted of 8 individuals from 24 to 73 years old who received 300 µA CES at 0.5 Hz for 20 minutes. Group B was 7 individuals from 26 to 70 who received 20 minutes of relaxation training which involved a hypnotic-like induction using the Speigal method of eye rotation and eye closure, with focus on breath control. Both groups were treated weekly for 4 weeks. The State Trait Anxiety Inventory (STAI) using form X to measure trait (constant) anxiety factors was used 1 week before, and again, 1 week after the treatments, along with electromyogram (EMG) measurements as an independent physiological measure and the Sexual Inventory (SI), a questionnaire that asks for information regarding fantasy and behavior relating to deviant and nondeviant activities. The SI is not yet qualified for validity and reliability, but serves a purpose of having a simple pencil/paper report tool. Two assumptions were made in this study: 1) anxiety is at the root of much of the deviant behavior, and 2) deviant behavior is an attempt to self-medicate anxiety. The CES group STAI was reduced from 41.63 pre-test to 27.38 post-test. The relaxation training group STAI was reduced from 41.29 to 36.86. EMG changes were 8.40 to 3.97 µV in the CES group, and 9.81 to 11.10 µV in the relaxation training group.

The authors stated that their results must be viewed cautiously due to the small sample size. Nevertheless they do reveal some important findings. Both groups were matched prior to STAI, and both improved significantly ($P=.01$ for CES group) in their trait anxiety with the clear advantage being demonstrated with CES. The EMG findings, attributable to changes in state anxiety, showed a significant decrease in the CES group while the relaxation group actually exhibited an increase in their muscle tension. The SI also demonstrated less behavior, both normal and deviant, in the CES group, suggesting that CES was effective in lowering sexual behavior/acting out. The authors were surprised by the findings between the groups, and believes that this study necessitates more testing in the distinction between state and trait anxiety as it relates to pedophilia. This research began looking at the feasibility of introducing a mechanism for reduction of trait anxiety among pedophiles. CES, according to the results of this study, has accomplished that task very well. No side effects were reported.

83. Weingarten, Eric. The effect of cerebral electrostimulation on the frontalis electromyogram. *Biological Psychiatry.* 16(1):61-63, 1981.

Device: Neurotone 101

This study of 24 alcoholic inpatients tested the idea that if the effects of CES can be attributed to general relaxation, reduction of arousal, or parasympathetic shift, then the effects of CES treatment should find a close correlation with the frontalis electromyographic score, since this measure also purports to reduce the central state of arousal, or sympathetic activity, by lowering the tension level of the frontalis muscle group in the forehead. The treatment was single-blind, at a subsensory current, for 40 minutes per day, Monday through Friday for 3 weeks. The EMG means were 8.03 ± 8.01 µV pretreatment and 8.01 ± 2.71 µV post-treatment for the active CES group, and 8.65 ± 2.31 µV pretreatment to 8.83 ± 1.86 µV post for the control group. While CES treated subjects (N = 12) improved significantly on the Tension/Anxiety (P<.05), Depression/Dejection, (P<.02) Fatigue/Inertia (P<.01), and Confusion/Bewilderment (P<.05) factors on the Profile Of Mood States, the controls (N = 12) improved insignificantly on only the

Confusion/Bewilderment factor (P<.10). 8 (33%) of the subjects left the study early, 6 (75%) of these being controls. As a group the initial EMG scores of those who left early were numerically higher than the initial scores of those who remained. It was concluded that while CES was an effective means of lowering stress levels, the EMG alone, without biofeedback training, did not show a correlated reduction. No side effects were reported.

84. Weiss, Marc F. The treatment of insomnia through use of electrosleep: an EEG study. *Journal of Nervous and Mental Disease.* 157(2):108-120, 1973.

Device: Electrodorn I, electrodes on forehead and neck

10 patients with objectively established insomnia were randomly selected from 40 volunteers solicited by newspaper ads. The subjects spent 3 initial nights in a sleep lab to establish baseline measurements, and then returned for 2 nights at the end of the study and again for follow-up. They were given 24, 15 minute CES treatments (N = 5) or simulated treatments (N = 5) in a double-blind manner and measured before and after treatment, and after a 14 day post-treatment period. The MMPI was used to establish equivalency of groups. EEG latencies of sleep onset for the CES group pretreatment means was 60.8 to 10.6 minutes post-treatment, and for the sham group 60.5 to 58.8 minutes. The CES group had a significant decline in latency of sleep onset (P=.00077), amount of bed time awake (CES pretreatment 19.334% to 4.192% post, and sham 17.296% pre to 18.500% post, P=.367), and percentage of total sleep time in stage 1 sleep. A significant increase in the total sleep time in stage 4 and total delta sleep was also found in the CES group. No significant improvement was found in the placebo group. All differences found were maintained at the 2 week and 2 year follow-up.

The author stated that we can now conclude that CES is effective in the treatment of chronic, sleep onset insomnia. No side effects were reported.

85. Wilson, Lawrence F. & Childs, Allen. Cranial electrotherapy stimulation for attention-to-task deficit: A case study. *American Journal of Electromedicine.* 5(6):93-99, 1988.

Device: RelaxPak, 100 Hz, 2 mS, 1 mA, sine wave, bilateral electrodes

4 patients with measurable attention-to-task deficit were studied. 2 had severe pain problems (27 year old female and 30 year old male) but no brain injury, while 2 had suffered from brain trauma (29 year old male, 25 year old female). One of the pain patients served as placebo control (the 30 year old male) for the other 3, each of whom served as his or her own control. CES was given for 50 minutes per day, 5 days a week for 3 weeks. Patients were pre- and post-tested on standardized cognitive measures (Trail Making Test, Digit Symbol Test, Porteus Mazes, Consonant Trigrams Test, Rey Auditory-Verbal Learning Test, Paced Serial Arithmetic Test) before and following CES, and again 3 weeks later. Patients were also tested on the Profile of Mood States Inventory.

The results among the CES treated patients showed striking and significant improvement in the post-treatment scores and in the associated extent of the neurological deficit. It was concluded that CES is an effective non-drug alternative in a cognitive rehabilitation model for treating attention-to-task deficit. No side effects were reported.

86. Winick, Reid L. Cranial electrotherapy stimulation (CES): a safe and effective low cost means of anxiety control in a dental practice. *General Dentistry.* 47(1):50-55, 1999.

Device: Alpha-Stim 100, 0.5 Hz, 50% duty cycle, 200 µA, biphasic asymmetrical rectangular wave, ear clip electrodes

This is a double-blind study of situational anxiety of 33 dental patients (9 males and 24 females, 20 to 59 years old). All patients completed informed consent. Patients were randomly assigned to an active CES group (N = 16), or placebo CES (N = 17) in the order they arrived for various dental procedures. All patients completed the study. A double-blinding box was used so neither the patient nor the dentist was aware who was receiving actual stimulation. 100 mm Visual Analogue Scales (VAS) of "not anxious" on the left to "very anxious" on the right were employed before, halfway through, and after various dental procedures by both the patient and dentist, and a 7 point Likert scale was used at the conclusion of each treatment. There was no significant difference in anxiety levels before the procedure between both groups. However, the anxiety level after the procedure was significantly lower in the treatment group than the control group.

Statistics were performed by the student's t-test (unpaired) comparing the active and placebo groups at specific time points. The results are considered statistically significant at P<.05. The mean value for the dentist's and patient's evaluations tended to be higher in the treatment group at the start probably due to the more severe procedures in that group compared to the placebo group. Nevertheless, the overall feelings of anxiety were decidedly less in the treatment group when considering both the differences found in the dentist's and patient's evaluations. The dentist's treatment assessment by the VAS was –24 ± 6.4 (SEM) and for placebo was -7.2 ± 3.2 (SEM) (P<.02). The difference was even seen at the midpoint where the mean change was -13.5 ± 5.0 (SEM) for treatment and -3.4 ± 2.9 (SEM) for placebo (P<.04). At the end of the study, the patient's evaluation by the VAS simulated the dentist's evaluation: differences were -30.1 ± 9.0 (SEM) for treatment and -4.2 ± 3.9 (SEM) for placebo (P<.02). However, no statistically significant differences were seen at the midpoint of the patient's evaluations: -5.6 ± 9.7 (SEM) for treatment and -2.8 ± 3.2 (SEM) for placebo. The use of the Likert scale corroborated these findings. The treatment group was less anxious as indicated by an increase in the scale values in both the dentist's and patient's evaluations: dentist 4.4 ± 0.4 (SEM) for treatment versus 2.3 ± 0.1 (SEM) for placebo (P<.01); patients 4.8 ± 0.4 (SEM) for treatment versus 2.5 ± 0.3 (SEM) for placebo (P<.01).

The author concluded that using CES during various dental procedures significantly comforts dental patients, who experience extreme levels of anxiety. Many members of the treatment group requested CES at subsequent visits, and none objected to it. The low cost, safety and ease of use of CES recommends its freer trial to enhance patient comfort during various routine dental procedures. There were no detectable adverse effects.

4

40 SUPPORTING SCIENTIFIC STUDIES OF CES

The following supporting scientific studies of CES fit the U.S. Food and Drug Administration's definition of valid scientific evidence, however, they have less reliable measurement vectors, and/or did not do reliability checks on the ratings used. Included in this section are published clinical evaluations and physicians' global analyses. Even though they sometimes appeared to have found highly positive results from CES, these studies have been separated because they tend to provide some degree of confusion to the CES literature.

Overall, based on the authors' conclusions of the outcomes of their studies, 85% (34) of the supporting scientific studies had positive outcomes.

1. Achte, K.A., Kauko, K. & Seppala, K. On "electrosleep" therapy. *Psychiatric Quarterly.* **42(1):17-27, 1968.**

Device: 5 - 10 Hz, .2 - .5 mS, 100 - 600 µA, electrodes from orbit to neck

In this uncontrolled study, 19 hospitalized patients and 5 outpatients with severe insomnia, half of who were drug abusers, were selected for CES because they were unresponsive to prior treatment. 6 (25%) fell asleep under the treatment, and the rest were relaxed. When the treatment was discontinued, 20 (83%) were subjectively content with it. On 2 month follow-up, 3 (12.5%) patients continued to be in good condition, 5 (21%) were fairly good, and in 13 (54%) no improvement was then observable. Complications were discovered in 5 (21%) cases, 2 complained of headaches, 3 felt aching in the eyes. 1 had hysterical convulsions during the treatment. Initially, experiments were done with eyes open and closed. If the duration exceeded 0.5 mS, there was a sensation of light in the eyes that was experienced as unpleasant and which prevented relaxation. Too strong currents caused headaches in healthy persons.

The authors stated that the currents were too weak to cause convulsions and too weak to bring about neuro-vegetative side effects. They concluded that the method is indicated for use chiefly in cases where neurotic patients suffer from chronic insomnia or are inclined to the abuse of drugs.

2. Alpher, Elliott J. & Kirsch, Daniel L. Traumatic brain injury and full body reflex sympathetic dystrophy patient treated with cranial electrotherapy stimulation. *American Journal of Pain Management.* **8(4):124-128, 1998. Presented at the Ninth Annual Clinical Meeting of the American Academy of Pain Management, Atlanta, Georgia, September, 1998.**

Device: Alpha-Stim 100, 0.5 Hz, 50% duty cycle, biphasic asymmetrical rectangular wave, ear clip electrodes

This is a case report of WHH, a 60 year old male with an intracranial traumatic brain injury (TBI) and full body reflex sympathetic dystrophy (RSD). In spite of severe disabilities of his brain and body, WHH continues to serve his country in his position on the Executive Staff of the President's Committee on Employment of People with Disabilities. Daily 20 minute treatments of CES provides satisfactory pain relief for WHH to complete his tasks and enjoy a relatively higher quality of life than he was able to have with drugs alone.

Prior to CES, WHH has been prescribed numerous medications including Prozac 20 mg q.i.d., Catapres Tab 20 mg q.d., Effexor 100 mg in AM and 50 mg at bedtime, Levo-Dromoran 1 mg b.i.d., Balofen 10 mg split AM and PM, Risperdal 7.5 mg at bedtime, Kolopin 0.5 mg 1 tab three to four times per day as needed, C-Dextromthrph 60 mg t.i.d. and Fentanyl patches for 4 years. This regime did little to reduce his whole body chronic intense critical pain and burning. Nor did it relieve his difficulty sleeping. Standard milliampere transcutaneous electrical nerve stimulation (TENS) did not help. WHH claims these treatments made him worse and is concerned about the short and long term side effects the drugs have on his ability to function.

WHH exhibited marked relaxation from CES, with a reduced anxiety level and a significantly enhanced pain threshold. Based on these positive results he was prescribed 20 minute CES treatments daily via ear clip electrodes. WHH credits the CES treatment for allowing him to return to work, and for improving his family and social life. Prior to CES he claimed that "life was not worth living to the degree that suicide was an attractive option." He found this treatment provided him a moderate improvement of 50 - 74% relief from his pain, anxiety, depression, headaches, and muscle tension, and a marked improvement of 75 - 99% in his insomnia.

A single CES treatment lasts for 6 to 8 hours, allowing him to get through the day, then the pain gradually returns, but never to his pre-CES pain levels prior to the next CES treatment. In his own words, "The Alpha-Stim 100 has given me short term relief from my pain levels that medications have not been able to accomplish. While the relief periods may only be for 8 hours or so, these near pain-free hours allow my body to recycle itself, granting me an improved quality of life. Without the Alpha-Stim 100, the constant 'level 10' debilitating pain levels leave me with no physical or emotional reserves to carry on daily life. The Alpha-Stim 100 has no side effects, whereas my medicines have profound, crippling and lasting side effects that have impaired my bowel and colon. These impairments can not be reversed." On a zero (no pain) to 10 (maximum pain) scale, He says CES reduces his pain level from a 10 to a 3 which he describes as "the difference between standing on a busy street in New York at 5 PM and fly fishing on a tranquil creek." He added "CES provides me with a measure of pain relief that brings me back from the depth of despair and gives me a wedge of hope."

CES reduces his pain level to a point where he can perform his daily exercise routine. He is also able to rest better at night, which he credits as creating a "positive emotional and physical self-environment." He now feels more rested in the morning. At present he is able to work 30 to 40 hours per week, up from a maximum of 15 hours prior to CES.

Following CES, his medication has been reduced to Prozac 10 mg q.d., Catapres Tab 0.1 mg b.i.d., Effexor 50 mg AM and 25 mg PM, Levo-Dromoran 1 mg b.i.d., Restoril 7.5 mg at bedtime, Kolopin p.r.n., and Neurontin 400 mg p.r.n.

3. Astrup, Christian. Follow-up study of electrosleep. *Biological Psychiatry.* **8(1):115-117, 1974.**

Device: Electrosleep 1 (from Russia)

51 patients, of which 41 were rather severe neurotic inpatients, and 10 neurotic outpatients were given 10 - 15, 1 hour treatments. The author followed the patients for as much as 18 years then concluded that their treatment had no long term effects in functional psychoses and improved only 1 of 24 neurotics. It was noted that CES increased the effects of verbal suggestions. No side effects were reported.

4. Barabasz, Arreed F. Hypnosis and cerebral electrotherapy in the treatment of sleep disturbances in mildly depressed patients. *Hypnosis Quarterly.* **19(2):321-34, 1976.** Also see next entry.

Device: Lafayette Model 7200 Somniatron, 12 Hz, 20 mA, cathodes over eyes, anodes behind ears

60 adult psychiatric outpatients with mild depressive neuroses complaining of sleep disturbances were divided into 4 groups and given 6, 2 hour CES treatments. A self-rating scale of 1 - 7 was used. Group A (CES only) reported significantly greater improvement than group B (CES placebo). Group C (CES and hypnosis) reported significantly greater improvement than group A, and group D (CES placebo and hypnosis) reported significantly greater improvement than group B. No significant differences were found between groups C and D, or A and D. No side effects were reported.

4a. Barabasz, A.F. Treatment of insomnia in depressed patients by hypnosis and cerebral electrotherapy. *American Journal of Clinical Hypnosis.* **19(2):120-122, 1976.**

This is the same study as in 4 above, rewritten for another publication.

5. Brand, J. Electrosleep therapy for migraine and headache. In Wageneder, F.M. and St. Schuy (Eds). *Electrotherapeutic Sleep and Electroanaesthesia.* **Excerpta Medica Foundation, Amsterdam, Pp. 113-115, 1970.**

Device: Dormed, 12 - 200 Hz

58 migraine and headache patients were treated and it is the author's conclusion that CES proved to be very useful. In 7 cases, CES was the only method that could prevent the onset of a migraine attack. In many cases it was possible to prevent the occurrence of headaches without any additional medication. No side effects were reported.

6. Boertien, André, H. The electrosleep apparatus as a device in an antismoking therapy. In *Electrotherapeutic Sleep and Electroanaesthesia.* **Masson, Pp. 103-104, 1978.**

Device: Electrodorm 1, 100 Hz, 1 mS, 500 μA

20 smokers were given 2 treatments per week for 5 weeks while simultaneously receiving hypnotic suggestion. Almost all of the subjects reported that it was very pleasurable and that they felt quite relaxed after a few sessions. 2 weeks after the last session the mean reduction in the smoking rate of the group was 65%.

7. Cartwright, Rosalind D. & Weiss, Marc F. The effects of electrosleep on insomnia revisited. *Journal of Nervous and Mental Disease.* **161(2):134-137, 1975.**

Device not specified

This is a double-blind study of 10 sleep onset insomnia patients with a 2 year follow-up done at the sleep laboratory at the University of Illinois. Of the 5 who received 24 CES treatments, 4 appeared to be able to fall asleep with little difficulty and to awake moderately to very well rested. Only 1 relapsed during the 2 year no-treatment period. Of those receiving sham treatment, 4 were having quite a bit of difficulty falling asleep, but 3 of the 5 awoke feeling moderately well rested.

The authors concluded that overall, the results appear to have remained positive for the actual treatment group, except for 1 who appears to be having as much or more difficulty as before being involved in the study, while those in the sham group appear to be still experiencing the difficulty of attaining sleep although they claim to be able to sleep a little longer and to wake up more refreshed. No side effects were reported.

8. Childs, Allen & Crismon, M. Lynn. The use of cranial electrotherapy stimulation in post-traumatic amnesia: a report of two cases. *Brain Injury.* **2(3):243-247, 1988.**

Device: Relaxpak, 100 Hz, 1 mA, electrodes behind each ear

Patient 1 is a 21 year old male injured 3 1/2 years prior to CES. He sustained a closed-head injury in a motor vehicle accident. Computerized tomography (CT) revealed a right lateral basal ganglia hemorrhage and hemorrhage into both ventricles. He was totally unresponsive for 10 days, semi-comatose for 10 days, and in a state of coma vigil for 20 days. 3 months after the accident he showed a dense left hemiparesis, and a Wechsler Memory Scale (WMS) score of 61, Full Scale IQ of 71. 6 months after the accident his IQ improved to 80, but the WMS score was essentially unchanged at 63. He showed marked deficits in short-term retention of visual and verbal information. By 8 months after the accident WMS was 83, but acquisition of new learning was significantly impaired. This patient was treated with CES 40 minutes daily for 3 weeks. He averaged 29 correct responses immediately after CES, and 30 correct responses (delayed recall) 30 minutes later. At the end of 3 weeks of CES immediate recall was in the 36 - 37 point range, while delayed recall increased to 40 (33% improvement). 10 days following discontinuation of treatment, he averaged 45 in immediate recall (55% improvement), and delayed recall improved to an average of 47 (56% increase over baseline).

Patient 2 is 58 year old orthopedic surgeon who sustained a closed head injury in a motor vehicle accident, with extensive lacerations and a broken leg, in 1984. Initial CT scan revealed intraventricular hemorrhages within the occipital horns of both ventricles. An area that appeared consistent with an infarction of the left anterior thalamus was also noted. An EEG 3 weeks later showed slowing consistent with diffuse encephalopathic process. CT scans 1 month later showed clearing of the hemorrhages and progressive dilation of the ventricles. From the day of injury, the patient was extremely confused, disoriented, and demonstrated severe memory deficits. 12 weeks after the injury he was transferred to a rehabilitation hospital where he exhibited disorientation, memory disturbance, and delusions of being dead. He had difficulty distinguishing between fantasy and reality, and experienced overwhelming anxiety during periods of disorientation. His problems was with new memory, exemplified by his successful completion of a state medical board exam, after which he was unable to find his way out of the building. He could not drive because he could not remember where he was going. He was diagnosed with diencephalic amnesia secondary to trauma. Baseline scores averaged 29 for immediate recall, and 23 for delayed recall. After 1 week of CES, immediate recall averaged 35 and delayed recall averaged 25. After 3 weeks of CES, immediate recall averaged 35 and delayed recall averaged 31. During 3 weeks following discontinuation of treatment, he was tested 3 times and averaged 37 on immediate recall (28% improvement), and 32 on delayed recall (39% improvement).

Subjective observations by staff indicated visible improvements in mood, spontaneity, and initiative in both patients, but deteriorated rapidly after the treatment was stopped. Nevertheless, the authors state that the clinical improvement in these 2 patients cannot be ignored. No side effects were reported.

9. Childs, Allen. Fifteen cycle cranial electrotherapy stimulation for spasticity. *Brain Injury*, 7(2):179-181, 1993.

Device: Liss Device, 15 Hz, <4mA, suboccipital electrodes

In this case history severe post-anoxic spasticity in a 25 year old female was significantly improved during an open trial of CES used for 40 minutes 3 times daily. CES also appeared to be very helpful for relaxation. A synergism appeared when dantrolene 50 mg b.i.d. was combined with CES, being greater than either therapy alone.

The author noted that he hoped that this preliminary report will stimulate interest in electromedical approaches to central nervous system induced spasticity. No side effects were noted.

10. Coursey, Robert D., Frankel, Bernard L., Gaarder, Kenneth R. & Mott, David E. A comparison of relaxation techniques with electrosleep therapy for chronic, sleep-onset insomnia: a sleep-EEG study. *Biofeedback and Self-Regulation.* 5(1):57-71, 1980.

Device: Electrosone 50, 15 and 100 Hz

22 chronic insomniacs were divided into 3 groups. 30, 45 minute CES treatments were given to 10 patients. Instead of a no-treatment control group for this study, there were EMG feedback and Autogenic training groups. Following treatments patients filled out the Taylor Manifest Anxiety Scale, Multiple Affect Adjective Check List, and Zung Depression Scale. 3 of 6 EMG feedback patients, 2 autogenic patients, and none of the CES patients succeeded in achieving a meaningful improvement in their difficulties sleeping. No side effects were reported.

11. Epifanov, V.A., Korableva, N.N. & Zhuravleva, N.V. The correction of the cardio-vascular system changes in patients with the spastic form of infantile cerebral palsy in the chronic residual stage by means of mesodiencephalic modulation. *Vopr Kurortol Fizioter Lech Fiz Kult.* **15-8, 1999. (Russia)**

Device not specified

CES, mesodiencephalic modulation on the basis of activation of the central regulatory structures induced by weak impulse current, proved effective in relief of clinical symptoms and mitral prolapse, correction of conduction, automatism, contractility, vegetative unbalance due to normalization of the sympathetic and parasympathetic components of the autonomic nervous system.

12. Evtiukhin, A.I., Dunaevski□, I.V., Shabut, A.M. & Aleksandrov, V.A. The use of trans-cranial electrostimulation for pain relief in cancer patients. *Vopr Onkol.* **44:229-33, 1998. (Russia)**

Device not specified

The report discusses whether CES in cancer patients can be accepted. A number of tumors were inhibited in an experiment using 120 rats. The procedure used in 80 cancer patients was followed by favorable changes in the concentration of several hormones. The antinociceptive action of CES is similar to that of narcotic analgesics.

13. Forster, S., Shapiro, A., Fine, L., Feldman, H.H., Berner, H. & Goldberg, M. In Wagen-eder, F.M. & St. Schuy (Eds). *Electrotherapeutic Sleep and Electroanaesthesia.* **International Congress Series No. 136. Excerpta Medica Foundation, Amsterdam, Pp. 169-171, 1967.**

Various devices are mentioned

6 patients were given up to 4 hours of treatment which resulted in an increased alertness, improved capacity for work, and decreased mental fatigue. Not all patients slept during the procedure. No side effects were reported.

14. Gigine□shvili, G.R., Dombrovskaia II, Orekhova, E.M., Radzievski□, S.A. The different-ial use of electrosleep for restoring the work capacity of athletes. *Vopr Kurortol Fizioter Lech Fiz Kult.* **31-4, 1995. (Russian)**

Device: 10 and 100 Hz square pulses

A comparative study has been made of the effects that might be produced on body functions of athletes by electric sleep (CES). The induction of the sleep was conducted using square electric pulses with 10 and 100 Hz frequencies. The 100 Hz (8 - 10 sleep procedures) stimulated the examinees somatically and psychologically, whereas CES procedures at 10 Hz displayed sedative effects and thus were indicated for overstrained sportsmen and in some diseases.

15. Glazer, I., Ashkenazxi, A. & Magora, F. Electrosleep therapy in bronchial asthma. *International Archives of Allergy.* **36(1):163-171, 1969.**

Device: 25 Hz, 4 mS, 1 ± 0.2 mA, monopolar, square waves, electrodes above hairline to occipital fossa

The study was interrupted by the six days' war in Israel. 13 patients were given 35 treatments. 6 patients had only 1 treatment, 1 had 2, 2 had 3, 3 had 4, and 1 had 9. All patients continued on their routine medication. The current produced objectively observed sleep or drowsiness in all of the 8 sessions when the patients were free of asthma. Even when there was wheezing, the current induced sleep on 19 occasions and brought about subjective improvement in 10 of them. In another 5 trials in patients with wheezing, sedation and a sense of improvement was noted on 2 occasions. The authors added that it is noteworthy that there was no objective significant change in physical status, particularly wheezing, immediately after the treatment. No ill-effect or aggravation was noted.

16. Kelley, J. Whitney, Kelley, Irene H. & Kaiman, Carman. Cerebral electric stimulation with thermal biomedical feedback. *Nebraska Medical Journal.* **62(9):322-326, 1977.**

Device: Neurotone, forehead to mastoid electrodes

5 cases are presented using a combination of CES, thermal biofeedback, and pychotherapeutical phrases concurrently. The authors concluded that with over 50 cases of this combined therapy there is a large enough statistical sample to allow them to infer some trends. Each of the 3 modalities has therapeutic value individually. Together they seem to synergize each other. The authors state they estimate they can replace 95 to 97% of electroconvulsive therapy with the combination treatment. They ended by stating that this method is pleasant to the patient, has practically no risk, has none of the bad side effects, and it is far less expensive to the patient. Also, hospitalization can generally be averted.

17. Klimke, A. & Klieser, E. Effectiveness of neuroelectric therapy in drug resistant endogenous psychoses. *Fortschr Neurol Psychiatry.* **59:53-9, 1991. (Germany)**

Device not specified

A retrospective chart review of 50 pharmacotherapeutically resistant patients was performed after treatment with CES in 1986 - 1988. 28 patients suffered from schizophrenia and 22 from affective psychosis. 60.7% of the treatment-resistant acute schizophrenics responded well to CES. 3 months after discharge from hospital 9 schizophrenics (32.1%) but only 3 patients with affective psychosis (13.6%) presented a 'good' outcome (full remission). A longer duration of schizophrenia (more than 5 years since first manifestation) and a good response to neuroleptics in history was predictive for a good actual CES response (14 of 17 patients), whereas 7 of 11 patients suffering from schizophrenia less than 3 years without any period of full remission on neuroleptics were non-responders to CES.

18. Koegler, Ronald R., Hick, Shelby M. & Barger, James H. Medical and psychiatric use of electrosleep (transcerebral electrotherapy). *Diseases of the Nervous System.* **32(2):100-104, 1971.**

Device: Electrosone 50, 25 Hz, 1 mS, 7 - 10 volts, eye electrodes

14 patients with a variety of symptoms and diagnoses, all with definite sleep problems, received 15 CES treatments. 12 had definite improvements in their sleep patterns. Symptoms of anxiety, depression, nightmares, and irritability disappeared in every case as

the sleep patterns improved. Some patients maintained their improvement 4 months later, while others had partial return of symptoms. None regressed completely. They also report good effects in 5 patients who were prior psychotherapy failures using "electro-psychotherapy" (combining CES with psychotherapy). 2 of 4 migraine patients improved significantly, 1 improved slightly, and 1 had no effect. The only side effects noted were blood pressure lowering during treatment, and a slight blurring of vision occurring due to eye electrodes, which stopped within a few minutes.

The authors concluded that the safety and ease of application of treatment makes it possible to use CES in a manner which would save time for the medical profession and money for the patient. They stated there is enough evidence already at hand from previous studies to justify the considered use of CES by physicians in clinical practice.

19. Komarova, L.A., Kir'ianova, V.V., Zabolotnykh II & Zabolotnykh, V.A. The use of transcranial electrotherapy in the rehabilitation of osteoarthrosis patients. *Vopr Kurortol Fizioter Lech Fiz Kult.* 27-9, 1999. (Russia)

Device: Transair, 77 Hz, frontal-retroauricular electrodes

Rehabilitation of 39 patients with osteoarthrosis deformans (OD) consisted of CES. There was a positive trend in clinical indices, pain intensity, and skin temperature. CES mechanism of action involves stimulation of endorphin brain structures which elevates blood levels of β-endorphins.

20. Kulkarni, Arun D. and Smith, Ray B. The use of microcurrent electrical therapy and cranial electrotherapy stimulation in Pain Control. *Clinical Practice of Alternative Medicine.* 2(2):99-102, 2001.

Device: Alpha-Stim SCS, 0.5 Hz, 50% duty cycle, <500 μA, biphasic asymmetrical rectangular waves, probes, self-adhesive silver electrodes and ear clip electrodes

This open clinical study, conducted by Dr. Kulkarni, an anesthesiologist working with orthopedic surgeons at a pain clinic at Nav-Durga hospital near Bombay, India, was designed to assess the effectiveness of Alpha-Stim microcurrent electrical therapy (MET), CES, or a combination of both therapies. 20 patients who had been refractory to previous treatments completed informed consent and joined the study in the order that they presented at the first author's hospital pain clinic. Ages ranged from 30 to 75 years (mean = 44). 15 were female. Treatments were provided for 1 hour daily, Monday through Friday, for 3 weeks. No pain medications were taken during the study period. MET was given via probes or self-adhesive electrodes at 600 microamperes, while the current for CES was regulated by each patient, ranging from 100 to 300 microamperes. Pain was scored on an 11 point self rating VAS scale, with 0 being no pain and 10 being the most intense pain they had experienced to date.

9 patients (45%) left the study early following reduction of their pain to a level between 0 and 1.5 on the 11 point scale. One had complete remission of her pain after only 2 treatments. Of 3 patients who received no relief, none returned for the final week of treatment. 7 patients (35%) who were treated with CES plus self-adhesive electrodes began at an average pain level of 7.7 (range 5 - 10) and ended with an average of 3.7 (range 0 - 10), or a 52% reduction in pain from an average of 12 days of treatment. 7 patients who were treated with CES plus probes fared even better beginning with a pain level of 7.1 (range 4 - 8) and ending at an average of 1.1 (range 1 - 6), or an 85% reduction of pain from an average of 8.1 days of treatment. 5 patients (25%) were treated with CES only.

They experienced an average of 50% drop in their pain level from 4.4 (range 3 - 7) to 2.2 (range 0.5 - 5) with an average of 10.6 days of treatment. No negative side effects were reported. The authors concluded that MET and CES are effective treatments for chronic pain patients.

21. Kuzin, M.I., Avrutski□, M.I., Shliuznikov, B.M., Lakhter, M.A. & Panchenko, L.F. Effect of transcutaneous transcerebral electrostimulation as electroanesthesia on the beta-endorphin content of the cerebrospinal fluid and blood plasma. *Biull Eksp Biol Med.* **97:515-6, 1984. (Russia)**

Device: 167 kHz modulated by 77 Hz, 250-300 mA, biphasic and rectangular waves

β-endorphin content was measured in the cerebrospinal fluid (CSF) and blood plasma of patients before and after 30 minutes of CES. Electrical stimulation resulted in an appreciable increase in the β-endorphin content in the CSF and blood plasma of patients. The data obtained attest to the intensification of the neuromodulator release to the CSF and blood plasma and to the involvement of the endorphinergic brain systems in the realization of the analgesic effect of CES.

22. Lett, Charles R., Wilson, James O. & Gambrell, Armanda. Effect of Neurotone therapy during methadone detoxification. *International Journal of the Addictions.* **11(1):187-189, 1976.**

Device: Neurotone 101, 100 Hz, 2 mS, <1.5 mA, forehead to mastoid electrodes

17 patients on methadone for 8 to 33 months with a stabilized dosage of 30 to 100 mg were given 15, 30 minute CES treatments. The following withdrawal symptoms were measured: anxiety, yawning, lacrimation, rhinorrhea, insomnia, cough, gooseflesh, tremors, hot/cold flashes, abdominal cramps, muscle cramps, muscle aches, nausea/vomiting, and diarrhea. Only 6 of the 17 patients completed the 15 treatments. Of 8 patients who completed 12 or more sessions, there were significant decreases in only 3 of 13 symptoms (tremor, rhinorrhea, and nausea). The authors stated that future studies should control for dosage level and duration of narcotics, include control groups, and have more accurate measurements of symptoms. No side effects were reported.

23. Long, Ray C. Electrosleep therapy. Some results with the use of electrically induced sleep in the treatment of psychiatric patients. *Journal of the Kansas Medical Society.* **67(2):81-85, 1966.**

Device: Somniatron Model 7200, 11 - 12 Hz, 55 - 80 μA

32 neuropsychiatric patients, including severe psychotics, with chronic anxiety, depression and insomnia, frequent conversion headaches and neuromuscular tension who failed to respond to medications, physiotherapy, and psychotherapy were given 5 - 10 daily, 50 minute CES treatments. One patient had 34 treatments. There was no control group. 69% reached a stage of somnolence while receiving CES. 22 patients who slept during treatment achieved somnolence after 1.5 (median) sessions. Another 31% became stuporously drowsy but never completely lost consciousness. There was 100% accomplishment of symptom relief; all 32 patients overcame nocturnal insomnia. 17 patients (53%) resumed occupational duties with increased efficiency and enthusiasm. 19 (59%) demonstrated more comfort and confidence in their social contacts. 18 (56%) were able to gain insight in regard to their psychodynamics' and to put their increased understanding to work in their best interests. The mean decrease in pulse rate was 10.5, and

3.8 for respiration reduction. The author concluded that the changes are due to physical changes, and not merely to suggestion. No patients were harmed as a result of treatment.

24. Lynch, Harold D. & Anderson, Milton H. Atropine coma therapy in psychiatry: clinical observations over a 20-year period and a review of the literature. *Diseases of the Nervous System.* **36(12):648-652, 1975.**

Device not specified

This is really a discussion of atropine coma therapy with mention of CES. The authors state, "Atropine alone is not enough for depressive illnesses, but in combination with CES, it is effective. This is particularly true in schizo-affective states where either treatment alone is apt to give disappointing results." No side effects of CES were reported.

25. McKenzie, Richard E., Costello, Raymond M. & Buck, Don C. Electrosleep (electrical transcranial stimulation) in the treatment of anxiety, depression and sleep disturbance in chronic alcoholics. *Journal of Altered States of Consciousness.* **2(2):185-196, 1976.**

Device: Electrosone 50, 1 mA, 25 Hz, forehead to mastoid electrodes

20 male alcoholic inpatients aged 26 - 61 (mean = 51) who were "dry" for at least 2 weeks, volunteered, and completed informed consent for this double-blind study. Random assignment into 4 equal groups was assured by throwing dice. Group 1 received 1 mA of current. Group 2 had the current turned up and then off. Group 3 had 1 mA of current. Group 4 was hooked up to the device, but turning it on was simulated (no current). All groups had 5, 30 minute treatments or simulated treatments. Results were analyzed by 2 pychometricians blinded to the conditions of each group. The Clinical Analysis Questionnaire (CAQ) and Self Report Scale (SRS) were utilized to measure the effects of treatment. Results were presented by group means in a graph form. Group 4 (sham) indicated no change or slight exacerbation of anxiety and sleep problems. The other groups reported an improvement over the 1 week period with the actual current groups (1 and 3) improving slightly more so. 2 group 4 subjects dropped out, while none of the others dropped out. No side effects were reported.

26. Miller, E.C. & Mathas, J.L. The use and effectiveness of electrosleep in the treatment of some common psychiatric problems. *American Journal of Psychiatry.* **122(4):460-462, 1965.**

Device not specified

27 patients were given 30 - 50 minute CES treatments 2 - 5 times per week. 15 patients managed a consistent sleeping state during the treatments. 56% of the CES group were adjudged improved, compared with a 66% improved rate in the control group. Daily drug use was weighed (literally). At the 5% level of confidence, t scores were not significant. The authors added, there appears to be no disturbing side effects; however, 1 patient did undergo a brief dissociative episode shortly after beginning his third treatment. Serial EEGs performed on the first 12 patients showed no alteration of the waking baseline after 6 treatments.

27. Padjen, A.L., Dongier, M. & Malec, T. Effects of cerebral electrical stimulation on alcoholism: a pilot study. *Alcohol Clin Exp Res.* **19:1004-10, 1995.**

Device not specified

Cerebral electrotherapy stimulation (CES), born from research on electroanesthesia in the 1970s, consists of the application of a pulsating current of small intensity (usually less than 1 mA, and below the threshold of perception) through the skull, in daily 30-minute sessions. Claims of biological effectiveness (neurochemical, hormonal and EEG changes, naloxone-reversible analgesia in rats, etc.) and of clinical effectiveness (anxiety, depression, cognitive functions in alcoholics) have often relied on poorly controlled data. A recent controlled study in the treatment of opiate withdrawal has been positive. The present double-blind controlled study compares active CES with sham stimulation in 64 alcohol-dependent males. Over 4 weeks, both treatment groups improved significantly in most aspects. In the active treatment group additional significant improvement was observed in week-end alcohol consumption, and in two psychological measures: depression and stress symptoms index, but not in general drinking behavior.

28. Patterson, M.A., Patterson, L. & Patterson, S.I. Electrostimulation: addiction treatment for the coming millennium. *Journal of Alternative and Complementary Medicine.* **2:485-91, 1998.**

Device not specified

At a period of fundamental review of the health care system, it is timely to re-assess one of medicine's most intractable problems; the treatment of addictions. The apparently insoluble dilemmas posed by the acute and chronic withdrawal syndromes underlie universally high drop-out and relapse rates. In a decade of HIV and AIDS infection, poly-substance addiction, potent street drugs, and ossified treatment strategies, it is urgent that policy formulators investigate seriously a flexible system of non-pharmacological CES treatment, based on its record of rapid, safe, and cost-effective detoxification in several countries, as one innovative contribution to the challenges presented by addiction in the 1990s. This is a brief report of the introduction of CES into Germany, describing the responses of the first 22 cases. The daily progress of a heroin addict and a methadone addict are detailed: both were treated as outpatients for 8 hours daily, for 7 and 10 days respectively.

29. Pickworth, Wallace B., Fant, Reginald V., Butschky, Marsha F., Goffman, Allison L. & Henningfield, Jack E. Evaluation of cranial electrostimulation therapy on short-term smoking cessation. *Biological Psychiatry.* **42(2):116-121, 1997.**

Device: 10 Hz, 30 μA, 2 mS, 3M pediatric red dot electrodes bilateral on mastoids

Unedited Medline Abstract: The effects of cranial electrical stimulation (CES) on short-term smoking cessation were evaluated in a double-blind study of cigarette smokers who wished to stop smoking. Subjects were randomly assigned to a CES- (N = 51) or a sham-treated group (N = 50). On 5 consecutive days subjects received CES treatments (30-microA, 2-msec, 10-Hz pulsed signal) or no electrical current (sham). There were no significant differences between groups on daily cigarettes smoked, exhaled carbon monoxide, urinary cotinine levels, treatment retention, smoking urges, or total tobacco withdrawal scores, although subjects in the CES group had less cigarette craving and anxiety during the first 2 experimental days. The ineffectiveness of CES to reduce withdrawal symptoms and facilitate smoking cessation are similar to results of other clinical studies of CES in drug dependence, although positive effects of CES in animal studies have been reported.

Reviewer's note: This government study, performed by the National Institute on Drug Abuse, Addiction Research Center, Clinical Pharmacology Branch, Baltimore, Maryland, used an unknown CES device that is not commercially available, with questionable electrodes never before used for CES, and at 30 μA which represents approximately 10% of the current that would be required for results. Also, 5 days of any therapy is inadequate to assist in smoking cessation. Accordingly, this reviewer believes that this study was predetermined to fail and should not be considered as science because of inadequate dosage at the very least, and possibly other intentional biasing factors. As an analogy, if a researcher were to open a Tylenol capsule, take all but a few grains out, use a good double-blind study design that showed ineffectiveness at 10% of the recommended dosage, would that prove Tylenol is not an effective analgesic; and would that be considered reliable science that would qualify for publication in a reputable medical journal?

A critical rebuttal of this study was published in a subsequent issue of *Biological Psychiatry* (43:468, 1998) by Drs. Nashaat N. Boutros and Evgeny M. Krupitsky of the Department of Psychiatry at Yale University.

30. Ramsay, John C. & Schlagenhauf, George. Treatment of depression with low voltage direct current. *Journal of the Southern Medical Association.* **59(8):932-934, 1966.**

Device: Self made, 90 - 500 μA, scalp anode electrodes, with a cathode on the leg

20 depressed patients, refractory to other therapies, several of whom were candidates for electroconvulsive therapy, were treated continuously for 4 to 6 hours per day for varying periods of time. 14 showed definite improvement, 4 had equivocal improvement, and 2 had no improvement. Very few side effects were noted. The authors concluded that the absence of serious side effects, the comfort to the patient, and the convenience of the patient being able to go about his business during treatment, all make this a treatment modality deserving of further study and consideration.

31. Rosenthal, Saul H. & Calverty, Lynn G. Electrosleep: Personal subjective experiences. *Biological Psychiatry.* **4(2):187-190, 1972.**

Device: 100 Hz, 1 mS, 0.5 - 1.5 mA, orbit to mastoid electrodes

7 subjects consisting of 1 male psychologist, 3 male medical students, 1 female psychiatry resident, 1 female research assistant, and 1 female secretary received a course of 5, 30 minute CES treatments over 1 week. The authors stated that they expected to find a mild sedative effect, but no particular effect on mood. Instead they found 1) activation of alertness seen in 5 subjects, 2) euphoric tranquillity in 4, and 3) not worrying in 4. 4 subjects described beneficial effects, such as feeling alert, bright and happy, unusual increased energy for household chores, feeling "very happy" all day, tranquil, alert, pleased, definitely sleeping better, and less anxious about work. 1 subject complained of mildly unpleasant experiences including visual disturbances lasting a maximum of 1 hour, tinnitus lasting several hours, hyperactivity, difficulty sleeping, and epigastric sensations. His hyperactivity and sleeping difficulty were gone 48 hours after the final treatment and after 1 week he reported, "I don't feel anxious, I feel fine." His previous mild transient reactive depression had not occurred and he was sleeping soundly. 2 subjects reported a headache lasting 1 hour. 2 subjects without any prior symptoms reported no significant effect. However, they reported feeling relaxed during the treatments and they did not have any significant side effects.

32. Rosenthal, Saul H. & Wulfson, Norman L. Electrosleep: A clinical trial. *American Journal of Psychiatry.* **127(4):175-176, 1970.**

Device: Electrosone 50, 100 Hz, 1 mS, 100 - 200 μA, orbit to mastoid electrodes

40 outpatients with chronic anxiety, depressive states, and associated insomnia, not responsive to medications, received 5 - 10, 30 minute treatments. The authors concluded that with this population of patients who were previously refractive to standard medical therapy, they found, to their surprise, that approximately two-thirds showed a rapid and relatively complete remission of symptoms. They added that it seems to be a humane treatment, and no significant side effects have been reported.

33. Scallet, Andrew, Cloninger, C. Robert & Othmer, Ekkehard. The management of chronic hysteria: A review and double-blind trial of electrosleep and other relaxation methods. *Diseases of the Nervous System.* **37(6):347-353, 1976.**

Device: Neurotone 101, 100 Hz, 2 mS, square waves, cathodes on orbits, anodes on mastoids

17 women diagnosed with chronic hysteria were given 12, 30 - 40 minute treatments and assessed by the National Institute of Mental Health Self-rating Symptom Scale (SRSS). All were instructed in relaxation techniques. 5 patients received central stimulation, 7 received peripheral stimulation, and 5 served as controls who had 30 seconds of stimulation. Electrical stimulation led to greater improvement in all types of symptomatology than did relaxing with a mask only, but the differences were only significant for anxiety. The women who had relaxation sessions without electrical stimulation had a consistent improvement in mood throughout treatment and did not relapse after treatment whereas the other patients became depressed again when electrical stimulation sessions were discontinued. No side effects were reported.

34. Singh, Jaabir M., King, Hugh A. & Super, William C. Effects of transcerebral electro-therapy (TCT) in stress related illness. *Pharmacologist.* **16(2):264, 1974.**

Device: Neurotone 101, 50 - 100 Hz, 2 - 4 mS, <1.5 mA

An unspecified number of selected alcoholics and non-alcoholic patients were given 3 - 5, 30 - 45 minute treatments, although some chronic cases received over 50 treatments. The patients were relaxed immediately after the treatment. Anxiety, tension headache and onset of sleep were improved in a majority of patients. The authors suggested from their findings that CES may be a useful treatment modality for stress related disorders. No side effects were reported.

35. Singh, Kirpal. Sleep inducing devices: a clinical trial with a Russian machine. *International Journal of Neuropsychiatry.* **3(4):311-318, 1967.**

Device: Portable Electric Sleep Apparatus, 50 - 200 μA, orbit to mastoid electrodes

15 anxiety patients, 9 of who also had disturbances of sleep, and 15 controls, were given 5 - 12, 30 minute to 2 hour treatments. Pulse, respiration, duration and quality of sleep, and side effects were measured or noted. The author concluded that the procedure was found to be more effective in the patient group than in the control group. He added that in his opinion, the application of low voltage electric current is helpful in reducing the tension found in patients who are morbidly anxious and is relatively ineffective in the subjects who are not abnormally tense. He was disappointed that the device was not universally successful in promoting sleep. The following side effects were noted: headache, giddiness, pains in tooth, heaviness around eyes, pain in eyes, pain behind the ears.

36. Sokolov, E.A., Tsvetkov, V.A. & Losev, I.F. Hemodynamics during epidural anesthesia in combination with transcranial electroanesthesia in pulmonary surgery. *Anesteziol Reanimatol.* **10-2, 1991. (Russia)**

Device not specified

Pulmonary surgery performed under epidural anesthesia (EA) combined with transcranial electrical anesthesia (CES) was characterized by minimum adverse hemodynamic reactions, typical of EA alone, and reduced overall dose of the local anesthetic with minimum volume of the infusion therapy and adequate anesthetic protection. The absence of marked hemodynamic reactions in this type of combined anesthesia made it possible to use it during pulmonary surgery in the most severely ill patients whose cardiovascular system is already compromised by the primary pulmonary disease.

37. Sornson, Robert, Liverance, Diane, Armstrong, George & Zelt, Beverly. Cerebral electrical stimulation neurotransmitter modulation benefits adolescent cerebral palsy students. *American Journal of Electromedicine.* **6(1):122-125, 1989.**

Device: Neurotransmitter Modulator, 1 mA, electrodes above ears

3 high school students with cerebral palsy were given CES twice daily on school days for 12 weeks. Lab results from plasma showed decreased ACTH in 2 of the 3 patients, increases in tryptophan, and decrease in cortisol in 2 of the 3. Self-esteem jumped at least 1 level on Battle's Culture Free Self Esteem Inventory. Increases in academic achievement over the 12 week period were remarkable. Subject 1 showed a 2.0 grade level increase in reading, and 1.2 in math on the Metropolitan Achievement Test. Subject 2 showed a 1.9 grade level increase in reading, and 0.6 in math. Subject 3 scored at the highest level of the testing form indicating a reading level beyond 9.9 and a 0.9 increase in math. All 3 also showed improvements in hand function. The authors concluded that the positive results of this short study increase the body of evidence that shows that CES can improve learning, self-esteem, and physical functioning in persons with spastic cerebral palsy. They added that since the devices are non-invasive and have few contraindications, they hope that more efforts will be made to understand how such devices can be most effective, and how they work. No side effects were reported.

38. Tomsovic, Milan & Edwards, Robert V. Cerebral electrotherapy for tension-related symptoms in alcoholics. *Quarterly Journal of Studies on Alcohol.* **34(4):1352-1355, 1973.**

Device: Neurotone 101, 100 Hz, 2 mS, <1.5 mA, orbit to mastoid electrodes

34 male alcoholic patients (aged 25 - 62, mean = 44) with anxiety, sleep problems, stomach disorders and headaches, volunteered, and were asked to rate their complaints on a 10 point scale. They were then given 5, 30 minute CES treatments. 18 patients received full course treatment, and a placebo group of 16 patients had the device turned up and then off at the beginning, and then again halfway through each treatment. Approximately 75% of each group reported some level of improvement. It is possible that the placebo group benefited from actual, brief treatments. No side effects were reported.

39. Turaeva, V.A. Treatment of eczema and neurodermatitis by electrosleep. In Wageneder, F.M. & St. Schuy (Eds). *Electrotherapeutic Sleep and Electroanaesthesia.* **International Congress Series No. 136. Excerpta Medica Foundation, Amsterdam, Pp. 203-204, 1967.**

Device: VNIIKhI, 100 - 800 mA, 1 - 20 Hz

158 patients were treated with CES alone (N = 20), or CES combined with other treatments. Out of the 158 total, 56 achieved a clinical cure, 45 had considerable improvement, 29 had some improvement, 5 had no effect, and 3 deteriorated. 12 months follow-up showed that the positive effects of CES were sufficiently stable. The authors repeated the experiments at several other locations with similar results. No complications from CES were seen.

40. Tyers, Steve & Smith, Ray B. A comparison of cranial electrotherapy stimulation alone or with chiropractic therapies in the treatment of fibromyalgia. *The American Chiropractor.* **23(2):39-41, 2001.**

Device: Alpha-Stim SCS, 0.5 Hz, 50% duty cycle, <500 μA, biphasic asymmetrical rectangular waves, ear clip electrodes

This study conducted at the Integrated Medical Centers of California, La Jolla, compared Alpha-Stim CES alone (N = 20) to Alpha-Stim CES and chiropractic treatment (N = 40). 60 patients diagnosed with fibromyalgia between the ages of 25 and 57 (mean of 45) completed informed consent, and were then evaluated on the Profile of Mood States along with self-ratings of their pain level, quality of sleep, feeling of well being, and quality of life, all on 10-point scales. Tender points were also evaluated. Patients were treated at 0.5 Hz, 1 hour per day for 3 weeks via ear clip electrodes. They were able to adjust the current to a comfortable level between 0 and 500 μA, with the majority choosing between 100 and 300 μA. No attempt was made to adjust medications.

One of the CES patients and 3 of the CES plus chiropractic patients dropped out leaving two groups of 19 and 37 patients. The patients who received CES alone achieved an average of 26% improvement in their pain levels, while the combined therapy group achieved 34% improvement. The combined therapy group exhibited an improvement of 32% in their tender point evaluations. The combined therapy group also fared better in 5 of the psychological measures. On the overall sleep self-rating scales, 87% of the patients entering the study rated their sleep as moderate to very poor. At the end of the study, 80% rated their sleep as moderate to excellent, an almost mirror image turn around in their quality of sleep. The authors concluded that CES is a valuable adjunct to chiropractic management of fibromyalgia patients. No negative side effects were reported.

5

2 META-ANALYSES OF CES

Meta-analyses is a statistical technique of pooling together scientific studies having common traits to reduce them to a single data point, as if the many smaller studies were one large study. Meta-analyses were conducted on the CES literature at the School of Public Health, Harvard University, and at the Graduate School of the University of Tulsa. Both found that CES is an effective means of treatment.

1. Klawansky, Sidney, Yeung, Albert, Berkey, Catherine, Shah, Nirav, Phan, Hai & Chalmers, Thomas C. Meta-analysis of randomized controlled trials of cranial electrostimulation: efficacy in treating selected psychological and physiological conditions. *Journal of Nervous and Mental Disease.* **183(7):478-485, l995.**

This study was conducted at the Harvard School of Public Health, Department of Health Policy and Management.

"To clarify the diverse published results of cranial electrostimulation (CES) efficacy, we conducted an extensive literature review that identified 18 of the most carefully conducted randomized controlled trials of CES versus sham treatment. For the 14 trials that had sufficient data, we used the techniques of meta-analysis to pool the published results of treating each of 4 conditions: anxiety (eight trials), brain dysfunction (two trials), headache (two trials), and insomnia (two trials). Because studies utilized different outcome measures, we used an effect size method to normalize measures which we then pooled across studies within each condition. The meta-analysis of anxiety showed CES to be significantly more effective than sham (P<.05). Pooling did not affect results that were individually positive (headache and pain under anesthesia) or negative (brain dysfunction and insomnia)..." (Authors' abstract).

The authors also noted that improvement occurred in 7 of the 8 studies for anxiety that used continuous measurement scales.

2. O'Connor, Mary Ellen, Bianco, Faust & Nicolson, Robert. Meta-analysis of cranial electro-stimulation (CES) in relation to the primary and secondary symptoms of substance with-drawal. Presented at the 12th annual meeting of the Bioelectromagnetics Society, June 14, 1991.

This study was conducted at the Graduate School of the University of Tulsa.

Initially 180 studies on CES from 1964 through 1987 were reviewed. 8 studies provided the necessary information to calculate means and standard deviations for meta-analysis of CES for chemical dependency. The largest effect sizes pertained to the primary withdrawal symptoms of drug use, drug craving, and anxiety specifically among methadone users. In addition the results showed effect sizes beyond that of a placebo effect in several studies relating to anxiety as a secondary withdrawal symptom. However, some studies that considered anxiety as a secondary withdrawal symptom were below the placebo effect level. The analysis displayed an average effect size of 0.940 SD units when comparing CES plus a standard treatment to a CES sham plus a standard treatment, and an effect size of 1.68 when comparing CES plus a standard treatment to standard treatments alone. The average effect sizes for the within groups studies were 0.534 SD units for CES treatments, 0.391 SD units for CES sham treatment plus the standard treatment and, 0.171 SD units for the standard treatment alone. The range of the effect sizes for the within group studies were between 0.25 and 0.83 units. The authors concluded that the statistical significance of the within group analysis is quite impressive. To put this into perspective, the average effect sizes of all psychotherapies are between 0.70 and 0.80 SD units when compared to no treatment (roughly 75% of the patients who receive psychotherapy improve in their condition relative to controls who receive no therapy). The average effect size for non-specific factors or placebo effects among psychotherapies as compared to wait-list controls is about 0.40 SD units (From Bianco, Faust. The efficacy of cranial electrotherapy stimulation for the relief of anxiety and depression among polysubstance abusers in chemical dependency treatment. Ph.D. dissertation, The University of Tulsa, 1994).

"We do not infer that CES is efficacious for primary and secondary symptoms based on only 8 studies, many of which were of questionable methodology. However, there was some degree of statistical significance in the within group analysis and a trend toward statistical significance in the between group analysis. Possibly more important from a therapeutic perspective, there appears to be a cluster of CES efficacy regarding the primary withdrawal symptoms and possibly secondary symptoms for opiate users. One potential therapeutic benefit of CES treatment is that it may be used to induce the addicted patient into therapy with the promise of minimal withdrawal discomfort. In addition, CES could eliminate the use of substitute psychoactive drugs during the detoxification phase of therapy. From both a psychological and medical perspective CES deserves to be thoroughly investigated, particularly given the current crisis of drug abuse that many cultures in the world face today."

6

CURRENT DENSITY MODEL OF CES

A model of the head was constructed by three biomedical engineers at the University of Texas at Austin to determine the pathways of current in CES. The conclusion, confirming prior reports, is that enough current from CES does indeed penetrate into the level of the thalamus and that could cause the changes reported in clinical studies.

1. Ferdjallah, Mohammed, Bostick Jr., Francis X. Jr. & Barr, Ronald E. Potential and current density distributions of cranial electrotherapy stimulation (CES) in a four-concentric-spheres model. *IEEE Transactions on Biomedical Engineering.* **43(9):939-943, 1996.**

This study was conducted at the Electrical Engineering Department, Biomedical Engineering Program of the University of Texas at Austin.

Cranial electrotherapy stimulation (CES) has been successfully used for treatment of many psychiatric diseases. Its noninvasive nature is its major advantage over other forms of treatments such as drugs. It is postulated that the low electric current of CES causes the release of neurotransmitters. However, the current pathways have not been extensively investigated. In this study, analytical and numerical methods are used to determine the distribution of potential and current density excited by 2 electrodes diametrically opposite to each other to mimic actual CES application, in a 4 zone concentric spheres model of the human head comprised of scalp, skull, cerebrospinal fluid and brain tissue. Because of the azimuthal symmetry, which is assumed in this study, a 2-dimensional (2-D) finite difference approximation is derived in the spherical grid. The current density distribution is projected around the center of the model, where the thalamus is modeled as a concentric sphere. All dimensions and electrical properties of the model are adapted from clinical data.

Results of this simulation indicate that from 1 mA of current, about 5 μA/cm^2 of CES reaches the thalamic area at a radius of 13.30 mm and may facilitate the release of neurotransmitters, which in turn could cause physiological effects such as relaxation.

7

29 ANIMAL STUDIES OF CES

Research conducted on six species of experimental animals did not reveal any significant long-term adverse side effects from CES. Positive findings were found in many of these studies that enhances our understanding of CES. These studies helped to determine the current density that actually enters the brain, neurochemical changes caused by CES, and the extent to which CES enhances pharmaceuticals, especially anesthetics.

INDEX TO ANIMAL STUDIES

C. BEHAVIORAL MEASURE OR OBSERVATION:

Alcohol or drug withdrawal syndrome: 9, 24

Analgesic/Anesthetic: 11, 18, 22, 25, 27

Epileptic activity: 23

Parkinson-like state: 14

Relaxation: 5

Reaction time: 3, 12, 22, 26

Sleep: 1, 2, 3, 6, 20, 21

D. INTRABRAIN ELECTRICAL PASSAGE: 1, 7

E. SAFETY: 5, 8, 10, 17, 20, 22

F. LOCUS OF CES MEASUREMENT:

Basal ganglia: 13

Brainstem: 20, 24

Caudate nucleus: 8

Hypothalamus: 1

Limbic system: 16

Motor Cortex: 7

Septum: 8

Striate cortex: 8

Subcortex: 6, 24

Thalamus: 7, 20

1. Austen, Burton G. Current distribution in subcortical regions of the cat's brain during electrosleep. In Reynolds, David V. & Anita Sjorberg (Eds), *Neuroelectric Research*. Springfield, Charles Thomas. 28:262-266, 1971.

Following up on earlier researchers who said that when the hypothalamus was electrically stimulated "natural sleep" resulted, the author stimulated the caudate nucleus and the preoptic region of the hypothalamus in 5 adult female cats. The stimulus was a 15 second train of rectangular pulses, each with a width of 0.3 mS, frequency of 5 Hz, and an amplitude of between 0.1 and 2 V. The resulting current density and distribution in the cats' brain was discussed.

2. Capel, I.D., Pinnock, M.H., Withey, N.J., Williams, D.C. & Patterson, M.A. The effect of electrostimulation on barbituate-induced sleeping times in rats. *Drug Development Research*, 2:73-79, 1982.

This study was conducted to determine the biochemical basis by which CES might induce drug detoxification. The time taken to regain righting reflex following barbiturate anesthesia (sleeping time) was investigated as a means to provide an in vivo estimate of hepatic function. Naloxone was administered prior to CES to determine whether the effects on barbiturate anesthesia was mediated by endorphins. Female rats were anesthetized by intraperitoneal administration of either hexobarbitol (100 mg/kg), thiopentone (56 mg/kg), or quinalbarbitone/amylobarbitone (25 mg/kg). Electrodes were attached to the rats ear via alligator clips to Michaels suture clips inserted through each pinna. Treated animals were stimulated until they regained their righting reflex with 1 volt at a 0.22 mS pulse width. A control group of rats were sham treated via the same connections without the CES device being turned on.

CES treated rats regained their righting reflex more rapidly than sham-treated controls following administration of anesthetics. The most effective frequencies in decreasing hexobarbital-induced sleeping time was 10 Hz (P<.001) or 500 Hz (P<.001). The treatment produced no significant difference in microsomal protein or cytochrome P450 levels. Paradoxically, two mixed function oxitase enzyme activities investigated, aminopyrine N-demethylase and aniline hydroxylase, were significantly lower (P<.001) in the CES treated rats than in the sham treated littermates.

Pretreatment with naloxone increased the hexobarbital-induced sleeping times of the non-CES rats. CES at 10 Hz was far less effective in reducing sleeping time following pretreatment with naloxone, whereas the reduction of sleeping time was greatly enhanced (P<.001) at 500 Hz.

Rats receiving CES at 10 Hz had significantly lower (P<.002) and those treated at 500 Hz had significantly higher (P<.025) serum cortisol levels than the sham treated controls.

3. Clark, Nancy, Mills, Daniel & Marchant, Jeremy. Evaluation of the potential efficacy of the Alpha-Stim SCS in the Horse. DeMontfort University Equestrian Centre and Field Station, Caythorpe, Lincolnshire, United Kingdom, January, 2000.

After completing a successful study of the stress reduction effects of the Alpha-Stim SCS in a 6 horse pilot study, a double-blind study was completed with 8 thoroughbred horses (2 fillies, 3 mares, 3 geldings) at the De Montfort University Equestrian Centre and Field Station at Caythorpe, Lincolnshire, United Kingdom. Alpha-Stim AS-Trode brand self adhesive electrodes were attached to shaved areas on each side of the neck beneath the collar. The devices were set to provide 0.5 Hz biphasic stimulation at 200 μA, or sham stimulation. Heart rate measurements (HR) were provided by an attached Polar Horse Trainer transmitter belt and a Polar Vantage receiver.

Observers blind to the treatment condition recorded duration behavior of body locomotion, head motion, ear position, oral behavior and the state of the lower lip at 15 second intervals for 15 seconds duration. 4 trials were carried out each day for a total of 8 days (4 testing days per week). The frequency of each behavior was calculated and divided by the total number of observations for statistical analysis. The time standing alert decreased significantly from trial 1 to trial 4 ($p<0.05$). The time spent standing alert also continued to decrease after the stimulation had stopped, suggesting an ongoing effect of CES following the period of actual stimulation. The horses spent significantly more time standing dozing between trials 1 and 4 ($p<0.05$), less time with lower lip tense between trials 1 and 2 ($p<0.05$), had less ear flicking from trial 1 to 3 ($p<0.05$), increased head wobbling between phases 1 and 4 ($p<0.05$), less time vocalizing between phase 1 and 4 ($p<0.05$), and less time shaking the head between phases 1 and 3 ($p<0.05$). All of these changes were highly intercorrelated and strongly indicated a reduction in the Horses' state of arousal following treatment but not sham treatment with Alpha-Stim CES. Finally, although not significant, there was a trend in which the variation in mean HR values decreased from the first to the latter phases of the study. HR fell more in the 3 horses with the highest mean HR going into the study.

4. Dougherty, P.M., Dong, W.Q., Faillace, L.A. & Dafny, N. Transcranial electrical stimulation attenuates abrupt morphine withdrawal in rats assayed by remote computerized quantification of multiple motor behavior indices. *Eur J Pharmacol.* 175:187-95, 1990. (Netherlands)

The goal of the present study was to assess the effects of CES on the behavioral signs of the abrupt withdrawal syndrome of rats. However, this goal also necessitated the introduction of an experimental model measuring animal behavior for prolonged periods of time using a computerized animal activity monitoring system to quantify spontaneous motor activities associated with abstinence behavior. Comparable withdrawal severity was obtained by both the activity monitoring system and investigator observation of motor signs of abstinence behavior. Moreover, using this system we demonstrate a time-dependent effect of electrical stimulation in reducing the severity of various indices of motor hyperactivity associated with abrupt morphine withdrawal in rats.

5. Geddes, L.A., Hoff, H.E. & McCrady, J.D. Electroanesthesia in the horse. In Wageneder, F.M. & St. Schuy (Eds). *Electrotherapeutic Sleep and Electroanaesthesia.* International Congress Series No. 136. Excerpta Medica Foundation, Amsterdam, Pp. 73-80, 1967.

The authors demonstrated the parameters of electrode size and current density necessary to produce burns via electrical stimulation of the skin. With electrodes similar to or smaller than those of most CES electrodes and with much greater current loads across the skin, they observed no burns. The discussion centered on the heat dissipation to be expected from polarized impedances when constant or controlled current sources are used.

6. Hornstein, S.R., Filho, R.A., Toledo, M. & Spirck, C.N. Preliminary data on a new method for lithium therapy. *Rev Bras Pesqui Med Biol.* 10:249-54, 1977. (Brazil)

Lithium therapy was assessed using CES on two dogs. Cotton swabs soaked in an aqueous isotonic lithium chloride solution were placed over the eyes and mastoids of the dogs, and connected to the CES apparatus. In 2 minutes, sleep was induced in both dogs, at

500 μA on the intensity scale (which runs 1 to 9 mA). After 2 hours, the apparatus was turned off. One of the dogs was put under continuous observation, and the other one was sacrificed. Parts of it's cortex, subcortex, and cerebellum were processed and fragments were assayed spectrophotometrically for Lithium. Lithium was found in all the material examined. These results suggest a possible technique for Lithium therapy using CES, the ion being carried directly to the CNS, avoiding systemic toxicity caused by oral administration.

7. Jarzembski, William B., Larson, Sanford J. & Sances Jr, Anthony. Evaluation of specific cerebral impedance and cerebral current density. *Annals of the New York Academy of Sciences.* 170:476-490, 1970.

Sensor electrodes were chronically implanted in the sagittal planes in the region of the medial thalamus and in sagittal and coronal planes in the region of the motor cortex of the brains of 30 monkeys. Electrodes were placed externally at the nasion and inion. Currents varying from 0.1 to 100 mA were generated with frequencies ranging from 10 to 5,000 Hz. They found that the current densities in the brain at all frequencies tested were linearly proportional to the applied currents, but with the thalamic current density slightly higher than the cortical current density. Calculations indicated that from 42% to 46% of the total applied current entered the brain.

8. Jordan, Eric J. & Morris, David. Evaluation of the electrosleep machine. *Diseases of the Nervous System.* 36(12):661-665, 1975.

9 littermate-male Beagle dogs were given 13 daily 1 hour treatments under anesthesia with eye to occipital electrodes and measured with EEG's, ERG's, blood pressure, temperature, respiration, blood and urine analysis. Photic stimulation was applied in addition to the CES. 3 dogs were given "normal" levels of 1 mA AC and .33 mA DC, another 3 received "high" levels of 5 mA AC and 1.33 mA DC, the third group of 3 had sham treatment. After the course of treatment, the dogs were sacrificed and examined. 2 dogs suffered direct trauma from the citernal puncture, causing spinal cord lesions. No neurologic signs were noted from the CES. It was noted that CES may cause mild EEG slowing. Suspicious findings were found in the striate cortex, caudate nucleus, and septum. Except for 1 case, these were small and of questionable significance. There were no changes that were unequivocally pathological. No acute or chronic changes were noted in BP, EKG, temperature or respiration. The authors concluded that evidence of CES-induced pathology is inconclusive.

9. Krupisky, E.M., Katznelson, Ya.S., Lebedev, V.P., Flood, N.V., Patterson, M.A., Lipton, J.M. & Kozlowski, G.P. Transcranial electrostimulation (TES) of brain opioid structures (BOS): experimental treatment of alcohol withdrawal syndrome (AWS) and clinical application. Presented at the Society for Neuroscience Annual Meeting, New Orleans, November 10-15, 1991.

Alcohol withdrawal syndrome (AWS) was induced in rats. Noninvasive CES increased the β-endorphin level in rat cerebrospinal fluid from 15.93 ± 2.17 to 53.25 ± 6.1 pmol/ml and met-enkephalin from 3.61 ± 1.39 to 7.86 ± 0.94 pmol/ml. Marked therapeutic effect of CES was also demonstrated in this animal model. Clinical double-blind placebo-controlled studies showed that CES was an effective method in the treatment of AWS in patients. After the CES treatment in AWS patients, the β-endorphin concentration in plasma rose from 5.86 ± 0.72 to 10.66 ± 0.65 pmol/L. There was a threefold increase in β-endorphin concentration after just 1 CES treatment.

10. Little, Bert & Patterson, Margaret A. Embryofetal effects of neuroelectric therapy (NET). *Electro and Magnetobiology*. 15(1):1-8, 1996.

After obtaining IRB approval by the University of Texas Southwestern Medical Center, virgin Spraque-Dawley female rats were mated with Spraque-Dawley male rats. All rats were fitted with 2 ear identification tags, including controls who did not receive any CES, to provide equal nociception and stress. All rats were permitted to move freely within their cages. The treated rats were divided into 3 groups and given CES 1 hour daily throughout their pregnancy at either 10, 100, or 1,000 Hz, 1 volt, 0.125 mA, at a 0.22 mS pulse width via alligator clips attached to the ear tags. On day 18 of pregnancy, the dams were killed by guillotine or with ether, and cesarean section was performed immediately. Fetuses were counted and the uteri were examined for evidence of embryo resorption. The fetuses were immediately placed in 10% fomalin. Xeroradiographic surveys of posteroanterior and lateral views of each fetus were taken and evaluated for cranial, rib, vertebral, or long bone abnormalities. After thorough external examination, autopsies were performed under a dissecting microscope to evaluate the palate, heart and major vessels, lungs, liver, kidneys, ureters, and bladder. Statistical analysis included the use of $x2$, analysis of variance, and Newman-Keuls multiple group comparisons test. 844 fetal rats were evaluated.

The detailed external examinations under light microscopy revealed no obvious neural tube defects, limb reduction deformities, or anterior abdominal wall abnormalities in the controls or any of the treatment groups. Skeletal surveys of the fetal rats revealed no vertebral column, rib, or long bone deformities. Comparison between groups revealed more pregnancy resorptions and fewer offspring in all treatment groups as compared to the control group, with the difference reaching significance in the 1,000 Hz treatment group. Average fetal weights were inversely proportional to frequency and were significantly different among groups. Fetal brain weight followed a similar pattern of reduction, except that weights were not significantly different between the medium and highest frequency treatment groups.

In their discussion, the authors stated that while the incidence of congenital anomalies was zero, the reason pregnancy resorptions were increased may be due to the CES treated rats being more complacent. Their behavior resembled the effects of CES in humans, even in this aggressive population well known for their violence. The treated rats were not as active as the controls, accordingly it is possible that food intake was lowered in the treatment group, a reasonable implication given the reduction in fetal weights. The authors concluded that CES may be embryolethal in the very early stages of pregnancy in the rat and might cause some miscarriages, but there is no evidence of fetotoxic effects. The relevance of these findings to humans is unknown.

11. Mantz, J., Azerad, J., Limoge, A. & Desmonts, J.M. Transcranial electrical stimulation with Limoge's currents decreases halothane requirements in rats. Evidence for the involvement of endogenous opioids. *Anesthesiology*. 76:253-60, 1992.

CES has been shown to facilitate anesthesia/analgesia in surgical patients. However, the neurobiologic substrate of this effect remains unknown. The present study was designed to analyze the influence of CES on halothane requirements in rats and the contribution of the central endogenous opioid, alpha 2-adrenergic and 5-hydroxytryptamine (5-HT1 and 5-HT2) serotonergic systems to this effect. The influence of CES on the MAC of halothane (MACH) and its reversibility by a subcutaneous 2 mg/kg naloxone injection were first determined in 20 rats using a randomized blinded protocol. MACH was decreased markedly in stimulated animals (CES, N = 10) in comparison with sham-operated nonstimulated rats (controls, N = 10): MACH = 0.60 ± 0.15, mean ± SD, versus 1.07 ± 0.05 vol%, P<.001. In CES animals, naloxone administration restored MACH values to the levels of controls but failed to affect MACH in controls. The influence of the duration of CES applied prior to MACH determination was further investigated in 30 animals. The magnitude of MACH reduction was significantly increased with the cumulative duration of stimulation. For each duration of stimulation tested, administration of a 5-micrograms intracerebroventricular (icv) dose of the enkephalinase inhibitor thiorphan significantly enhanced CES effects (P<.05). Finally, the icv administration of a 15-micrograms naloxone dose appeared to completely reverse the MACH reduction elicited by CES (N = 8, P<.01).

12. Pocta, J., Lebl, M. & Hanka, R. The autonomic and stress reactions during electrosleep. In Wageneder, F.M & St. Schuy (Eds) *Electrotherapeutic Sleep and Electroanaesthesia.* **International Congress series, No. 136. Excerpta Medica Foundation, Amsterdam, Pp. 342-344, 1967.**

The authors completed 45 experiments in dogs, saying that dogs are known to respond to exogenous stimuli by developing disturbances of the autonomic system. The oculocardiac reflex, the carotid sinus reflex, the solar plexus reflex, leukocyte count, hemoglobin, hematocrit, segmented cells, and eosinophil count were obtained. They found that CES elicited firm and reliable stabilization of the organism. No features of instability of the autonomic nervous system were observed.

13. Pozos, Robert S., Richardson, Alfred W. & Kaplan, Harold M. Electroanesthesia: A proposed physiologic mechanism. In Reynolds, David V. & Anita Sjoberg (Eds.) *Neuro-electric Research.* **Charles Thomas, Springfield, Pp. 110-113, 1971.**

The authors used both electoanesthesia and CES current levels along with reserpine, anoxia, L-dopa, atropine and physostigmine in mongrel dogs to elucidate the mechanisms of action from electrical stimulation to the head. Their findings suggested that CES releases dopamine in the basal ganglia, and that the overall physiological effects appear to be anticholinergic and catecholamine-like in action, and that some form of acidosis or a concomitant of this state is implicated in the mechanism of action.

14. Pozos, Robert S., Strack, L.E., White, R.K. & Richardson, Alfred W. Electrosleep versus electroconvulsive therapy. In Reynolds, David V. & Sjoberg, Anita E. (Eds), *Neuroelectric Research.* **Charles Thomas: Springfield, 23:221-225, 1971.**

This is a report of a series of 5 studies that involved a complex examination of physiologic changes in pharmacologically altered experimental animals (dogs), 20 experimental and 20 controls. The animals were prepared with 0.2 mg/kg reserpine intramuscularly. After 1 hour those given either CES, electroconvulsive stimulation or lithium chloride, developed Parkinson-like symptoms. Dogs given electroconvulsive levels of stimulation while in the Parkinson-like state experienced evoked hypersynchrony persisting for 3 - 7 minutes, while stimulated controls showed a discharge pattern lasting for only 20 - 40 seconds. The evoked hypersynchrony in the electroconvulsively stimulated animals could be returned to the duration of hypersynchrony found in the control dogs by giving them atropine (0.4 mg/kg), L-dopa (2.5 mg/kg), or CES.

The authors conclude: "It is proposed that CES, electroconvulsive stimulation, and lithium salts may share a common mechanism... Based on this study alone, the net effects of CES stimulation and electroconvulsive stimulation seem quite similar."

15. Reigel, D.H., Dallmann, D.E., Christman, N.T., Hamilton, L.H., Zuperku, E.J., Henschel, E.O., Larson, S.J., & Sances Jr, A. Physiological effects of electrotherapeutic currents in the primate and man. In Wageneder, F.M., & St. Schuy (Eds.), *Electrotherapeutic Sleep and Electroanesthesia*. Vol. II, Amsterdam, Excerpta Medica, Pp. 158-165, 1970.

Studies were completed on squirrel monkeys, macaque monkeys and 15 human volunteers. Measures studied were somatosensory evoked potentials, visual evoked potentials, electroretinograms, electrocorticograms, electromyographic potentials, electro-cardiograms, respiratory rate, and gastric acid. For the animal studies pulse type currents from 2.5 to 80 Hz were used. For the human studies, pulsed currents of 100 - 200 µA intensity and 5 Hz were used. They summarized: "Neurophysiologic, cardiorespiratory and gastric secretory physiology was observed in man and primate during CES. Visual and somatosensory evoked potentials were not significantly altered during and after CES in the primates. The EMG and ECG suggested changes compatible with relaxation in the primates. Respiration and EKG remained stable in both humans and primates. Total gastric acid output in primates is significantly reduced by CES. These studies suggest that CES may be of therapeutic value." Abstract courtesy of Ray B. Smith, Ph.D., M.P.A.

16. Reigel, D.H., Larson, Sanford J., Sances Jr., Anthony, Christman, Norbert, Dallmann, Donald & Henschel, Ernest O. Effects of electrosleep currents on gastric physiology. In Reynolds, David V. & Sjoberg, Anita (Eds.) *Neuroelectric Research*. Springfield, Charles Thomas. 24:226-229, 1971.

Gastric cannulas were placed in the dependent portion of the stomach of seven stump-tailed monkeys. After recovery from surgery, CES currents of 20 to 100 µA, 2.5 to 70 Hz, were applied between the nasion and inion for periods of 1 hour. The maximal change in gastric secretion occurred during the last half of the 60 minute period of CES. The mean volume decreased 28.3%, the mean concentration decreased 38%, and acid production decreased 60%. Acid production returned to normal within 1 to 2 hours after CES. The authors found that nocturnal gastric acid levels without CES were similar to those during application of CES or during in-depth stimulation of various limbic structures, and concluded that these two types of stimulation may affect similar structures.

17. Richter, Ward R., Zouhar, Raymond L., Tatsuno, Jiro, Smith, Robert H. & Cullen, Stuart C. Electron microscopy of the macaca mulatta brain after repeated applications of electric current. *Anesthesiology*. 36(4):374-377, 1972.

2 immature Rhesus monkeys and a control were studied to assess safety of electric currents applied to the brain. 1 monkey received only sine wave current up to 50 mA, another received only square wave, up to 13 mA. They received 10, 1 hour treatments. Following the course of treatment, the monkeys were sacrificed and brain tissue was analyzed. They examined neurons, neuroglia, myelinated and nonmyelinated fibers,

capillaries and nearby astrocytes, synaptic endings and the general architecture of the neurophil. Special attention was given to the structure of the synapse and the size, location, and distribution of synaptic vesicles. The authors concluded that all of these structures were within normal limits, that there is no generalized evidence of injury, and that they have greatly increased their confidence in the safety of repeated application of electric currents.

18. Robert, Claude, Limoge, Aymé & Stinus, Luis. Transcranial electrical stimulation (Limoge's currents) potentiates the inhibition of righting reflex induced by droperidol in rats. *Brain Research.* **822(10-2):132-141, 1999. (France)**

The effects of CES on droperidol-treated rats were evaluated using the righting reflex latency (RRL) test. CES was shown to potentiate the inhibition of righting reflex induced by droperidol. This potentiation was found to depend on the dose of the drug, the characteristics of the current delivered and the duration of stimulation. The author's also observed that CES-induced potentiation of inhibition of righting reflex produced by droperidol injection was not reversed after naltrexone administration, or when measures were performed on p-chlorophenylalanine (pCPA)-treated animals. These results suggest that, under the experimental conditions: (i) CES does not interact with endogenous opioids to potentiate droperidol effects, (ii) the effect of CES on dopaminergic system prevails against CES action on serotonergic system. Though these findings enlarge the comprehension of CES effects on the central nervous system, further investigations are necessary to elucidate CES mechanisms.

19. Siegesmund, K.A., Sances Jr, A. & Larson, S.J. The effects of electrical currents on synaptic vesicles in monkey cortex. In Wageneder, F.M. & St. Schuy (Eds.), *Electrotherapeutic Sleep and Electroanaesthesia.* **International Congress Series No. 136. Excerpta Medica Foundation, Amsterdam, Pp. 31-33, 1967.**

Biased rectangular current pulses of 2.5 mS duration, 75 Hz, and 5 mA were delivered through electrodes on the nasion and inion of 4 squirrel monkeys. Electron photo-micrographs were made of neural tissue biopsies prior to, during, and post stimulation and the number of synaptic vesicles in close apposition to the presynaptic membranes were counted for at least 200 synapses in each group. They found that in the control specimen 65% of the presynaptic terminals contained 14 ±2 vesicles near the cleft. Shortly after maximum stimulation was reached, there was an increase of terminals with less than 9 vesicles and corresponding decrease in those with 14. After 5 minutes at an applied current of 5 mA, a further decrease in terminals with 14 vesicles and a corresponding increase in terminals with more than 24 vesicles were found. Shortly after discontinuation of stimulation, the number of terminals with 24 or more vesicles returned to control levels while the number with 9 vesicles or less remained at a higher level than in the controls.

20. Singh, Baldev, Chhina, G.S., Anand, B.K., Bopari, M.S. & Neki, J.S. Sleep and consciousness mechanism with special reference to electrosleep. *Armed Forces Medical Journal India* **(New Delhi). 27(3):292-297, 1971.**

4 normal human subjects showed increased alpha index on EEG immediately following CES (30 to 45 minutes), which culminated in spindle and slow sleep after a variable interval. In 6 patients suffering from subjective insomnia the passage of current

resulted in increased alpha activity and a subjective feeling of well-being but was not accompanied by either slow or paradoxical sleep. No side effects were reported.

In 10 monkeys with electrodes implanted in the brain the results showed that the cortical EEG activity either had increased spindle or it gave high voltage slow wave paroxysmal activity following CES induction. The increased slowing was also observed in the periaqueductal grey of the brain stem and lateral geniculate nucleus of the thalamus. The caudate, intralaminar thalamic nuclei and hippocampus showed no consistent changes. The tentative conclusion drawn by the authors was: 1) The EEG record tends to show more alpha activity after CES in human subjects, 2) Monkeys go into slow sleep showing sleep spindles and slow waves, 3) No paradoxical sleep has been recorded in animals. The authors also stated that the depth electrodes in monkeys seem to favor the contention that CES has an initial effect on the periaqueductal region and then it spreads to other regions of the brain.

21. Sommer, H. & Kriebel, J. Neuropathological investigations of electrosleep in animal experiments (Rabbits). In Wageneder, F.M. & St. Schuy (Eds.) *Electrotherapeutic Sleep and Electroanesthesia.* **Vol. II, Amsterdam, Excerpta Medica, Pp. 169-174, 1970.**

Finding that the electrical parameters indicated for CES in humans did not produce sleep in rabbits, they gave 700 Hz square wave pulses with a pulse width of 0.4 mS, an average current of 0.5 mA, with a peak value of 4 mA. The animals were put into a sleep-like state 5 times per week for 15, 30, 45, or 60 minutes. Histological sections of the brains were made after 20 sessions. They found numerous pathological changes that were related to intensity of stimulation. One discussant noted that he had found such pathological changes in cats following CES experiments. At the end of the conference discussion, the authors stated that these results cannot be extrapolated to humans because these current parameters are not usually used in humans, and the conditions within the human brain are quite different from those encountered in the rabbit brain. No control animals were used.

22. Stinus, Louis, Auriacombe, Marc, Tignol, Jean, Limoge, Aimé & Le Moal, Michel. Transcranial electrical stimulation with high frequency intermittent current (Limoge's) potentiates opiate-induced analgesia: blind studies. *Pain.* **42(3):351-363, 1990.**

CES with high frequency (166 kHz) intermittent current (100 Hz: 2 μS positive and 4 μS negative pulses, 100 mA peak-to-peak current corresponding to 17.5 mA effective current, "Limoge" current) has been used for several years in cardiac, thoracic, abdominal, urological and micro-surgery in France. The main benefits are a reduced requirement for analgesic drugs, especially opiates, and a long-lasting postoperative analgesia. This study confirmed these clinical observations using an Anesthelec MPO3 device with 213 male Sprague-Dawley rats using the tail-flick latency (TFL) test to measure pain threshold. CES was not found to modify the pain threshold in drug-free rats, but it potentiated morphine-induced analgesia (systemic injection). To obtain a maximal effect, the stimulation must be initiated 3 hours before the drug injection and be maintained throughout the duration of its pharmacological action. CES potentiation was found to depend on the dose of the drug, the intensity of the current and the polarity of electrodes. Blind tests of the efficiency of CES on several opiate analgesic drugs currently used in human surgery (morphine, fentanyl, alfentanil and dextromoramide) confirmed these findings. The analgesic effect of these 4 opiates (TFL as % of baseline without or with CES) were respectively: 174%, 306%; 176%, 336%; 160%, 215%; and 267%, 392%. The results were obtained not only after systemic opiate treatment, but also after intracerebroventricular injection of morphine (10 micrograms; analgesic effect 152%, 207% with CES) suggesting that CES potentiation of opiate-induced analgesia is centrally mediated. These findings confirm clinical observations on the potentiation of the analgesic properties of opiates by CES.

Non-quantitative observations indicated that CES did not affect the behavior of the rats. They ate, drank, and slept as well as the control rats. Under 100 mA CES, the rats moved normally in the cages, during handling they seemed reactive, motor strength and movements were not affected, catalepsy and sedation were absent and their tail-flick reaction was vigorous. This observation suggests the asymptomatic nature of CES, which can be applied for several days without causing any adverse reactions.

23. Tatsuno, Jiro, Marsoner, Hermann J. & Fukuda, Hiroshi. The effects of diffuse currents on focal epileptic discharges. In Wageneder, F.M. & St. Schuy (Eds.) _Electrotherapeutic Sleep and Electroanesthesia_. Vol. II, Amsterdam, Excerpta Medica, Pp. 93-101, 1970.

In a study using 15 rabbits in which the skull was exposed via a burr hole and focal discharges engendered by painting the exposed brain surface with penicillin solution, the authors found that no currents of CES intensity were effective in suppressing epileptic activity, but some evidence was obtained which suggested that the more intense currents (30 mA, 1,000 Hz) altered the frequency of firing in the epileptic focus. They noted that while no CES study had found problems in grand mal epilepsy patients with CES (often finding positive results instead), this study suggested that focal epilepsy may react differently to CES, though the authors admit that "from the intensity of the currents used in this experiment it was not possible to conclude that the current in the CES therapy has such effects on the seizure activity of the epileptic patients." Abstract courtesy of Ray B. Smith, Ph.D., M.P.A.

24. Titaeva, M.A. Changes in the functional state of the central nervous system under the influence of a pulse current as used in electrosleep. In Wageneder, F.M. & St. Schuy (Eds.) _Electrotherapeutic Sleep and Electroanaesthesia_. International Congress Series, No. 136. Excerpta Medica Foundation, Amsterdam, Pp. 175-180, 1967.

This was an uncontrolled set of clinical observations of 110 patients, including 85 with schizophrenia and 25 with "asthenohypochondriacal syndromes of varied etiology." For CES they used a pulsed current of 5 - 10 Hz, and duration of 0.2 msec, at an unspecified amperage. Treatment lasted from 40 minutes to 2 hours and continued for 16 - 25 days. They deduced that their observations indicated that the principal changes arising during CES can be attributed most probably to its direct action on the brain.

They then did a series of 35 experiments on 9 rabbits with the same pulse characteristics but with 0.7 to 2.0 V. Again they concluded that their observations indicated that CES has its effects via stimulation of the nonspecific structures of the subcortex and brain stem.

25. Warner, R., Hudson-Howard, L., Johnston, C. & Skolnick, M. Serotonin involvement in analgesia induced by transcranial electrostimulation. _Life Sciences_. 46:1131-8, 1990.

The experiments described here were intended to investigate whether serotonin (5HT) may be involved in analgesia induced by low current CES. The CES stimulus is a 10 μA, 10 Hz, pulsed current transmitted via electrodes in the pinnae. Combinations of the following were given as intraperitoneal injections: 300 mg/kg p-chlorophenylalanine (pCPA) 48 hours before testing, 100 mg/kg 5-hydroxytryptophan (5HTP) 30 minutes before testing and the saline vehicle for these drugs. Rats were tested prior to and 30 minutes after CES or sham CES. Testing for analgesia consisted of putting progressively increasing pressure on the rat tail 1/4 inch from the tip with a pneumatically driven, right angle wedge. The amount of pressure at which the rat moved its tail was measured both before and after CES, or sham CES, and recorded as the difference in tolerated peak pressure (DTPP). CES produced analgesia as manifested by a 613% increase in DTPP compared with sham CES treatment values. Among CES treated rats, pretreatment with pCPA decreased DTPP 91.5% compared with saline control values, indicating 5HT involvement. 5HTP restored CES induced analgesia in pCPA treated rats to the level of saline treated control animals, confirming 5HT involvement.

26. Wilson, A.S., Reigel, D., Unger, G.F., Larson, S.J. & Sances Jr., A. Gastric secretion before and after electrotherapeutic sleep in executive monkeys. In Wageneder, F.M. & St. Schuy (Eds.), *Electrotherapeutic Sleep and Electroanesthesia*. Vol. II, Amsterdam, Excerpta Medica, Pp. 198-206, 1970.

The authors produced a demonstrable increase in gastric acid secretion as a result of learned avoidance behavior in 6 stump-tailed macaques. CES (100 μA, 15 Hz) markedly reduced gastric hypersecretion (50% - 75%) associated with shock avoidance behavior in these animals. The authors concluded that CES may be of clinical importance in acid hypersecretion in humans. There was no alteration in efficient behavioral performance during or after CES in these animals.

27. Wilson, O.B., Hamilton, R.F., Warner, R.L., Johnston, C.M., deFriece, R., Harter, L., Schweitzer, C., Talaverra, J., Hymel, C.M. & Skolnick, M.H. The influence of electrical variables on analgesia produced by low current transcranial electrostimulation of rats. *Anesth Analg*. 68:673-81, 1989.

Pulsed low current CES has been shown to induce analgesia in rats as measured by the wet tail flick test. This study investigates the effect of varying stimulus frequency, pulse width, charge balance and polarity, as well as the influence of electrode placement and time of day at which stimulus occurred. A biphasic, charge balanced waveform with a first phase duration of 2 mS, 10 μA and 10 Hz was found to induce maximum tail flick latency changes. The effects of morning or nighttime stimulation were statistically indistinguishable, as were the differences between monophasic and biphasic stimulation. Analgesia was maximized when a positive first phase was delivered into the right ears of the rats, but monolateral stimulation with both electrodes on either the left or the right ear produced no measurable effect. Examination of CES responses in sham and stimulated populations reveals normal response distributions with the stimulated group skewed toward a positive effect.

28. Wulfsohn, N.L. & Waldron, L. The importance of trains of current producing electrosleep. In Wageneder, F. M. & St. Schuy (Eds.), *Electrotherapeutic Sleep and Electroanesthesia*. Vol. II, Excerpta Medica, Amsterdam, Pp. 212-216, 1970.

In an early attempt to see what parameters of CES would more likely yield sleep in subjects, 5 cats were implanted subdurally, bitemporally and occipito-frontally. The researchers applied numerous stimulation parameters, and concluded that EEG modulated trains produced better sleep effects than non-modulated trains, and were better than EEG modulated current without trains when compared with controls.

29. Zuperku, E.J., Hosek, R.S., Larson, Sanford J., Reigel, D.H., Sances Jr, Anthony & Henschel, Ernest O. Studies during electrotherapeutic sleep. In Reynolds, David V. & Anita Sjoberg (Eds.) *Neuroelectric Research***. Charles Thomas, Springfield, Pp. 235-241, 1971.**

CES currents from 2.5 to 80 Hz, with amplitudes from 20 µA to 1.5 mA were applied to stump-tail macaque and squirrel monkeys and various physiological recordings made. It was found that visual and somatosensory evoked potentials were not significantly altered during and after CES. A reduction in EMG amplitude occurred during CES, and the EEG showed a greater tendency toward slower, high-voltage activity. Respiration and EKG were stable.

8

31 PUBLISHED CES REVIEWS

Some of the early reviewers in the 1960s and 1970s were disappointed that sleep could not be readily induced. Reviewers who mixed studies containing reliable measures and studies with measures of unknown reliability into their reviews tended to end up confused about the effectiveness of CES. Those who did not mix the two kinds of studies had few problems discerning areas of CES treatment effectiveness, such as anxiety. There are five reviews published in the past decade. They are all positive about the beneficial effects of CES. No reviewer found any significant negative side effects from the use of CES.

1. Alling, Frederic A., Johnson, Bruce D. & Elmoghazy, Elsayed. Cranial electrostimulation in the detoxification of opiate-dependent patients. *Journal of Substance Abuse Treatment.* **7:173-180, 1990.**

In spite of the difficulties and confusing reports in both the clinical and theoretical areas, this review concludes that there seems to be enough evidence from extensive animal and human studies to show that CES has a significant effect in reducing feelings of discomfort during opiate withdrawal, and that there are biochemical changes that correlate with the clinical symptomatic relief.

2. Appel, Claus-Peter. Effect of electrosleep: review of research. *Göteborg Psychological Reports.* **2(1):1-23, 1972.**

The technique of CES was reported and difficulties were discussed. The major hypotheses in the field were presented and analyzed. Effects and concomitants were presented. Some diseases treated were mentioned. The discussion concluded that prior work with CES would have benefited from employing better experimental designs and making use of statistical analysis. A classification of variables, some of which have not been investigated thoroughly enough hitherto was attempted.

3. Boblitt, William Edgar. Electrosleep as a sleep induction method. *Psychiatric Forum.* **1(1):9, 1969.**

This early review concluded by stating, "Much of the investigation of the instrument's therapeutic potential has been conducted without benefit of experimental controls. The likely possibility of a sort of 'electronic placebo effect' has been inadequately investigated."

4. Brown, Clinton C. Electroanesthesia and electrosleep. *American Psychologist.* **30(5):402-410, 1975.**

This review paper that includes a chart of 7 early CES devices begins with a discussion that since no chemical agent satisfies 5 attributes sought after in anesthesia, attention has turned to electrical means. It ends with "The efficacy of CES in physical and emotional disorders remains a question to be resolved."

5. DeFelice, Eugene A. Cranial electrotherapy stimulation (CES) in the treatment of anxiety and other stress-related disorders: a review of controlled clinical trials. *Stress Medicine.* **13:31-42, 1997.**

This CES review covers published and to be published trials in the English language and reported to be controlled in some fashion and completed from January 1963 to January 1996. Cranial electrotherapy stimulation is defined as the application of low-level pulsed electrical current through skin surface electrodes on the head for treatment of anxiety and other stress-related disorders. A total of 34 controlled clinical trials concerning the efficacy of CES in the treatment of anxiety and other stress-related disorders were evaluated. Overall the results suggest that CES may be capable of producing significant (P<.05) benefit in the short-term symptomatic relief of anxiety and other stress-related disorders. CES may be effective alone and as an adjunct to other conservative measures of treatment. The primary mechanism of action of CES appears to be a direct effect on the brain followed by secondary responses. While adverse effects are reported to occur in less than 3% of patients, it is believed they are substantially underreported (*although the author gives no reasoning or reference for this speculation*). The short- and long-term ef-ficacy, adverse effects, safety and mechanism of action of CES remain to be established in rigorous, well-controlled clinical trials. Results reported in this review suggest that CES warrants further study.

6. The Editors. Electrosleep and cerebral electrotherapy. *Medical Letter on Drugs and Therapeutics.* **13(20):81-82, 1971.**

CES has been an officially recognized treatment in the Soviet Union for more than 20 years for the treatment of neuroses, depression, schizophrenia, insomnia, essential hypertension, peptic ulcer, and neuralgic syndromes. The authors suggest that CES should not be confused with electroanaesthesia, and that until well controlled clinical studies have established its value, there is justification only for experimental use of electrotherapy for the relief of insomnia, and common mental or psychological disorders or symptoms. They suggest that it is possible that the apparent effects are the result of suggestion.

7. Flemenbaum, A. Cerebral electrotherapy (electrosleep): A review. In Masserman, J.H. (Ed.), *Current psychiatric therapies.* **Grune & Stratton, New York. 45:195-202, 1975.**

Since CES is economical, safe, and superior to self-treatment with alcohol or other abused drugs, the author feels that CES should be included in the psychiatrist's regular modes of treatment, regardless of the negative reports and although improved research is still clearly indicated.

8. Frankel, Bernard L. Research on cerebral electrotherapy (electrosleep): some suggestions. *American Journal of Psychiatry.* **131(1):95-98, 1974.**

The author discusses methodological problems with previous studies and suggests some better design procedures for future studies.

9. Iwanovsky, Arsen & Dodge, Chritopher H. Electrosleep and electroanesthesia - theory and clinical experience. *Foreign Science Bulletin.* **4(2):1-64, 1968.**

CES and electroanesthesia have been widely accepted in clinical and surgical practice in the USSR for over 10 years. In the past few years these approaches, especially CES, have begun to gain favor in Austria, West Germany, and other Western countries. Both approaches are generally regarded with skepticism or extreme caution in the U.S., although some active theoretical research is being conducted. The authors review Soviet, European, their own, and U.S. clinical and theoretical experience with CES. They conclude that little doubt should remain that electroanesthesia, and especially CES, are firmly entrenched in Soviet medicine as widely accepted electroneural modes. Though still in the formative stages of development, even by Soviet admission, the experimental and clinical experience with CES already accumulated by the Soviet biomedical community is enormous and the trend shows no sign of abating. The evolution of CES and other electroneural approaches is already underway in Austria, West Germany, and other Western countries whose individual and collective ingenuity will undoubtedly lead to new advances in this area. It seems likely, therefore, that the volume of both Soviet and Western literature on this subject will increase and that "electrosleep" and "electroanesthesia" will join the ranks of other accepted biomedical terms.

10. Jarzembski, W.B. Electrical stimulation and substance abuse treatment. *Neurobehavioral Toxicology and Teratology.* **7:119-123, 1985.**

The findings of many studies indicate that CES treatment, when of sufficient duration, yields a significant increase in the ability of the subjects to respond to stress in a positive manner. This appears to be true for subjects in a psychiatric institution, a scholarly environment, or a hospital environment as inpatients or outpatients. Different types of anxiety have been studied, using as many as 6 psychological testing instruments. All of these studies indicate a significant positive response to CES and a lack of response to sham treatments. Situational anxiety, in which a person responds to stress created by his personal situation as a short-term event, responds to CES treatment within a relatively short time. Thus positive results were reported within a week to 10 days after treatment started. On the other hand, patients who present trait anxiety, which is a chronic anxiety regardless of the current personal situation, require significantly longer periods of treatment. In such cases daily CES treatments for several weeks are required before evidence of improvement appears.

11. Kirsch, Daniel L. Cranial electrotherapy stimulation: a safe and effective treatment for anxiety. *Medical Scope Monthly.* **3(1):1-26, 1996.**

This is a review of all known CES studies, with an emphasis on the treatment of anxiety. The history and mechanisms are discussed. 103 human and 18 animal studies are reviewed for comments on side effects and follow-up.

When restricted to anxiety populations or studies that measured for physiological and/or psychological changes in anxiety, there are 40 scientific studies of CES, involving 1,835 patients. 34 of the 40 (85%) studies reported efficacious results in the treatment of anxiety. Five of the studies on CES (all using the Alpha-Stim) support the effectiveness for managing anxiety during or after a single treatment (Gibson, 1983; Heffernan, 1995; Smith, 1993; Voris, 1995; Winick, 1995).

Of the 6 of 40 (15%) anxiety studies categorized by the authors as having negative or indeterminate results, 5 were done in the 1970s, and 1 in 1980. 3 showed both actual treatment and sham groups to improve significantly, most likely because both groups were also taking medications (Levitt, 1975; Passini, 1976; Von Richtofen, 1980). One was a depression study in which the author noted that acute anxiety was not relieved and again, the study did not control for medications (Hearst, 1974). One reported no significant change on anxiety or depression scales, but subjective insomnia improved (P<.05) during active treatment (Moore, 1975). Only one study conducted on a population of insomniacs with an average duration of symptoms for almost 20 years did not show any significant change at all in any parameters (Frankel, 1973).

The author reviewed all the aforementioned 103 CES studies for comments on side effects and safety. The most common area of complaint, reported in 5 studies, was transient blurring of vision lasting no more than 1 hour from the mechanical pressure caused by eye electrodes used in the 1960s and early 1970s. The incidence of this problem was seen equally in active CES groups and sham CES, indicating the problem was due to mechanical pressure over the orbits, and not electrically-induced. This problem does not apply to modern CES devices in the U.S. because none use eye electrodes. There was 7 reports of headaches (0.2%), and 3 cases of skin irritation or electrode burns at the electrode sites (0.09%). A table is provided that lists all comments on side effects and safety in the English language literature on CES.

A postmarketing survey of health care practitioners using Alpha-Stim CES technology is included. It was conducted during October, 1995. A total of 313 individual patient report forms were received. 112 males, and 199 women were identified, ranging from 5 to 85 years old. 20 of the forms were completed on inpatients, the balance on outpatients. 57.84% of the patients were reported to have completed CES treatment, and 42.16% were still receiving treatment at the time of the survey. 4 patients discontinued treatment because it was not efficacious, 3 discontinued due to undesirable side effects, and 24 for other reasons. significant results (>25% improvement) were reported in 97% of anxiety (N = 207), stress (N = 162), depression (N = 102), pain (N = 125), and headache patients (N = 74), 96% in insomnia (N = 74), and 99% in muscle tension (N = 110).

12. Kirsch, Daniel L. & Smith, Ray B. The use of cranial electrotherapy stimulation in the management of chronic pain: A review. *NeuroRehabilitation,* **14(2):85-95, 2000.**

This is the first published review of cranial electrotherapy stimulation (CES) for the treatment of pain. CES has a growing history of applications in rehabilitation medicine in the United States dating back to early 1970. As a recognized non-drug treatment of anxiety, depression and insomnia, CES gained its first major application in the field of addiction treatment and rehabilitation. By the mid 1980s research was showing additional important uses of CES in the treatment of closed head injured patients, and in paraplegic and quadriplegic patients. The most recent research is showing CES to be highly effective in the management of chronic pain patients. It may be elevating the pain threshold due to its stress reducing effects when anxiety and depression are reduced below clinical levels. Modern theorists of a pain neuromatrix in the cerebral cortex may provide an additional basis for understanding CES mechanisms in the control of pain related disorders.

This comprehensive review article covers the following areas in which CES is now in use. Research in rehabilitation medicine: 1) rehabilitation of addicted persons; the use of CES in paraplegic and quadriplegic patients; the use of CES in closed head injured patients; the use of CES in physical therapy. 2) research in chronic pain patients: research in spinal pain; research in fibromyalgia; research in headaches; research in dental pain. 3) studies of anesthetic equivalency.

13. Lewis, J.A. Electrosleep. In Williams, R.L. & Webb, W.B. (Eds.), *Sleep Therapy.* **Charles C. Thomas, Springfield, IL, Pp. 26-39, 1966.**

This author starts out by saying, "Profound alterations in the normal state of consciousness of men and animals are possible through the application of electric current." He then, like all early reviewers, suggests we need more research.

14. Montgomery, Iain., Perkin, Graham & Wise, Deirde. A review of behavioral treatments for insomnia. *Journal of Behavior Therapy and Experimental Psychiatry.* **6(2):93-100, 1975.**

This review discusses various treatments for insomnia, including hypnosis, relaxation training, systematic desensitization, classical conditioning, biofeedback, CES, and the use of attribution techniques.

15. National Research Council, Division of Medical Sciences. An evaluation of electro-anesthesia and electrosleep. FDA Contract 70-22, Task Order No. 20 (NTIS PB 241305), Pp. 1-54, 1974.

This FDA study concluded, "Review of these reports reveals that significant side effects or complications attributable to the procedure is virtually nonexistent."

16. Nias, David K.B. Therapeutic effects of low-level direct electrical currents. *Psychological Bulletin.* **83(5):766-773, 1976.**

The results presented in this paper, derived from research often carried out without an awareness of previous work, appear sufficiently consistent to warrant the conclusion that direct currents do have psychological effects. Only 2 adverse effects have been consistently reported for these treatments. The first is the tendency for some people to feel worse after treatment; with constant current, at least, it appears that these people will benefit from the opposite direction of current. The second is the risk of skin burning at the site of the electrodes; however, this occurs only if the electrodes are not adequately covered with lint. Prolonged treatment with CES is generally claimed to be harmless and without side effects.

17. Obrosow, Alexandre N. Electrosleep therapy. In Licht, Sidney (Ed.), *Therapeutic electricity and ultraviolet radiation.* **Vol. 4, Physical Medicine Library, Elizabeth Licht, Publisher: New Haven Connecticut, Chapter 5:179-187, 1969.**

In 1836, the Russian physiologist A.W. Ilomafitcky began to study the response of the human nervous system to the electric current. He was the first to show the inhibitory effect of the electric current on the nervous system. The author states that "we are now convinced that the mechanism of CES is neurohumoral." Several possible mechanisms, treatment techniques and tips are discussed in this entusiastic review paper.

18. Patterson, Meg, Krupitsky, Evgeny, Flood, Noel, Baker, Denise & Patterson, Lorne. Amelioration of stress in chemical detoxification by transcranial electrostimulation. *Stress Medicine.* **10:115-126, 1994.**

Psychic distress and aggression traditionally experienced as a substantial part of the withdrawal syndrome is a major obstacle to the successful detoxification and rehabilitation of the chemical dependent. CES significantly ameliorates these affective components resulting in a lowered drop-out rate while enhancing the patient's ability to benefit from relapse-prevention modalities. CES has been demonstrated as efficacious in both inpatient and outpatient settings; and used appropriately, has no unwanted side effects. Correct application of CES, influencing the neuromediatory mechanisms involved in addiction and affective disorders has been established to result in significant amelioration of stress. This ability has been demonstrated in differing medical and social contexts, and with different cultural groups within Europe, the USA, and Russia.

The work of the authors in relevant animal and clinical studies over the past 20 years is summarized. Various representative psychological assessments are reported.

The authors conclude by stating that the principal benefits emerging from these and other clinical results are threefold: First is the rapidity of effect of treatment. All successful clinical applications report this therapeutic effect. The benefits offered to both patient and physician by this rapid therapeutic effect are obvious and manifold – including its cost-effectiveness. The amelioration of depression within such a short period of time is particularly significant when contrasted with the initial 3 - 6 week period before antidepressant medication begins to show effect. Secondly, CES demonstrates that medication is no longer an essential aspect to a humane detoxification from opioids, tranquilizers, stimulants or alcohol. CES has demonstrated a substantial reduction in withdrawal distress. The majority of patients treated with CES experience withdrawal relief of between 50 and 75% of the assessed symptomatology; while a minority experiences relief of between 75 and 90%. However, even at 50% relief, CES negates the necessity to implement medication -- anxiolytic, antidepressive, hypnotic, anticonvulsant, or antiwithdrawal. Further, the mental and emotional clarity provides greater opportunity for the patient to derive benefit from relapse prevention modalities and discourages reliance on psychoactive chemicals as a coping strategy. Thirdly, the unexpectedly low drop-out rates found with CES would seem to suggest that the psychological distress experienced in detoxification is far more pivotal to a poor treatment outcome than is generally believed. CES-supported treatments in particular suggest that when this distress is substantially ameliorated, treatment outcome is significantly enhanced even in the presence of physical discomfort. A new positive and hopeful attitude towards life is frequently observed and recorded by the end of most treatments, possibly derived from normalization of endorphins, dopamine, and monoamine levels.

19. Phillips, Philip B. Notes on Russian psychiatry. *Journal of the Florida Medical Association.* **63(9):715-717, 1976.**

The author was 1 of 160 psychiatrists to visit the Soviet Union where CES is often used in treating children. CES was being used at the children's hospital in Kiev in an effort to calm the disturbed behavior of the children and habituate them to an afternoon nap. Children in this hospital were said to be victims of childhood encephalitis or meningitis and some had minimal brain dysfunction. Others were epileptic and some were mental retardates. There were also juvenile schizophrenic and autistic children.

20. Pleitez, Jose A. New Frontier: Electrosleep therapy. *Nebraska Medical Journal.* **58(1):9-11, 1973.**

"In summary, CES therapy is highly effective in a wide range of well selected clinical conditions. It is a new approach to the treatment of so many patients for whom we are now prescribing hypnotics, sedatives, and addictive tranquilizers. In my opinion, since it is a harmless, nontoxic, nonaddictive, quite safe and inoffensive procedure, its discovery brought into the medical armamentarium is one of the most effective, powerful therapeutic weapons ever known for the treatment of chronic insomnia."

21. Rosenthal, Saul H. A qualitative description of the electrosleep experience. In Wulfsohn, N.L. & Sances, A. (Eds.), *The nervous system and electric currents.* **Plenum, New York, 2:153-155, 1971.**

In our normal, intelligent, verbal subjects we expected to find a mild, sedative or tranquilizing effect and no particular effect on mood or affect. On the contrary we found the following: 1) Activation of alertness, 2) Euphoria, and 3) Not worrying. Some typical illustrative comments include the following: "Anxiety about capability seems reduced, as it does about much that is external - getting into the correct freeway lane for an exit, for example - so what? I can always go back - I think that this provides for better handling of myself in daily situations." "During the day I would find myself smiling for no real reason." "Euphoric and extremely happy as though I have been given a happy pill. Sort of a floaty, smiley feeling, very pleasant. This is quite a change of moods." "I feel as though I have almost been conditioned not to worry. It is almost as if my mind won't function in that area." And when a serious situational problem intervened, "although I feel depressed, it is nothing like what I would expect from past experience, even though the problem is large."

22. Rosenthal, Saul H. Electrosleep therapy. *Current Psychiatric Therapies.* **12:104-107, 1972.**

The best results are probably seen when anxiety is not clearly related to environmental stress but has persisted chronically with only partial and temporary remissions over a long period of time. As with many other psychiatric treatments, CES works much more effectively in patients with otherwise good ego strength and without serious major personality disorders. As the treatment takes several days, it cannot be used for the immediate management of acute anxiety attacks or hyperventilation syndrome. It may, however, prevent recurrences in chronically anxious patients. CES is probably contra-indicated in severe endogenous or psychotic depressions or involutional melancholia. We have seen 2 hospitalized patients with these diagnoses become more agitated. Blurring of vision for 5 or 10 minutes following the removal of electrodes is ascribed to the pressure of the anterior electrodes on the eyes as it is observed whether or not there is any application of electrical current. Occasionally, patients report a mild headache following treatments lasting several hours, and usually relieved by aspirin. Some patients find the increased dreaming uncomfortable.

The remission of symptoms has been maintained for variable times ranging from 1 week to 1 year. There have been over 20 years of experience in the Soviet bloc countries, which seem to indicate a remarkable absence of serious side effects. CES may indeed have fewer side effects than most of the medications currently in use and certainly has fewer obvious CNS side effects than electroshock therapy.

As a substitute for medication, CES has several advantages. It is possibly more effective. It avoids the common medication side effects as well as problems of medication abuse, incorrect dosage, and suicidal and accidental overdoses.

23. Rosenthal, Saul H. & Briones, David F. Hormonal studies in cerebral electrotherapy. Presented at the Third International Symposium on Electrosleep and Electroanesthesia. In Wageneder, F.M. & Germann, R.H. (Eds). *Electrotherapeutic Sleep and Electroanaesthesia.* **Excerpta Medica Foundation, Amsterdam, 3:156-157, 1972.**

After completing a number of clinical studies using CES during the past 3 years, the hypothesis suggested itself that one of the actions of CES is to stimulate the hypothalamus and/or pituitary. This conclusion was reached from observations of the effects of CES including a marked rise in sexual libido. To seek further evidence of CES, the authors studied thyroxine, which exhibited a definite transient rise, 10 of 20 males had increases of 0.5 μgm% or more and 15 females had increases, while 6 had falls. There were also increases in catecholamines, but not as significant increases in 17 keto-steroids. The authors concluded that there are definite hormonal changes seen with CES.

24. Smith, Ray B. Cranial Electrotherapy Stimulation. In Myklebust, Joel B., Cusick, Joseph F., Sances Jr, Anthony & Larson, Sanford J. (Eds), *Neural Stimulation.* **Vol. II, 8:129 -150, 1985.**

There are 40 studies of CES readily available in the U.S. in which the dependent variable is reliable. When these are examined alone it becomes apparent that CES is effective in alleviating symptoms of anxiety, depression, and insomnia. From the study results, it can be stated with confidence that CES alleviates anxiety as measured by the tension-anxiety factor of the Profile of Mood States (POMS), the state anxiety scale of the State-Trait Anxiety Index (STAI), the anxiety scale score, and the anxiety index score. CES requires at least 5 - 7 days of at least 30 minutes of treatment per day for the later 3 measures. To improve anxiety as measured by the Taylor Manifest Anxiety Scale (TMAS), the Hamilton Anxiety Scale (HAS), and the trait anxiety scale of the STAI takes more than a week. These do not respond in fewer than 2 weeks or more of treatment.

The safety or nonsafety of CES will remain anecdotal until some real harm is found in 1 or more patients and then approached in a controlled study. For example, CES therapists learn to expect headaches in about 3 patients out of 100. CES researchers know to expect the rate to be the same in both CES-treated and sham-treated controls. One cannot design a study to show that something is safe, in a generic sense, of course, so initially one must fall back on anecdotal evidence of lack of safety. Below is a summary of what several researchers have said after researching or reviewing CES:

"The technique appears to be entirely safe. Follow-up of patients up to one year after treatment has not revealed any harmful effects."

"No ill effects were observed after repeated experiments in the same and different individuals."

"CES is safe; no patients were harmed as a result of treatment."

"In CES, therefore, the safety factor seems to be as close to 100% as one could expect with a potent therapy. Headaches were not observed in our series..."

"Many investigations on animals and man during and after CES have failed to uncover any ill effect from the treatment."

So run the comments when authors make them, which is not often. In practice, each physician tends to make up his own list of proscribed disorders in which CES must not be used. At an alcoholics treatment center where this reviewer once worked the rule was that no patient known to have withdrawal seizures was to have CES, only to discover that a large hospital in New Orleans was using CES as a specific treatment for this condition. We also determined early on not to use it on any patient known to have suffered brain damage, only to discover after researching it that CES is quite possibly the best treatment available for several forms of what we then called permanent brain damage.

25. Templer, Donald I. The efficacy of electrosleep therapy. *Canadian Psychiatric Association Journal.* **20(8):607-613, 1975.**

The Summary states, "A review of the literature on the efficacy of CES is presented. The vast majority of non-double-blind based reports are very optimistic about its effectiveness, but the inferences from the double-blind based research are much less positive. It is concluded that the efficacy of CES therapy has not yet been demonstrated."

26. Van Poznak, Alan. Advances in electrosleep and electro-anesthesia during the past decade. *Clinical Anesthesia.* **Vol. 3, 19:501-520, 1969.**

The author of this early negative review states that we have known for thousands of years that electricity can produce instant unawareness of the environment, but that little progress has been made since Leduc reported all of the good and bad features of electroanesthesia in 1903.

27. Von Richthofen, Carmen L. & Mellor, Clive S. Cerebral electrotherapy: Methodological problems in assessing its therapeutic effectiveness. *Psychological Bulletin.* **86(6):1264-1271, 1979.**

After reviewing the research, suggestions are made for better methodology in future CES research.

28. Wageneder, F.M. The application of electrosleep therapy in people of advanced age. *American Journal of Proctology*. 20(5):351-358, 1969. Also presented at the 20th Annual Congress and Teaching Seminar, The International Academy of Proctology, Montreux, Switzerland, May 4-8, 1968.

The author, who is from the Department for Electrosleeptherapy of the Chirurgische Universitaetsklinik, Graz, Austria, discusses various CES devices used in research from 1956 through 1967. He discusses central and peripheral nervous system effects, the controversy over the terminology of "electrosleep", and procedures. Case histories are reviewed, especially a 56 year old bronchial asthma patient who had significant improvement in various pulmonary tests after CES. This review concludes with, "No matter what will be the explanation of the mechanism of action of CES one day, we can confidently state now that a current applied to the skull flows through the brain and has an influence on the central nervous system. We hope that we were able to show that the results of CES can be striking and are therefore sure that CES as a new method of therapy should not be underestimated.

29. Wageneder, F.M., Iwanovsky, A., and Dodge, C.H. Electrosleep (cerebral electro-therapy) and electroanesthesia -- the international effort at evaluation. *Foreign Science Bulletin*. 5(4):1-104, 1969.

This is a comprehensive early review by the Chief of Surgery at the University of Graz, the Head, Science and Technology Section, Aerospace Technology, Library of Congress, and the Deputy Head, Biosciences Division Department of the Navy. It reflects the efforts of the international biomedical and bioengineering communities to critically approach and quantitatively evaluate CES and electroanesthesia, and to improve the understanding of the physiological mechanisms of these electroneural techniques.

30. Weinberg, Abraham. Clinical observations in the use of electrosleep. *Journal of the American Society of Psychosomatic Dentistry and Medicine*. 16(2):35-39, 1969.

The author wrote, "The claims of the CES investigators intrigued me, and I decided to attempt to reproduce these claims. I was disappointed in the results. I could duplicate but a very few. In further pursuing the matter, I decided that I would first hypnotically induce the patient preceding the application of the CES stimulation. The results were quite gratifying. Using hypnoelectrosleep therapy many psychosomatic complaints were helped, such as neurotic headaches, some neurodermatitis, tics, insomnia, impotency and in the reconditioning of habit control in obesity, smoking and alcoholism. In continuing to use direct hypnosis altering with CES, I found that many patients who previously had been difficult to hypnotize were able to enter into a quicker, smoother hypnotic relationship, either directly or through verbal 'as if' associations. I then began to use CES as a routine method for the conditioning of previously hypnotically resistant patients.

"It would seem that electrical sleep can be a safe, non-toxic, easily controlled and efficient method for the induction of pure sleep therapy, and as a preconditioning technique for the induction of hypnosis and hypnotherapy in some refractory patients.

"Hypnosis can be used to decrease the anxiety concerning the use of CES procedures, possibly enhancing the results and the CES method can be used to reduce the anxiety concerning hypnosis as a result of pre-conceived ideas and to facilitate hypnotic induction."

31. Woods, Lawrence W., Tyce, Francis A.J. & Bickford, Reginald G. Electric sleep producing devices: an evaluation using EEG monitoring. *American Journal of Psychiatry.* **122(4):153-158, 1965.**

This review of early CES EEG research concludes with "When tested on normal subjects with various psychiatric disorders, the electric 'sleep-inducing' devices have been found to be ineffective from a practical standpoint, although behavioral observations and EEG monitoring have indicated the onset of normal drowsiness and sleep patterns in some subjects and patients. No clinically evident EEG disturbances of a pattern attributed to injury have resulted from the use of the devices. There is some question whether currents of the magnitude employed would penetrate the cranium in sufficient intensity to produce the complex changes theorized in the Russian literature."

9

COMMENTS ON SIDE EFFECTS AND SAFETY FROM ALL CES RESEARCH STUDIES

Of 126 studies encompassing 4,541 subjects who had CES treatment, side effects reasonably associated with the use of CES were 9 headaches (0.20%, 1:506), and 5 cases of skin irritation (0.11%, 1:910), 2 of which were the result of a "home-made" CES device. Eye electrodes were discontinued in the USA in the early 1970s so transient blurred vision is no longer considered an adverse effect although it is included in these tables because it is mentioned in the early CES literature.

FROM PIVOTAL SCIENTIFIC STUDIES:

Study No. First Author, Year	N	Subject Description	Authors' Comments on Safety and Side Effects
12 England, Ronald R. 1976	18	migraine patients	1 subject in the placebo group developed a skin irritation at the location of the electrode. She suggested that sensations felt during the treatment were responsible.
13 Feighner, John P. 1973	23	long term psychiatric patients, unresponsive to meds, ECT, psychotherapy	4 of 6 long term depressed patients were dropped from the study because of massive worsening of depressive symptoms.
14 Flemenbaum, A. 1974	28	anxiety, depression, insomnia patients unresponsive to medications	An insignificant trend towards worsening was seen by the 24th week. 5 of 25 patients were not improved or had become worse. The author added that side effects are virtually nonexistent.
15 Forster, Sigmund 1963	23	inducing sleep	Although as current amplitude was increased to 20 volts a feeling of slight dizziness approaching a headache was noted, the authors concluded that the technique appears to be entirely safe.
16 Frankel, Bernard 1973	17	insomniacs	A commonly reported innocuous side effect was mild blurring of vision lasting 15-30 minutes, which resulted from sustained mechanical pressure of the electrodes on the eyeballs.
19 Gomez, Evaristo 1979	28	14 heroin patients, 7 placebo and 7 controls	It was noted that with a higher current the patients felt uncomfortable, but there were no skin burns.
20 Hearst, E.D. 1974	28	psychotherapy outpatients	No patient with primary affective disorder was adversely effected by CES.
24 Hochman, Richard 1988	600	dental patients	From the results obtained during 1 year of treating a variety of patients requiring a broad scope of dental treatments, CES was found to provide a safe, noninvasive, readily acceptable, adjunctive analgesic modality to maintain patient comfort through the majority of dental procedures for most patients.
28 Kirsch, Daniel L. 1998	500	anxiety, depression, insomnia, pain, and stress patients	Side effects: 6 (1.2%) reported dizziness, and 2 (0.4%) reported nausea, both of which normally occur when the current is set too high, 3 (0.6%) reported skin irritation, 1 each (0.2%) reported, anger, a metallic taste, a heavy feeling, or intensified tinnitus.
30 Krupitsky, E.M. 1991	20	alcoholic patients with affective disorders	CES was not accompanied by side effects or complications and was well tolerated by patients. CES tends to avoid side effects and complications sometimes observed in antidepressant therapy and tranquilizers.
31 Levitt, Eugene 1975	13	psychiatric inpatients	Subjects in both groups reported slight blurring of vision lasting 30 - 45 minutes following treatments. This supports the findings of other researchers that the blurred vision effect was mechanically caused by pressure from eye electrodes, and not electrical current.
34 McKenzie, Richard 1971, 1976	12	8 chronic anxiety, depression and insomnia patients and 4 controls	Blurring of vision due to eye electrode pressure was fairly uniform over the small control sample and was not especially uncomfortable.
36 Magora, F. 1967	A: 20 B: 9	A: hospitalized polysubstance abusers, and B: asthmatic children	No ill-effects were noted on prolonged and repeated observations in dogs and in humans.

Study No. First Author, Year	N	Subject Description	Authors' Comments on Safety and Side Effects
37 Magora, F. 1965	31	inducing sleep	No ill effects were observed after repeated experiments in the same and different individuals.
39 Marshall, Alan 1974	40	depressive inpatients	Although no patients were burned, the author and 1 pilot subject suffered second degree burns behind 1 ear at the point of electrode contact.
40 Matteson, Michael 1986	62	graduate students	4 subjects left the study due to complaints of headaches.
45 Overcash, Stephen 1995	197	anxiety outpatients	There were no reported side effects (short or long term)
48 Patterson, M. 1984	186	hospitalized alcohol and polysubstance abusers	There were 8 deaths over an 8 year period. All were drug addicts. The average time between CES and death was 22 months, with only 1 being less than 1 year. None were associated with CES. This 6.1% death rate compares favorably with 12% reported in a representative sample of 128 patients of London Drug Dependence Clinics over 10 years, or 23% in New York City over 20 years. There was a 75% overall improvement in the health of these patients, with no long-term illnesses or negative physical effects on health which could have resulted from CES.
49 Philip, P. 1991	21	psychiatric depressive inpatients	In 2 cases, benodiazepine withdrawal induced epileptic seizures in patients devoid of epileptic history. These seizures did not occur during CES.
53 Rosenthal, Saul H. 1970	13	psychiatric patients unresponsive to meds	There was no side effects reported by any of the patients other than a transient blurring of vision reported by several of the patients, probably associated with the forced closure of the eyes by the eyepads for 1 hour, which cleared 15-30 minutes after treatment.
54 Rosenthal, Saul H. 1970	18	outpatients with chronic anxiety, depression & insomnia	The only side effect was the transient blurring of vision reported by several of the patients, which cleared within 15 minutes after treatment. It was probably due to the forced closure of the eyes and the pressure of the eye pads. It was seen less often with later patients, and this may be due to less tight placement of the electrodes.
67 Smith, Ray B. 1993	23	psychiatric outpatients with anxiety, depression, ADD	There did not seem to be any pattern of addiction to or over dependence on the CES device. There was no side effects except 1 patient who cried during treatments, and 1 was sore behind the ears when the electrode gel began drying out.
70 Smith, Ray B. 1994	21	closed head injury inpatients	1 patient on sham CES was seen to have a seizure. No negative effects from CES treatment was seen.
72 Solomon, Seymour 1989	112	tension headache patients	6 of 7 in the active group, and 7 of 55 in the placebo group had 1 or more adverse events. The incidence of adverse events was not significantly different between the active and placebo groups for any of the reported symptoms.

FROM SUPPORTING SCIENTIFIC STUDIES:

Study No. First Author, Year	N	Subject Description	Authors' Comments on Safety and Side Effects
1 Achte, K.A. 1968	24	severe insomnia patients and drug abusers	Complications were discovered in 5 cases, 2 complained of headaches, 3 felt aching in the eyes, 1 had hysterical convulsions during the treatment. Too strong currents caused headaches in healthy persons. The currents were too weak to cause convulsions.
18 Koegler, R.R. 1971	14	insomnia patients	The only side effects noted were blood pressure lowers during treatment, and a slight blurring of vision occurs due to eye electrodes, which stops within a few minutes.
26 Miller, E.C. 1965	27	sleep induction	There appears to be no disturbing side effects; however, 1 patient did undergo a brief dissociative episode shortly after beginning his third treatment.
31 Rosenthal, Saul H. 1972	7	1 psychologist, 3 medical students, 1 psychiatry resident, 1 secretary	1 subject complained of mildly unpleasant experiences including visual disturbances lasting a maximum of 1 hour, tinnitus lasting several hours, hyperactivity, difficulty sleeping, and epigastric sensations. His hyperactivity and sleeping difficulty were gone 48 hours after the final treatment and 1 week later he reported, "I don't feel anxious, I feel fine." His previous mild transient reactive depression had not occurred and he was sleeping soundly. 2 subjects reported a headache lasting 1 hour.
35 Sing, K. 1967	30	anxiety patients with sleep disturbances	The following side effects were noted: headache, giddiness, pain in tooth, heaviness around eyes, pain in eyes, pain behind the ears.

10

COMMENTS ON FOLLOW-UP FROM ALL CES RESEARCH STUDIES

One hundred percent of the 17 studies that included follow-up showed CES to have positive long term, cumulative effects. None of these studies revealed any long term negative adverse effects.

FROM PIVOTAL SCIENTIFIC STUDIES:

Study No. First Author, Year	N	Subject Description	Authors' Comments on Follow-up
4 Brotman, Philip 1986	36	classical migraine patients	The CES group responded significantly better than the other 2 groups over the 3 month follow-up. Only the CES group showed significant carry-over effects in finger temperature.
5 Brovar, Alan 1984	25	Cocaine abusers	A follow-up of the 3 groups from 6 to 8 months later showed that no CES patients had returned for treatment, while 50% of the CES refusers and 39% of the controls had recidivated.
14 Flemenbaum, A. 1974	28	anxiety, depression, insomnia outpatients unresponsive to medications	Those who had beneficial results maintained them throughout the 6 month follow-up.
15 Forster, Sigmund 1963	23	inducing sleep	Follow-up of patients up to 1 year after treatment did not reveal any harmful side effects.
20 Hearst, E.D. 1974	28	Psychotherapy outpatients	3 patients showed continued improvement for 2 weeks to 2 months.
21 Heffernan, Michael 1995	20	generalized stress >1 year, unresponsive to meds	1 week follow-up measures in the CES group showed significant carryover effects in EMG and HR, but were not significant at the .05 level for finger temperature or capacitance.
22 Hochman, Richard 1988	600	dental patients	From the results obtained during 1 year of treating a variety of patients requiring a broad scope of dental treatments, CES was found to provide a safe, noninvasive, readily acceptable, adjunctive analgesic modality to maintain patient comfort through the majority of dental procedures for most patients.
36 Magora, F. 1967	A: 20 B: 9	A: anxiety, depression, insomnia hospitalized polysubstance abusers, and B: asthmatic children	A: Follow-up has continued for 8-12 months after treatment and has revealed no relapse. B: The asthmatic attacks stopped completely in 3 children and 4 months later the children felt well without taking any drugs.
40 Matteson, Michael 1986	62	32 CES graduate students, 22 controls	A follow-up measure 2 weeks post study found that 11 of the 13 variables were still significantly improved in the treatment group.
42 Moore, J.A. 1975	17	anxiety and insomnia patients	Despite largely negative findings several subjects reported "a remarkable improvement" in their symptoms 2 - 3 weeks after CES.
45 Overcash, Stephen, 1998	197	anxiety outpatients	At 6 - 8 month follow-up, 73% of the patients were "well satisfied with their treatment and had no significant regression or other anxiety disorder, 18% were "satisfied" but had some problem with anxiety since they stopped the treatment, and 9% chose not to respond, had significant symptoms since stopping the treatment, or in 1 case, "was not satisfied."
48 Patterson, M. 1984	186	hospitalized alcohol and polysubstance abusers	Of a 50% response to follow-up, 78.5% were addiction-free (80.3% of drug addicts) 1 to 8 years after CES, with an average time in rehabilitation of only 16 days. Alcohol, marijuana and cigarette use were decreased in 64%. Diminished drug use was reported in 76% of recidivists. 17% had 1 treatment after CES (another CES treatment or other hospital treatment), and 1% had 2 treatments. This compares favorably with a U.S. government survey showing that 26% to 43% had repeat treatments every year after the initial treatment, for up to 6 years.

Study No. First Author, Year	N	Subject Description	Authors' Comments on Follow-up
67 Smith, Ray B. 1999	23	psychiatric outpatients with anxiety, depression, ADD	On 18 month follow-up the patients performed as well or better than in the original study.
84 Weiss, Marc F. 1973	10	insomnia patients	All differences found were maintained at the 2 week and 2 year follow-up.

FROM SUPPORTING SCIENTIFIC STUDIES:

7 Cartwright, R.D. 1975	10	sleep onset insomnia patients	Only 1 of 4 responders relapsed during the 2 year no-treatment period.
17 Klimke, A. 1991	50	schizophrenic and psychotic patients unresponsive to medications	3 months after discharge from hospital 9 schizophrenics (32.1%) but only 3 patients with affective psychosis (13.6%) presented a "good outcome" (full remission).
18 Koegler, R.R. 1971	14	insomnia patients	Some patients maintained their improvement 4 months later, while others had partial return of symptoms. None regressed completely.
39 Turaeva, V.A. 1967	156	eczema and neuro-dermatitis patients	12 months follow-up revealed that the positive effects of CES was sufficiently stable.

11

NUMBER OF SUBJECTS AND AUTHORS' EVALUATION OF OVERALL RESULTS FROM ALL CES STUDIES

Of 126 total human studies of CES, 89% (112) had positive outcomes and 11% (14) were seen as having negative or indeterminate outcomes.

PIVOTAL SCIENTIFIC CES STUDIES:

	Study No. First Author	Year	Total N	Active CES N	Authors' Evaluation of Overall Results	CES Device
1.	Bianco, Faust	1994	65	29	+	LB2000
2.	Braverman, Eric	1990	15	15	+	HealthPax
3.	Briones, David F.	1973	7	6	+	(not specified)
4.	Brotman, Philip	1989	36	12	+	Alpha-Stim
5.	Brovar, Alan	1984	25	5	+	Alpha-Stim
6.	Chanpagne, C.	1984	20	10	+	Anesthelec
7.	Childs, Allen	1995	1	1	+	(not specified)
8.	Clark, Morris S.	1987	50	30	+	(not specified)
9.	Cox, Aris	1975	1	1	+	Neurotone 101
10.	Dymond, A.M.	1975	1	1	+	Grass S88
11.	Empson, J.A.C.	1973	8	8	+	Somlec
12.	England, Ronald R.	1976	18	6	+	Neurotone 101
13.	Feighner, John P.	1973	23	23	+	Electrosone 50
14.	Flemenbaum, A.	1974	28	28	+	Electrosone 50
15.	Forster, Sigmund	1963	23	23	+	(not specified)
16.	Frankel, Bernard L.	1973	17	17	-	Electrosone 50
17.	Gibson, Thomas H.	1983	64	32	+	Alpha-Stim
18.	Gold, M.S.	1982	not specified		+	(not specified)
19.	Gomez, Evaristo	1979	28	14	+	(not specified)
20.	Hearst, E.D.	1974	28	14	-	Neurotone 101
21.	Heffernan, Michael	1995	20	10	+	Alpha-Stim
22.	Heffernan, Michael	1996	30	20	+	Alpha-Stim
23.	Heffernan, Michael	1997	50	30	+	Alpha-Stim, Liss
24.	Hochman, Richard	1988	600	600	+	Neuro. Modulator
25.	Hozumi, S.	1996	27	14	+	Hess-100
26.	Itil, T.	1971	10	10	+	Electrosone 50
27.	Jemelka, Ron	1975	28	14	+	Neurotone 101
28.	Kirsch, Daniel L.	1998	500	500	+	Alpha-Stim
29.	Kotter, Gary S.	1975	23	23	+	Electrodorn
30.	Krupitsky, E.M.	1991	20	10	+	(not specified)
31.	Levitt, Eugene A.,	1975	13	5	-	Dormed
32.	Lichtbroun, Alan S.	2001	60	43	+	Alpha-Stim
33.	Logan, Michael P.	1988	36	18	+	Pain Supressor
34.	McKenzie, Richard E.	1976	12	12	+	Electrosone 50
35.	Madden, Richard	1987	103	39	+	Alpha-Stim
36.	Magora, F.	1967	29	29	+	(not specified)
37.	Magora, Florella	1965	31	31	+	(not specified)
38.	Malden, Joan W.	1985	20	20	+	Neuro. Modulator
39.	Marshall, Alan G.	1974	40	20	-	(not specified)
40.	Matteson, M.T.	1986	62	32	+	RelaxPak
41.	May, Brad	1993	14	14	+	Alpha-Stim
42.	Moore, J.A.	1975	17	17	-	Neurotone 101
43.	Naveau, S.	1992	50	50	+	(not specified)
44.	Okoye, Renee	1986	16	10	+	Neuro. Modulator
45.	Overcash, Stephen J.	1999	197	182	+	Alpha-Stim
46.	Overcash, Stephen J.	1989	32	16	+	Alpha-Stim
47.	Passini, Frank G.	1976	60	30	-	Neurotone 101
48.	Patterson, Margaret A.	1984	186	186	+	(not specified)
49.	Philip, P.	1991	21	10	+	Diastim
50.	Romano, Thomas	1993	100	100	+	Pain Supressor
51.	Rosenthal, Saul H.	1972	22	11	+	(not specified)
52.	Rosenthal, Saul H.	1973	41	41	+	(not specified)
53.	Rosenthal, Saul H.	1970	13	13	+	Electrosone 50
54.	Rosenthal, Saul H.	1970	18	12	+	Electrosone 50
55.	Ryan, Joseph J.	1976	42	12	+	Neurotone 101
56.	Ryan, Joseph J.	1977	40	20	+	Neurotone 101

Study No. First Author	Year	Total N	Active CES N	Authors' Evaluation of Overall Results		CES Device
57. Sausa, Alan De.	1975	160	80	+		Somlec
58. Schmitt, Richard	1984	60	20	+		Neurotone 101
59. Schmitt, Richard	1986	60	30	+		Neurotone 101
60. Schroeder, Mark J.	1999	12	12	+		Alpha-Stim
61. Shealy, C. Norman	1989	48	34	+		Liss Stimulator
62. Shealy, C. Norman	1998	10	10	+		Liss Stimulator
63. Singh, Baldev	1971	10	10	+		LRDE/HB-1705
64. Smith, Ray B.	1982	100	50	+		Neurotone 101
65. Smith, Ray B.	1979	53	53	+		Neurotone 101
66. Smith, Ray B.	1977	227	198	+		Neurotone 101
67. Smith, Ray B.	1999	23	23	+		Alpha-Stim, Liss
68. Smith, Ray B.	1975	72	36	+		Neurotone 101
69. Smith, Ray B.	1992	31	30	+		Alpha-Stim
70. Smith, Ray B.	1994	21	10	+		CES Labs
71. Smith, Ray B.	1991	146	39	+		(not specified)
72. Solomon, Seymour	1989	112	57	+		Pain Supressor
73. Southworth, Susan A.	1999	52	31	+		Liss Stimulator
74. Stanley, Theodore, H.	1982	50	50	+		(not specified)
75. Stanley, Theodore, H.	1982	120	60	+		(not specified)
76. Straus, Bernard	1964	34	34	+		Electrosom
77. Taaks, H.	1968	7	7		-	(not specified)
78. Taylor, Douglas, N.	1991	210	100	+		Neurometer
79. Tomaszek, David E.	2002	38	28	+		Alpha-Stim
80. Von Richthofen, C.L.	1980	10	10		-	Neurotone 101
81. Voris, Marshall, D.	1995	105	40	+		Alpha-Stim
82. Voris, Marshall, D.	1996	15	8	+		Alpha-Stim
83. Weingarten Eric	1981	24	12	+		Neurotone 101
84. Weiss, Marc F.	1973	10	5	+		Electrodorn
85. Wilson, L.F.	1988	4	3	+		RelaxPak
86. Winick, Reid L.	1999	33	16	+		Alpha-Stim
SUBTOTALS:		**4,898**	**3,575**	**78**	**8**	

78 positive (91%) and 8 negative (9%) outcomes out of 86 studies

SUPPORTING SCIENTIFIC CES STUDIES:

Study No. First Author	Year	Total N	Active CES N	Authors' Evaluation of Overall Results		CES Device
1. Achte, K.A.,	1968	24	24	+		(not specified)
2. Alpher, Elliott J.	1998	1	1	+		Alpha-Stim
3. Astrup, C.A.	1974	51	51		-	Electrosleep 1
4. Barabasz, Arreed F.	1976	60	30	+		Somniatron 7200
5. Brand, J.	1970	58	58	+		Dormed
6. Boertien, Andre, H.	1975	20	20	+		Electrodorm
7. Cartwright, Rosalind	1975	10	5	+		(not specified)
8. Childs, Allen	1988	2	2	+		Relaxpak
9. Childs, Allen	1993	1	1	+		Liss Device
10. Coursey, Robert D.	1980	22	10		-	Electrosone 50
11. Epifanov, V.A.	1999	not specified		+		(not specified)
12. Evitukhin, A.I.	1998	80	80	+		(not specified)
13. Forster, S.	1967	6	6	+		various devices
14. Gigineishvili, G.R.	1995	not specified		+		(not specified)
15. Glazer, I.	1969	13	13	+		(not specified)
16. Kelley, J.W.	1977	50	50	+		Neurotone
17. Klimke, A.	1991	50	50	+		(not specified)
18. Koegler, R.R.	1971	14	14	+		Electrosone 50
19. Komarova, L.A.	1999	39	39	+		Transair
20. Kulkarni, Arun D.	2001	20	20	+		Alpha-Stim
21. Kuzin, M.I.	1984	not specified		+		(not specified)
22. Lett, C.R.	1976	17	17		-	Neurotone 101
23. Long, R.C.	1966	32	32	+		Somniatron 7200
24. Lynch, Harold D.	1975	not specified		+		(not specified)
25. McKenzie, R.E.	1975	20	10	+		Electrosone 50
26. Miller, E.C.	1965	27	27		-	(not specified)
28. Patterson, M.A.	1998	22	22	+		(not specified)
29. Pickworth, W.B.	1997	101	51		-	(not specified)
30. Ramsay, John C.	1966	20	20	+		(self made)
31. Rosenthal, S.H.	1972	7	7	+		(not specified)
32. Rosenthal, S.H.	1970	40	40	+		Electrosone 50
33. Scallet, A.	1976	17	12	+		Neurotone 101
34. Singh, J.M.	1974	not specified		+		Neurotone 101
35. Singh, K.	1967	30	15	+		(not specified)
36. Sokolov, E.A.	1991	not specified				(not specified)
37. Sornson, Robert	1989	3	3	+		Neuro. Modulator
38. Tomsovic, M.	1973	34	18		-	Neurotone 101
39. Turaeva, V.A.	1967	158	158	+		VNIIKhI
40. Tyers, Steve	2001	60	60	+		Alpha-Stim
SUBTOTALS:		**1,109**	**966**	**34**	**6**	

34 positive (85%) and 6 negative (15%) outcomes out of 40 studies

	Total N	Active CES N	Authors' Evaluation of Overall Results	
TOTALS OF ALL CES STUDIES:	**6,007**	**4,541**	**112 pos.**	**14 neg.**

12

AN ANALYSES OF ALL CES STUDIES WITH NEGATIVE OR INDETERMINATE OUTCOMES

Fourteen (11%) out of the total 126 human studies of CES had negative or indeterminate outcomes. All studies with negative or indeterminate outcomes were published between 1965 and 1980, except one suspicious U.S. government study that used less current than ever before attempted with CES. No Alpha-Stim CES studies had negative or indeterminate outcomes.

DEVICES:

Devices used in studies that had negative or indeterminate outcomes:

2 Electrosone   1 Electrosleep 1 (Russian)
6 Neurotone   4 not specified
1 Dormed

Note: None of the specified devices are still commercially available.

GENERAL OBSERVATIONS:

Some of the possible reasons for researchers finding negative or indeterminate outcomes are:

1. Some of the studies categorized as having negative or indeterminate outcomes <u>did not control for medications</u>.

2. In the early days of CES when it was called "electrosleep" studies were considered to have negative outcomes because CES <u>failed to actually put people to sleep</u>.

3. Some used actual treatment of short duration as "placebo", although no one has ruled out the possibility that <u>brief treatment could produce a positive therapeutic outcome</u>, as is often seen clinically.

4. One US government study used only 30 µA in an attempt to get people to stop smoking cigarettes, which would be approximately <u>10% of the minimum reasonable dosage</u> and is unprecedented in the literature.

5. It is possible that some of the older devices malfunctioned. A <u>device malfunction</u> would be the most logical explanation for the complete lack of results unique to Frankel's study.

In some of these studies there were some significant positive changes, but the author did not consider them significant. For example, Hearst found the CES group to be significantly ($P<.05$) less depressed than the sham group, but the results were only temporary. In this case, it is probable that <u>5 treatments were not enough treatments to provide long term relief of depression</u>.

Finally, some of the patient populations studied were <u>too severely afflicted</u> for CES, such as <u>chronic inpatient schizophrenics</u>, and <u>severe neurotic inpatients</u>.

SPECIFIC REASONS:

See the underlined comments in the following complete listing of studies having negative or indeterminate outcomes for more details. *Note: The numbers preceding the following abstracts are from the CES Bibliographies.*

16. Frankel, Bernard L., Buchbinder, Rona & Snyder, Frederick. Ineffectiveness of electro-sleep in chronic primary insomnia. *Archives of General Psychiatry.* 29:563-568, 1973.

Device: Electrosone 50: 100 or 15 Hz, 1 mS, 100 - 700 µA, square waves, cathodes over orbits, anodes over mastoids

17 insomniacs referred from local physicians with an average duration of symptoms for almost 20 years were given 15, 45 minute CES treatments Monday through Friday at 100 or 15 Hz, a week off, then 15 more treatments at 15 or 100 Hz in a cross-over design with each group split in half. Both the 100 Hz and 15 Hz groups appeared to be combined for the 3rd week and 7th week measurements. There were no changes in the EEG, sleep onset time, sleep efficiency, total number and duration of awakenings, etc. The Taylor Manifest Anxiety Scale did not change (Pretreatment means of 21.0 ± 9.3, after 15 treatments 19.9 ± 10.1, after 30 treatments 19.2 ± 10.1, at 1 month follow-up 20.5 ± 9.6) nor did the Zung depression scale. 17-hydroxycorticosteroid levels did not change. All of these changes have been found in other controlled studies, so Frankel's findings stand virtually alone in the literature. Note: From the write up, it is not clear that the authors did not combine the two groups for the final statistical analysis, even though Frankel noted in his introduction the comment made by Obrosov in the European literature that hertz of different levels should not be mixed when treating the same patient, as was done in this study, since beneficial effects can be eliminated or canceled out. We also now know that beneficial gains from CES treatment tend to increase following the initial treatment. Such effect, when present, would nullify the expected effect in crossover designs involving sham (or other) treatment.

20. Hearst, E.D., Cloninger, R., Crews, E.L. & Cadoret, R.J. Electrosleep therapy: A double-blind trial. *Archives of General Psychiatry.* 30:463-66, 1974.

Device, Neurotone 101, 100 Hz, 2 mS, alternating and direct current, forehead to mastoid electrodes

28 psychiatric outpatients on medication and undergoing psychotherapy were divided into 4 groups, 22 received CES treatments or sham treatments using alternating current, and 6 more were divided into an alternating or direct current, or sham treatment group. A total of 14 received actual CES. All had 5, 30 minute treatments or sham treatments. Assessment was by the National Institute of Mental Health self rating scale (SRSS) and by physician and patient global ratings for sleep, anxiety, depression, and overall status. The groups did not differ substantially in the number of days they were symptomatic following treatment. However, the patients receiving active treatment were confirmed by Fisher's exact test for 2 x 2 contingency tables to be significantly (P<.05) less depressed than the sham group (79% vs. 21%). Other positive findings showed a trend (P<.10) towards improvements in the CES group over the sham in feeling lonely (64% vs. 21%), having feelings easily hurt (64% vs. 21%), and difficulty falling or staying asleep (71% vs. 29%). Physicians and patients global ratings showed an insignificant tendency towards improvement on the last day of treatment. There was no significant differences between the groups 2 weeks post-treatment, and only 2 patients continued improvement, 1 relapsed after 1 month, while another relapsed in 2 months. A third patient showed marked improvement for 1 week, relapsed for 3 weeks, then responded again to biweekly treatments for 2 months. All 3 patients with sustained improvement had active treatment. Self rating scales did not indicate a significant improvement for anxiety, insomnia, or somatic complaints.

31. Levitt, Eugene A., James, Norman McI & Flavell, Philippa. A clinical trial of electro-sleep therapy with a psychiatric inpatient sample. *Australia and New Zealand Journal of Psychiatry.* **9:287-290, 1975.**

Device: Dormed: 100 Hz, 50 - 200 µA, square pulses, cathodes over orbits, anodes over mastoids

This is a double-blind study of 13 chronically distressed patients, 6 male and 7 female, 23 - 63 years old, in an inpatient psychiatric hospital (length of stay, 2 months to 16 years). All were on anti-depressant and/or tranquilizing medication, with 9 on sleep medication. They were diagnosed with schizophrenia (N = 4), alcoholism (N = 2), psychotic depression (N = 2), and mixed neurosis and disorders of personality (N = 5). 5 received CES treatment and 6 received simulated treatment for 10 sessions over 2 weeks, 30 minutes per session. Instrument malfunction made it impossible to complete the treatment program with 2 active CES patients. There were no significant changes between groups on the Taylor Manifest Anxiety Scale or the Zung Self-Rating Depression Scale. Clinician ratings of anxiety and insomnia were "found to agree to an extremely limited extent" with results on the anxiety and depression scales. 4 of 5 of the active CES patients showed a decrease on Taylor, while the 5th remained constant, for an average drop of 4.4. 5 patients improved with placebo while the remaining 1 got worse, an average drop of 3.2. Therapist ratings of anxiety showed 2 patients to be improved, 2 unchanged, and 1 worse following active CES. Of those receiving sham treatment, 1 was rated improved, 2 unchanged, and 3 more anxious. The Zung depression scores for 2 CES patients showed improvement while the other 3 showed an increase. 5 of 6 sham patients showed a decrease in depression, and 1 was more depressed. Clinician ratings of depression noted improvement in 3, no change in 1, and increased depression in 1 receiving active CES, while 3 sham CES patients improved, and 3 were unchanged. The authors noted that since nightly sedatives were administered the fact of a nonsignificant increase in sleep was hardly surprising.

39. Marshall, Alan G. & Izard, Carrol E. Cerebral electrotherapeutic treatment of depressions. *Journal of Consulting and Clinical Psychology.* **42(1):93-97, 1974.**

Device: 100 Hz, 1 mS, 0.5 - 1.5 mA, cathodes over orbits, anodes over mastoids

40 depressive inpatient volunteers without a chronic psychotic history (30 females and 10 males, aged 25 - 70 years) in a state psychiatric hospital were given 30 minute CES treatments for 5 successive days while on the regular hospital regimen. All of the patients were taking medication, part of the effect of which was usually sedative. Both active CES (N = 20), and simulated CES controls (N = 20) improved significantly on the DES+D II modification of Izard's Differential Emotion Scale. Heart rate, blood pressure and sleep records were also maintained, but they were largely invalidated by sources of variability associated with hospital routine. Note: The first author made the CES device used in this study.

42. Moore, J.A., Mellor, C.S. Standage, K.F. & Strong, H. A double-blind study of electro-sleep for anxiety and insomnia. *Biological Psychiatry.* **10(1):59-63, 1975.**

Device: Neurotone, 100 Hz, 2 mS, mean of 480 µA

17 persistent anxiety and insomnia patients (21 - 60 years old, mean of 37.7), without evidence of psychosis, were given 5, 30 minute CES treatments or simulated treatments in a cross-over design after providing informed consent. The patients were told not to make any changes in their medication. There was improvement in all measures but one during

the first week, but no significant difference between groups on the Taylor Manifest Anxiety Scale, Beck's Depression Inventory, or Eysenck's Lie, Neuroticism, or Extraversion scales, except that subjective insomnia improvement (P<.05) was noted during active treatment. The mean change in ratings over the first week for clinical anxiety was 0.62 for active CES and .61 for sham, for subjective anxiety was 0.37 for active and 0.55 for sham, and on Taylor was -0.75 for active and 2.55 for sham. Over the second week for clinical anxiety the mean was 0.27 for active CES and 0.31 for sham, for subjective anxiety was 0.00 for active and 0.88 for sham, and on Taylor was 1.87 for active and 2.25 for sham. The authors concluded that five, 30 minute sessions might not be sufficient to elicit the effects studied. Also the current was unusually low for the device used. Curiously, the authors noted up front, in the abstract, that despite largely negative findings, several subjects reported a remarkable improvement in their symptoms some 2 - 3 weeks after CES. Note: While this was called a double-blind study, only the patients, and not the therapist were blind to treatment conditions.

47. Passini, Frank G., Watson, Charles G. & Herder, Joseph. The effects of cerebral electric therapy (electrosleep) on anxiety, depression, and hostility in psychiatric patients. *Journal of Nervous and Mental Disease.* **163(4):263-266, 1976.**

Device: Neurotone 101, 100 Hz, 2 mS, cathodes over orbits, anodes over mastoids

60 inpatient volunteers (59 males, 1 female) in a V.A. hospital suffering from either anxiety or depression were randomly assigned to CES treatments or simulated treatments. The diagnoses included alcohol addiction, depressive neurosis, manic-depression, anxiety neurosis, drug dependence, organic brain syndrome, schizophrenia, psychotic depressive reaction, hypochondriacal neurosis, hysterical neurosis, adult adjustment reaction, social maladjustment, acute alcohol intoxication, personality disorder, passive-aggressive personality, and situational disturbance. Both groups were given 10, 30 minute treatments. All subjects in both groups improved significantly (P<.001) on the Multiple Affect Adjective Check List (for anxiety, active CES means was 12.06 pre-test to 8.67 post-test, for placebo CES 11.47 to 7.90) and on both the State Scale of the STAI (active: 64.93 to 45.20, placebo: 52.17 to 44.10) and Trait Scale of the STAI (active: 52.10 to 46.67, placebo: 50.47 to 43.77). The authors noted that no attempt was made to control the amount or type of psychotropic medication administered to the patients and most of the subjects on the study were on psychoactive drugs.

77. Taaks, H. & Kugler, J. Electrosleep and brain function. *Electroencephalograpy and Clinical Neurophysiology.* **24:62-94, 1968.**

Device: 100 Hz, 600 µA, cathodes on orbits and anodes on neck

In this early study attempting to put people to sleep, 7 female depressives (17 - 65 years old) were given CES for 20 minutes or a sham CES (actually 5 minutes of CES) for 20 minutes, 3 or 4 times on 7 successive days and measured for sleep or wakefulness with EEG, EOG, respiratory abdominal movements and body movements recorded for 20 minutes. The stages of sleep according to Loomis were determined visually for 40 second periods. Some slept under either or neither condition, some did not.

80. Von Richthofen, C.L. & Mellor, C.S. Electrosleep therapy: a controlled study of its effects in anxiety neurosis. *Canadian Journal of Psychiatry.* **25(3):213-229, 1980.**

Device: Neurotone 101, 100 Hz, 2 mS, <1.5 mA, anodes on forehead, cathodes on mastoid

10 patients with anxiety neurosis (6 males, 4 females, 17 - 52 years old) on medication, were given 5, 30 minute sessions of CES or simulated CES in a double-blind, cross-over design. Results were made by psychiatric clinical assessment using a 0 - 7 scale, Eysenck Personality Inventory, State-Trait Anxiety Inventory, and Complaint Checklist. Both groups improved significantly and were not different from each other either before or following the study. It should be noted that the placebo group received actual current across their foreheads, which may have accounted for their results.

FROM SUPPORTING SCIENTIFIC STUDIES:

3. Astrup, C.A. Follow-up study of electrosleep. *Biological Psychiatry*. 8(1):115-117, 1974.
   Device: Electrosleep 1 (from Russia)
   51 patients, of which 41 were rather severe neurotic inpatients, and 10 neurotic outpatients were given 10 - 15, 1 hour treatments. The authors followed the patients for as much as 18 years then concluded that their treatment had no long term effects in functional psychoses and improved only 1 of 24 neurotics. It was noted that CES increased the effects of verbal suggestions.

10. Coursey, Robert D., Frankel, Bernard L., Gaarder, Kenneth R. & Mott, David E. A comparison of relaxation techniques with electrosleep therapy for chronic, sleep-onset insomnia: a sleep-EEG study. *Biofeedback and Self-Regulation*. 5(1):7-73, 1980.
   Device: Electrosone 50, 15 and 100 Hz
   22 chronic insomniacs were divided into 3 groups. 30, 45 minute CES treatments were given to 10 patients. Instead of a no-treatment control group for this study, there were EMG feedback and Autogenic training groups. Following treatments patients filled out the Taylor Manifest Anxiety Scale, Multiple Affect Adjective Check List, and Zung Depression Scale. It seems that 3 of 6 EMG feedback patients, 2 autogenic patients, and none of the CES patients succeeded in achieving a meaningful improvement in their sleep difficulties.

22. Lett, C.R., Wilson, J.O. & Gambrell, A. Effect of Neurotone therapy during methadone detoxification. *International Journal of the Addictions*. 11(1):187-189, 1976.
   Device: Neurotone 101, 100 Hz, 2 mS, <1.5 mA, forehead to mastoid electrodes
   17 patients on methadone for 8 to 33 months with a stabilized dosage of 30 to 100 mg were given 15, 30 minute CES treatments. The following withdrawal symptoms were measured: anxiety, yawning, lacrimation, rhinorrhea, insomnia, cough, gooseflesh, tremors, hot/cold flashes, abdominal cramps, muscle cramps, muscle aches, nausea/vomiting, and diarrhea. Only 6 of the 17 patients completed the 15 treatments. Of 8 patients who completed 12 or more sessions, there was significant decreases in only 3 of 13 symptoms (tremor, rhinorrhea, and nausea). The authors stated that future studies should control for dosage level and duration of narcotics, include control groups, and have more accurate measurements of symptoms.

26. Miller, E.C. & Mathas, J.L. The use and effectiveness of electrosleep in the treatment of some common psychiatric problems. *American Journal of Psychiatry*. 122(4):460-462, 1965.

Device not specified

27 patients were given 30 - 50 minute CES treatments 2 - 5 times per week. 15 patients managed a consistent <u>sleeping</u> state during the treatments. <u>56% of the CES group were adjudged improved, compared with a 66% improved rate in the control group</u>. Daily drug use was weighed (literally). At the 5% level of confidence, t scores were not significant. The authors added, there appears to be no disturbing side effects; however, 1 patient did undergo a brief dissociative episode shortly after beginning his third treatment. Serial EEGs performed on the first 12 patients showed no alteration of the waking baseline after 6 treatments.

29. Pickworth, Wallace B., Fant, Reginald V., Butschky, Marsha F., Goffman, Allison L. & Henningfield, Jack E. Evaluation of cranial electrostimulation therapy on short-term smoking cessation. *Biological Psychiatry.* **42(2):116-121, 1997.**

Device: 10 Hz, 30 µA, 2 mS, 3M pediatric red dot electrodes bilateral on mastoids

Unedited Medline Abstract: The effects of cranial electrical stimulation (CES) on short-term smoking cessation were evaluated in a double-blind study of cigarette smokers who wished to stop smoking. Subjects were randomly assigned to a CES- (N = 51) or a sham-treated group (N = 50). On 5 consecutive days subjects received CES treatments (<u>30-microA, 2-msec, 10-Hz pulsed signal</u>) or no electrical current (sham). There were no significant differences between groups on daily cigarettes smoked, exhaled carbon monoxide, urinary cotinine levels, treatment retention, smoking urges, or total tobacco withdrawal scores, <u>although subjects in the CES group had less cigarette craving and anxiety during the first 2 experimental days</u>. The ineffectiveness of CES to reduce withdrawal symptoms and facilitate smoking cessation are similar to results of other clinical studies of CES in drug dependence, although positive effects of CES in animal studies have been reported.

Reviewer's note: This study, performed by the National Institute on Drug Abuse, Addiction Research Center, Clinical Pharmacology Branch, Baltimore, Maryland, used an unknown CES device that is not commercially available, with questionable electrodes never before used for CES, and at <u>30 µA which represents approximately 10% of the current that would be required for results</u>. Also, 5 days of any therapy is inadequate to assist in smoking cessation. Accordingly, this reviewer believes that this study was predetermined to fail and should not be considered as science because of inadequate dosage at the very least, and possibly other factors. As an analogy, if a researcher were to open a Tylenol capsule, take a few grains out, use a good double-blind study design that showed ineffectiveness at 10% of the recommended dosage, would that prove Tylenol is not an effective analgesic; and would that be considered reliable science that would qualify for publication in a decent medical journal?

<u>A critical rebuttal of this study was published in a subsequent issue of *Biological Psychiatry* (43:468, 1998) by Drs. Nashaat N. Boutros and Evgeny M. Krupitsky of the Department of Psychiatry at Yale University.</u>

38. Tomsovic, M. & Edwards, R.V. Cerebral electrotherapy for tension-related symptoms in alcoholics. *Quarterly Journal of Studies on Alcohol.* **34(4):1352-1355, 1973.**

Device: Neurotone 101, 100 Hz, 2 mS, <1.5 mA, orbit to mastoid electrodes

34 male alcoholic patients (aged 25 - 62, mean = 44) with anxiety, sleep problems, stomach disorders and headaches, volunteered, and were asked to rate their complaints on a

10 point scale. They were then given 5, 30 minute CES treatments. 18 patients received full course treatment, and <u>a placebo group of 16 patients had the device turned up and then off at the beginning, and then again halfway through each treatment. Approximately 75% of each group reported some level of improvement. It is possible that the placebo group benefited from actual, brief treatments.</u>

13

POSTMARKETING SURVEY OF ALPHA-STIM CES WITH WARRANTY CARD VALIDATION

A postmarketing survey of 500 patients using Alpha-Stim CES technology was conducted in 1995 and 1998. The results were quite impressive. Some of the survey questions were also asked of patients completing warranty cards. The 2,500 patient warranty card analysis validated the postmarketing survey, with the patient's self-reports tending to be just slightly more optimistic than the physicians. A great deal of information was culled from these questionnaires. This postmarketing survey and warranty card analysis adds a multitude of practical outcome data to the scientific literature on CES.

POSTMARKETING SURVEY

A postmarketing survey was originally conducted for the FDA during October, 1995 of all known health care practitioners using Alpha-Stim CES technology. A total of 313 individual patient report forms were received. Another survey was conducted in 1998 ending in April 1998 when 187 more forms were received providing combined data from 47 physicians on a total of 500 patients. Reports on 174 males, and 326 females were identified, ranging from 5 to 92 years old. Outpatients accounted for 423 of the forms, while 21 were hospitalized at time of treatment. 197 (41%) of the patients were reported to have satisfactorily completed CES treatment, and 207 (43%) were still receiving treatment at the time of the survey, so the final outcomes of these were not yet known.

While the exact treatment procedures can not be known for each case, only 10 patients discontinued treatment because they thought it was not helping them, and 3 more discontinued due to undesirable side effects. An additional 13 terminated treatment when their insurance ran out and they could no longer pay for treatment. Twenty patients moved out of the area while treatment was in progress or discontinued treatment for other, unstated reasons.

Negative adverse effects were all rare, mild and self-limiting, with 472 (94.4%) reporting none. Six (1.2%) reported vertigo as a side effect and 2 (0.4%) reported nausea, either of which normally occur when the current is set too high or in patients with a history of vertigo. Only 3 (0.6%) reported skin irritation, and 1 (0.2%) each reported, anger, a metallic taste, a heavy feeling, or intensified tinnitus. These generally recede or disappear as soon as the current is reduced.

The most important aspect of this survey was the results reported as a degree of improvement in the seven symptoms present in most patients for which CES is prescribed; *i.e.,* pain, anxiety, depression, stress, insomnia, headache, and muscle tension. The treatment outcome was broken down into response categories beginning with [it made my condition] "Worse", and progressing up to "Complete" improvement or cure. As in pharmaceutical studies, a degree of improvement of 25% or more was considered to be clinically significant. The combined data for all 500 patients reporting on multiple symptoms is summarized below:

Condition	N	Worse	No Change	Slight <24%	Fair 25-49%	Moderate 50-74%	Marked 75-99%	Complete 100%	Significant >25%
Pain	286	1 0.35%	5 1.75%	20 6.99%	48 16.78%	77 26.92%	108 37.76%	27 9.44%	260 90.90%
Anxiety	349	0 0.00%	8 2.29%	14 4.01%	39 11.17%	89 25.50%	181 51.86%	18 5.16%	327 93.71%
Depression	184	0 0.00%	8 4.35%	11 5.98%	31 16.85%	38 20.65%	82 44.57%	14 7.61%	165 89.68%
Stress	259	0 0.00%	6 2.32%	12 4.63%	37 14.29%	70 27.03%	124 47.88%	10 3.86%	241 93.06%
Insomnia	135	0 0.00%	16 11.85%	12 8.89%	17 12.59%	34 25.19%	45 33.33%	11 8.15%	107 79.26%
Headache	151	1 0.66%	8 5.30%	6 3.97%	25 16.56%	32 21.19%	63 41.72%	16 10.60%	136 90.07%
Muscle Tension	259	2 0.77%	6 2.32%	6 2.32%	42 16.22%	76 29.34%	111 42.86%	16 6.18%	245 94.60%

WARRANTY CARDS

To further validate the results of the survey, some of the same data was asked of patients completing Alpha-Stim warranty cards. The table appearing on the following page is a peer-reviewed analysis[1] of 2,500 consecutive survey forms from warranty cards completed as of July, 2000 by patients who were prescribed Alpha-Stim microcurrent electrical therapy (MET) and cranial electrotherapy stimulation (CES). Most had multiple diagnoses. The only inclusion criteria were that the patients used their Alpha-Stim for at least 3 weeks. 1,949, or 78% of the total listed pain as their primary diagnosis. Of those, 93% claimed significant pain reduction of greater than 25% improvement, ranging from a low of 82% in chronic regional pain syndrome (reflex sympathetic dystrophy) to a high of 98% in those suffering from migraine headaches and 100% in carpal tunnel syndrome. Of the various psychological diagnoses, 92% of 723 reporting claimed significant improvement. 72% of the patients were female. The age ranged from 15 to 92 years with a mean of 50 years. The length of use ranged from the 3 week minimum cutoff period to 5 years in 2 cases. The average period of use was 14.68 weeks, or just over 3 1/2 months. Unlike the practitioner survey, the patients completing warranty cards were not asked how they used their Alpha-Stim, what settings they used, how often they used it, nor for what length of time. What was found, however, is that the patients who use Alpha-Stim CES at home find it to be a very effective treatment for a wide range of physical and emotional disorders. The results reported by these patients were only 2% off the previous physician survey of 500 patients (the patients self-reports giving slightly higher ratings overall). None of these listed any significant adverse effects even though asked about that on the cards.

In addition, an analysis of warranty cards delineated the type of practitioners who prescribe the Alpha-Stim from those that purchase them for use in their practice. The following table compares prescriptions with clinical usage:

Practitioner	Prescriptions	Clinical Use
Medical Doctor	46%	16%
Chiropractor	15%	34%
"Doctor"	9%	-----
Dentist	8%	6%
Osteopath	6%	2%
Physical Therapist	4%	3%
Miscellaneous	4%	15%
Psychologist	3%	9%
Acupuncturist	3%	15%
Registered Nurse	1%	0.2%
Podiatrist	1%	0.3%
Occupational Therapist	0.4%	0.7%

---

[1] Smith, Ray B. Is microcurrent stimulation effective in pain management? An additional perspective. *American Journal of Pain Management*, 11(2):62-66, 2001.

Peer-Reviewed Outcomes on 2,500 Alpha-Stim Patients Self-Reports

Condition	N	Slight <24%	Fair 25-49%	Moderate 50-74%	Marked 75-100%	Significant >25%
Pain (all cases)	**1949**	**136** 6.98%	**623** 31.97%	**741** 38.02%	**449** 23.04%	**1813** 93.02%
Back Pain	403	20 4.96%	109 27.05%	157 38.96%	117 29.03%	383 95.04%
Cervical Pain	265	18 6.79%	69 26.04%	125 47.17%	53 20.00%	247 93.21%
Hip/Leg/Foot Pain	160	6 3.75%	43 26.88%	53 33.13%	58 36.25%	154 96.25%
Shoulder/Arm/Hand Pain	150	13 8.67%	41 27.33%	63 42.00%	33 22.00%	137 91.33%
Carpal Tunnel	25	0 0.00%	5 20.00%	17 68.00%	3 12.00%	25 100.00%
Arthritis Pain	188	11 5.85%	51 27.13%	88 46.81%	38 20.21%	177 94.15%
TMJ Pain	158	17 10.76%	60 37.97%	60 37.97%	21 13.29%	141 89.24%
Myofascial Pain	62	6 9.68%	18 29.03%	18 29.03%	20 32.26%	56 90.32%
Reflex Sympathetic Dystrophy	55	10 18.18%	16 29.09%	19 34.55%	10 18.18%	45 81.82%
Fibromyalgia (alone)	142	13 9.15%	53 37.32%	52 36.62%	24 16.90%	129 90.85%
Fibromyalgia (with other)	363	33 9.09%	131 36.09%	152 41.87%	47 12.95%	330 90.91%
Migraine	118	2 1.69%	49 41.53%	30 25.42%	37 31.36%	116 98.31%
Headaches (all other)	112	20 17.86%	30 26.79%	24 21.43%	38 33.93%	92 82.14%
Psychological (all cases)	**723**	**61** 8.44%	**175** 24.20%	**237** 32.78%	**250** 34.58%	**662** 91.56%
Anxiety (alone)	128	13 10.16%	29 22.66%	42 32.81%	44 34.38%	115 89.84%
Anxiety (with other)	370	33 8.92%	85 22.97%	122 32.97%	130 35.14%	337 91.08%
Anxiety/Depression	58	3 5.17%	19 32.76%	19 32.76%	17 29.31%	55 94.83%
Depression (alone)	53	7 13.21%	11 20.75%	23 43.40%	12 22.64%	46 86.79%
Depression (with other)	265	29 10.94%	61 23.02%	93 35.09%	82 30.94%	236 89.06%
Stress	123	6 4.88%	30 24.39%	39 31.71%	48 39.02%	117 95.12%
Chronic Fatigue	50	3 6.00%	30 60.00%	10 20.00%	7 14.00%	47 94.00%
Insomnia	163	10 6.13%	47 28.83%	47 28.83%	59 36.20%	153 93.87%

Chart represents results of using Alpha-Stim™ technology for MET and CES *at least 3 weeks* from consecutive warranty cards. Total N = 2,500 patients with multiple symptoms.

POSTMARKETING SURVEY DETAILS

The following comprehensive summary data details the findings and results of the postmarketing survey. The first data set is an overview of the 500 individual patient reports. Tables and graphs are provided for the results of prior treatment plotted against the efficacy of Alpha-Stim CES for anxiety, depression, stress, insomnia and pain. Efficacy on additional symptoms of pain, headache, and muscle tension are also provided in the table. Following that are two major sub-categories, one for primary psychiatric and psychological diagnoses, and the other reporting on the efficacy of Alpha-Stim CES on symptoms of anxiety, depression, stress, and insomnia in primary pain-related disorders and other diagnoses. Then the data is further broken down into 22 diagnostic sub-categories.

Several observations were evident from this data. Overall, the results of Alpha-Stim CES are highly significant and consistent for all seven symptoms in all diagnostic categories. While Alpha-Stim provides consistently safe and effective results well beyond the previous therapies used, it works slightly better for patients with primary psychiatric and psychological diagnoses. The efficacy is greatest for anxiety and stress patients, and then for depression and insomnia. The results also indicate that Alpha-Stim actually works best for muscle tension, and it is as efficacious for relieving headaches as it is for the other indications.

The majority of people used the Alpha-Stim for 10 - 60 minutes, with only 6.74% reporting using it for more than one hour. The recommended frequency setting of 0.5 Hz was used 92% of the time. It is no surprise that a variety of current strengths were used as people have variable sensory tolerances.

Far more people reported that their anxiety relief lasted days (67.93%) than those who said it only lasted hours (18.87%). While 12.26% of 106 reports stated their anxiety was relieved for more than a week, half that many (6.60%) stated it never returned. 68.42% of the people reported that they would use Alpha-Stim again, and nearly half (48.87%) said it was the most efficacious treatment for their diagnosis. Quality of life measures were also significantly improved with 85% reporting it helped overall.

Of 151 reports, 58.94% stated Alpha-Stim CES reduced or eliminated medications.

There were 22 diagnostic sub-categories for which Alpha-Stim CES was analyzed. These 22, two page analyses are useful in evaluating the potential outcome in a given patient population, and they also provide additional confirmation of the consistency in which Alpha-Stim technology is able to control anxiety, depression, insomnia, and other symptoms in any patient population. The 22 sub-categories are:

Psychiatric/Psychological Diagnoses		Pain-Related and Other Diagnoses	
76	anxiety	50	back pain
61	dental anxiety	35	joint pain
18	depression	24	cervical pain
7	mixed anxiety depressive disorder	38	headache (including migraines)
21	stress	32	fibromyalgia and chronic fatigue
48	mood disorder due to a medical condition		syndrome
14	insomnia disorder due to a medical	5	complex regional pain syndrome (RSD)
	condition	4	closed head injury
20	substance abuse and withdrawal	3	temporomandibular disorder
	(alcohol, drugs, and/or nicotine)	3	carpal tunnel syndrome
1	post traumatic stress disorder	17	chronic pain and pain not otherwise
1	attention deficit disorder		specified
		3	other
		19	not specified

SUMMARIES OF SURVEY RESULTS

SUMMARY FOR ALL DIAGNOSTIC CATEGORIES

500 total N   174 male (age range 5-87, mean 41)   21 inpatients
                     326 female (age range 9-92, mean 44)   423 outpatients

Treatment(s) used prior to Alpha-Stim:

36 ECT	122 physical therapy	46 sedative-hypnotics
111 psychotherapy	46 surgery	6 psychostimulants
41 behavior modification	51 other non-drug	49 major tranquilizers
55 milliampere TENS	36 alcohol	52 analgesics
39 chiropractic	51 anxiolitics	122 NSAIDs
26 nerve blocks	148 anti-depressants	105 muscle relaxants
13 biofeedback	87 narcotics	73 other drugs

Reason(s) for discontinuing prior treatment:

44 still using	10 exacerbated	23 negative drug effects	2 moved
140 not efficacious	12 too expensive	9 uses Alpha-Stim	38 other

Side effects of prior treatment:

74 none	25 felt drugged	20 sedation
10 pain	9 drug sensitivity/allergy	17 GI discomfort
6 addiction	12 mental cloudiness	26 other

Treatment results obtained by using Alpha-Stim

Chief Complaints	# Reported	Worse (neg)	None (no change)	Slight (<24%)	Fair (25 - 49%)	Moderate (50 - 74%)	Marked (75 - 99%)	Complete (100%)	Significant Improvement (>25%)
Pain	286	1	5	20	48	77	108	27	260
		0.35%	1.75%	6.99%	16.78%	26.92%	37.76%	9.44%	90.91%
Anxiety	349	0	8	14	39	89	181	18	327
		0.00%	2.29%	4.01%	11.17%	25.50%	51.86%	5.16%	93.70%
Depression	184	0	8	11	31	38	82	14	165
		0.00%	4.35%	5.98%	16.85%	20.65%	44.57%	7.61%	89.67%
Stress	259	0	6	12	37	70	124	10	241
		0.00%	2.32%	4.63%	14.29%	27.03%	47.88%	3.86%	93.05%
Insomnia	135	0	16	12	17	34	45	11	107
		0.00%	11.85%	8.89%	12.59%	25.19%	33.33%	8.15%	79.26%
Headache	151	1	8	6	25	32	63	16	136
		0.66%	5.30%	3.97%	16.56%	21.19%	41.72%	10.60%	90.07%
Muscle Tension	259	2	6	6	42	76	111	16	245
		0.77%	2.32%	2.32%	16.22%	29.34%	42.86%	6.18%	94.59%
Treatment results obtained prior to use of Alpha-Stim									
Prior Treatments	389	24	95	116	75	51	28	0	154
		6.17%	24.42%	29.82%	19.28%	13.11%	7.20%	0.00%	39.59%

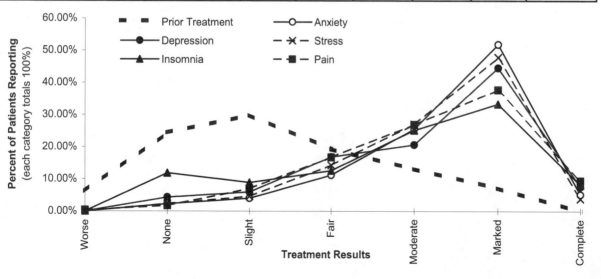

SUMMARY FOR ALL DIAGNOSTIC CATEGORIES

#	Number of Alpha-Stim treatments								Received in:	
									Doctor's	Patient's
Reported	1	2	3 - 5	6 - 10	11 - 15	16 - 20	21+	Ongoing	Office	Home
379	55	40	68	63	29	24	63	37	172	79
	14.51%	10.55%	17.94%	16.62%	7.65%	6.33%	16.62%	9.76%	68.53%	31.47%

Alpha-Stim settings used

#	Intensity (µA)						Frequency (Hz)			Time (minutes/treatment)			
Reported	100	200	300	400	500	600	0.5	1.5	100	0 - 10	11 - 20	21 - 60	>60
474	113	112	85	61	95	87	436	40	15	37	150	173	26
	24%	24%	18%	13%	20%	18%	91.98%	8.44%	3.16%	9.59%	38.86%	44.82%	6.74%

Alpha-Stim treatment course

#	Treated With			Completed	Still	Discontinued treatment because:			
Reported	Earclips	Probes	Electrodes	Satisfactory	Receiving	Not Efficacious	Side Effects	Insurance ran out	Other
482	421	106	83	197	227	12	3	13	20
	87.34%	21.99%	17.22%	40.87%	47.10%	2.49%	0.62%	2.70%	4.15%

Average residual relief received with a single Alpha-Stim treatment

	#		Hours			Days				Never
	Reported	None	<1	1 - 8	9 - 23	1	2	3 - 6	7+	Returned
Pain	150	18	2	39	9	16	14	32	12	9
		12.00%	1.33%	26.00%	6.00%	10.67%	9.33%	21.33%	8.00%	6.00%
Anxiety	106	7	2	18	0	28	5	26	13	7
		6.60%	1.89%	16.98%	0.00%	26.42%	4.72%	24.53%	12.26%	6.60%

Medication use:				#	Other concomitant therapy received with Alpha-Stim						
In-creased	No Change	Re-duced	Elimi-nated	Reported	None	Psycho-therapy	Chiro-practic	Acu-puncture	Bio-feedback	Physical Therapy	Other
1	61	64	25	427	142	66	63	35	34	58	57
0.66%	40.40%	42.38%	16.56%		33.26%	15.46%	14.75%	8.20%	7.96%	13.58%	13.35%

Eliminated use of these drugs: Acetaminophen (1), Advil (3), Ambien (1), Amitriptyline (1), Aspirin (3), Excedrin (1), Flexeril (1), Lidocaine (1), Lorcet (1), Paxil (2), Tylenol (1), Xanax (2), analgesics (5), anti-convulsants (1), anti-depressants (3), NSAIDs (5), muscle relaxants (1), narcotics (3)

Reduced use of these drugs: Ambien (1), Amitriptyline (2), Baclofen (1), DHE (1), Demerol (1), Depakote (1), Desril (1), Excedrin (1), Flexeril (2), Ibuprofen (4), Imitrex (3), Inderal (1), Methadone (1), Motrin (2), Naproxin (2), Neurontin (1), Nicotine (1), Oxycontin (1), Percocet (3), Prozac (1), Soma (2), Trazodone (1), Tylenol (2), Tylenol #3 (3), Ultram (2), Valium (2), Vicodin (1), Xanax (1), analgesics (4), anti-depressants (3), barbiturates (1), muscle relaxants (8), narcotics (4), NSAIDS (4), sedatives (2)

Increased use of this drug: Zoloft (1)

Side effects reported with use of Alpha-Stim:

472 (94.40%) "None" reported   Specify: anger (1), better concentration (1), calming effect (1), dizziness (6), heavy feeling (1), marked decrease in food consumption of compulsive overeater (1), metallic taste (1), nausea (2), ringing in ears (1), skin irritation (3)

Doctor's evaluation of Alpha-Stim

#			Reasonably
Reported	Efficacious	Safe	Well Tolerated
450	410	402	267
	91.11%	89.33%	59.33%

Doctor's evaluation of Alpha-Stim ('98 survey only)

#	Would Use	Most Efficacious	
Reported	Alpha-Stim Again	for this Diagnosis	Other
133	91	65	11
	68.42%	48.87%	8.27%

Quality of life ('98 survey only)

Lose of Work		Return to Work		Work Comp		Improve Family Life		Improve Social Life		Overall QOL		Rx by:						
YES	NO	YES	NO	YES	NO	YES	NO	YES	NO	YES	NO	MD/DO	PhD	DDS	DC	PT	Other	Not Specified
74	79	32	56	12	31	107	34	102	33	131	24	96	4	70	22	3	9	0
48%	52%	36%	64%	28%	72%	76%	24%	76%	24%	85%	15%							

SUMMARY FOR PSYCHIATRIC & PSYCHOLOGICAL DIAGNOSTIC CATEGORIES

267 total N   100 male (age range 5-67, mean 39)   16 inpatients

167 female (age range 9-86, mean 42)   225 outpatients

Treatment(s) used prior to Alpha-Stim:

36 ECT	6 physical therapy	15 sedative-hypnotics
67 psychotherapy	10 surgery	5 psychostimulants
22 behavior modification	31 other non-drug	27 major tranquilizers
2 milliampere TENS	34 alcohol	9 analgesics
12 chiropractic	28 anxiolitics	6 NSAIDs
1 nerve blocks	61 anti-depressants	10 muscle relaxants
2 biofeedback	24 narcotics	33 other drugs

Reason(s) for discontinuing prior treatment:

18 still using	5 exacerbated	13 negative drug effects	1 moved
55 not efficacious	9 too expensive	1 uses Alpha-Stim	16 other

Side effects of prior treatment:

33 none	7 felt drugged	9 sedation
0 pain	3 drug sensitivity/allergy	5 GI discomfort
5 addiction	5 mental cloudiness	12 other

Treatment results obtained by using Alpha-Stim

Chief Complaints	# Reported	Worse (neg)	None (no change)	Slight (<24%)	Fair (25 - 49%)	Moderate (50 - 74%)	Marked (75 - 99%)	Complete (100%)	Significant Improvement (>25%)
Pain	89	0	0	3	17	26	36	7	86
		0.00%	0.00%	3.37%	19.10%	29.21%	40.45%	7.87%	96.63%
Anxiety	206	0	1	3	22	59	111	10	202
		0.00%	0.49%	1.46%	10.68%	28.64%	53.88%	4.85%	98.06%
Depression	102	0	0	3	14	25	55	5	99
		0.00%	0.00%	2.94%	13.73%	24.51%	53.92%	4.90%	97.06%
Stress	141	0	0	4	20	41	69	7	137
		0.00%	0.00%	2.84%	14.18%	29.08%	48.94%	4.96%	97.16%
Insomnia	70	0	3	2	7	20	30	8	65
		0.00%	4.29%	2.86%	10.00%	28.57%	42.86%	11.43%	92.86%
Headache	55	0	2	0	5	13	29	6	53
		0.00%	3.64%	0.00%	9.09%	23.64%	52.73%	10.91%	96.36%
Muscle Tension	87	0	0	1	17	19	42	8	86
		0.00%	0.00%	1.15%	19.54%	21.84%	48.28%	9.20%	98.85%
Treatment results obtained prior to use of Alpha-Stim									
Prior Treatments	175	10	36	51	37	31	10	0	78
		5.71%	20.57%	29.14%	21.14%	17.71%	5.71%	0.00%	44.57%

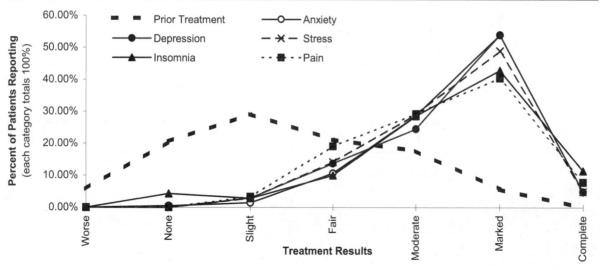

SUMMARY FOR PSYCHIATRIC & PSYCHOLOGICAL DIAGNOSTIC CATEGORIES

# Reported	Number of Alpha-Stim treatments								Received in:	
	1	2	3 - 5	6 - 10	11 - 15	16 - 20	21+	Ongoing	Doctor's Office	Patient's Home
230	40	22	38	33	18	17	43	19	64	9
	17.39%	9.57%	16.52%	14.35%	7.83%	7.39%	18.70%	8.26%	87.67%	12.33%

Alpha-Stim settings used

# Reported	Intensity (µA)						Frequency (Hz)			Time (minutes/treatment)			
	100	200	300	400	500	600	0.5	1.5	100	0 - 10	11 - 20	21 - 60	>60
264	90	48	65	49	68	27	249	15	7	11	100	122	18
	34%	18%	25%	19%	26%	10%	94.32%	5.68%	2.65%	4.38%	39.84%	48.61%	7.17%

Alpha-Stim treatment course

# Reported	Treated With			Completed Satisfactory	Still Receiving	Discontinued treatment because:			
	Earclips	Probes	Electrodes			Not Efficacious	Side Effects	Insurance ran out	Other
266	247	1	1	136	106	3	0	7	8
	92.86%	0.38%	0.38%	51.13%	39.85%	1.13%	0.00%	2.63%	3.01%

Average residual relief received with a single Alpha-Stim treatment

	# Reported	None	Hours			Days				Never Returned
			<1	1 - 8	9 - 23	1	2	3 - 6	7+	
Pain	1	0	0	1	0	0	0	0	0	0
		0.00%	0.00%	100.00%	0.00%	0.00%	0.00%	0.00%	0.00%	0.00%
Anxiety	10	0	1	2	0	4	0	0	2	1
		0.00%	10.00%	20.00%	0.00%	40.00%	0.00%	0.00%	20.00%	10.00%

Medication use:					Other concomitant therapy received with Alpha-Stim						
In-creased	No Change	Re-duced	Elimi-nated	# Reported	None	Psycho-therapy	Chiro-practic	Acu-puncture	Bio-feedback	Physical Therapy	Other
0	3	2	7	238	94	58	29	12	25	13	26
0.00%	25.00%	16.67%	58.33%		39.50%	24.37%	12.18%	5.04%	10.50%	5.46%	10.92%

Eliminated use of these drugs: Ambien (1), Xanax (2), anti-depressants (2), NSAIDs (1)

Reduced use of these drugs: analgesics (1), NSAIDs (1)

Increased use of this drug:

Side effects reported with use of Alpha-Stim:
253 (94.76%) "None" reported   Specify: better concentration (1), calming effect (1), dizziness (2), heavy feeling (1), marked decrease in food consumption of compulsive overeater (1), metallic taste (1), skin irritation (1)

Doctor's evaluation of Alpha-Stim

# Reported	Efficacious	Safe	Reasonably Well Tolerated
254	241	228	157
	94.88%	89.76%	61.81%

Doctor's evaluation of Alpha-Stim ('98 survey only)

# Reported	Would Use Alpha-Stim Again	Most Efficacious for this Diagnosis	Other
8	7	1	0
	87.50%	12.50%	0.00%

Quality of life ('98 survey only)

Lose of Work		Return to Work		Work Comp		Improve Family Life		Improve Social Life		Overall QOL		Rx by:						
YES	NO	YES	NO	YES	NO	YES	NO	YES	NO	YES	NO	MD/DO	PhD	DDS	DC	PT	Other	Not Specified
3	5	4	2	1	3	5	3	6	2	7	1	7	1	61	1	0	2	0
38%	63%	67%	33%	25%	75%	63%	38%	75%	25%	88%	13%							

SUMMARY FOR PAIN & OTHER DIAGNOSTIC CATEGORIES

233 total N   74 male (age range 14-87, mean 43)   5 inpatients

                            159 female (age range 11-92, mean 46)   198 outpatients

Treatment(s) used prior to Alpha-Stim:

ECT	116 physical therapy	31 sedative-hypnotics
44 psychotherapy	36 surgery	1 psychostimulants
19 behavior modification	20 other non-drug	22 major tranquilizers
53 milliampere TENS	2 alcohol	43 analgesics
27 chiropractic	23 anxiolitics	116 NSAIDs
25 nerve blocks	87 anti-depressants	95 muscle relaxants
11 biofeedback	63 narcotics	40 other drugs

Reason(s) for discontinuing prior treatment:

26 still using	5 exacerbated	10 negative drug effects	1 moved
85 not efficacious	3 too expensive	8 uses Alpha-Stim	22 other

Side effects of prior treatment:

41 none	18 felt drugged	11 sedation
10 pain	6 drug sensitivity/allergy	12 GI discomfort
1 addiction	7 mental cloudiness	14 other

Treatment results obtained by using Alpha-Stim

Chief Complaints	# Reported	Worse (neg)	None (no change)	Slight (<24%)	Fair (25 - 49%)	Moderate (50 - 74%)	Marked (75 - 99%)	Complete (100%)	Significant Improvement (>25%)
Pain	197	1	5	17	31	51	72	20	174
		0.51%	2.54%	8.63%	15.74%	25.89%	36.55%	10.15%	88.32%
Anxiety	143	0	7	11	17	30	70	8	125
		0.00%	4.90%	7.69%	11.89%	20.98%	48.95%	5.59%	87.41%
Depression	82	0	8	8	17	13	27	9	66
		0.00%	9.76%	9.76%	20.73%	15.85%	32.93%	10.98%	80.49%
Stress	118	0	6	8	17	29	55	3	104
		0.00%	5.08%	6.78%	14.41%	24.58%	46.61%	2.54%	88.14%
Insomnia	65	0	13	10	10	14	15	3	42
		0.00%	20.00%	15.38%	15.38%	21.54%	23.08%	4.62%	64.62%
Headache	96	1	6	6	20	19	34	10	83
		1.04%	6.25%	6.25%	20.83%	19.79%	35.42%	10.42%	86.46%
Muscle Tension	172	2	6	5	25	57	69	8	159
		1.16%	3.49%	2.91%	14.53%	33.14%	40.12%	4.65%	92.44%

Treatment results obtained prior to use of Alpha-Stim

Prior Treatments	214	14	59	65	38	20	18	0	76
		6.54%	27.57%	30.37%	17.76%	9.35%	8.41%	0.00%	35.51%

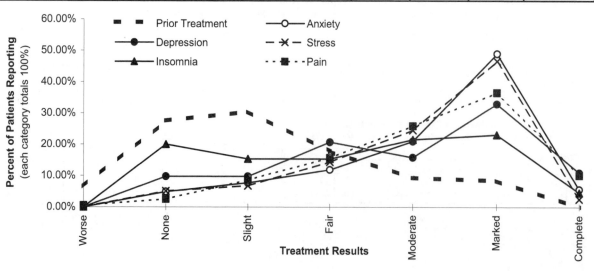

SUMMARY FOR PAIN & OTHER DIAGNOSTIC CATEGORIES

# Reported	\#1	2	3 - 5	6 - 10	11 - 15	16 - 20	21+	Ongoing	Doctor's Office	Patient's Home
	Number of Alpha-Stim treatments								**Received in:**	
149	15	18	30	30	11	7	20	18	108	70
	10.07%	12.08%	20.13%	20.13%	7.38%	4.70%	13.42%	12.08%	60.67%	39.33%

Alpha-Stim settings used

# Reported	Intensity (µA)						Frequency (Hz)			Time (minutes/treatment)			
	100	200	300	400	500	600	0.5	1.5	100	0 - 10	11 - 20	21 - 60	>60
210	23	64	20	12	27	60	187	25	8	26	50	51	8
	11%	30%	10%	6%	13%	29%	89.05%	11.90%	3.81%	19.26%	37.04%	37.78%	5.93%

Alpha-Stim treatment course

# Reported	Treated With			Completed Satisfactory	Still Receiving	Discontinued treatment because:				
	Earclips	Probes	Electrodes			Not Efficacious	Side Effects	Insurance ran out	Other	
216	174	105	82	61	121	9	3	6	12	
	80.56%	48.61%	37.96%	28.24%	56.02%	4.17%	1.39%	2.78%	5.56%	

Average residual relief received with a single Alpha-Stim treatment

	# Reported	None	Hours				Days				Never Returned
			<1	1 - 8	9 - 23	1	2	3 - 6	7+		
Pain	149	18	2	38	9	16	14	32	12	9	
		12.08%	1.34%	25.50%	6.04%	10.74%	9.40%	21.48%	8.05%	6.04%	
Anxiety	96	7	1	16	0	24	5	26	11	6	
		7.29%	1.04%	16.67%	0.00%	25.00%	5.21%	27.08%	11.46%	6.25%	

Medication use:					Other concomitant therapy received with Alpha-Stim						
In-creased	No Change	Re-duced	Elimi-nated	# Reported	None	Psycho-therapy	Chiro-practic	Acu-puncture	Bio-feedback	Physical Therapy	Other
1	58	62	18	189	48	8	34	23	9	45	31
0.72%	41.73%	44.60%	12.95%		25.40%	4.23%	17.99%	12.17%	4.76%	23.81%	16.40%

Eliminated use of these drugs: Acetaminophen (1), Advil (3), Amitriptyline (1), Aspirin (3), Excedrin (1), Flexeril (1), Lidocaine (1), Lorcet (1), Paxil (2), Tylenol (1), analgesics (5), anti-convulsants (1), anti-depressants (1), NSAIDs (4), muscle relaxants (1), narcotics (3)

Reduced use of these drugs: Ambion (1), Amitriptyline (2), Baclofen (1), DHE (1), Demerol (1), Depakote (1), Excedrin (1), Flexeril (2), Ibuprofen (4), Imitrex (3), Inderal (1), Methadone (1), Motrin (2), Naproxin (2), Neurontin (1), Nicotine (1), Oxycontin (1), Percocet (3), Prozac (1), Soma (2), Trazodone (1), Tylenol (2), Tylenol #3 (3), Ultram (2), Valium (2), Vicodin (1), Xanax (1), analgesics (3), anti-depressants (3), barbiturates (1), muscle relaxants (8), narcotics (4), NSAIDS (3), sedatives (2)

Increased use of this drug: Zoloft (1)

Side effects reported with use of Alpha-Stim:

219 (93.99%) "None" reported   Specify: anger (1), dizziness (4), nausea (2), ringing in ears (1), skin irritation (2)

Doctor's evaluation of Alpha-Stim

# Reported	Efficacious	Safe	Reasonably Well Tolerated
196	169	174	110
	86.22%	88.78%	56.12%

Doctor's evaluation of Alpha-Stim ('98 survey only)

# Reported	Would Use Alpha-Stim Again	Most Efficacious for this Diagnosis	Other
125	84	64	11
	67.20%	51.20%	8.80%

Quality of life ('98 survey only)

Lose of Work		Return to Work		Work Comp		Improve Family Life		Improve Social Life		Overall QOL		Rx by:						
YES	NO	YES	NO	YES	NO	YES	NO	YES	NO	YES	NO	MD/DO	PhD	DDS	DC	PT	Other	Not Specified
71	74	28	54	11	28	102	31	96	31	124	23	89	3	9	21	3	7	0
49%	51%	34%	66%	28%	72%	77%	23%	76%	24%	84%	16%							

SURVEY RESULTS FOR
PSYCHIATRIC AND PSYCHOLOGICAL INDICATIONS

Summary for Diagnostic Category: ANXIETY

97 total N   40 male (age range 5-62, mean 40)   0 inpatients
                  57 female (age range 12-78, mean 43)   82 outpatients

Treatment(s) used prior to Alpha-Stim:

2 ECT	10 physical therapy	7 sedative-hypnotics
37 psychotherapy	7 surgery	2 psychostimulants
16 behavior modification	20 other non-drug	12 major tranquilizers
3 milliampere TENS	11 alcohol	5 analgesics
6 chiropractic	14 anxiolitics	9 NSAIDs
2 nerve blocks	32 anti-depressants	7 muscle relaxants
3 biofeedback	13 narcotics	10 other drugs

Reason(s) for discontinuing prior treatment:

11 still using	2 exacerbated	5 negative drug effects	0 moved
23 not efficacious	4 too expensive	0 uses Alpha-Stim	10 other

Side effects of prior treatment:

21 none	3 felt drugged	6 sedation
1 pain	1 drug sensitivity/allergy	2 GI discomfort
3 addiction	4 mental cloudiness	6 other

Treatment results obtained by using Alpha-Stim

Chief Complaints	# Reported	Worse (neg)	None (no change)	Slight (<24%)	Fair (25 - 49%)	Moderate (50 - 74%)	Marked (75 - 99%)	Complete (100%)	Significant Improvement (>25%)
Pain	33	0 0.00%	0 0.00%	2 6.06%	6 18.18%	12 36.36%	12 36.36%	1 3.03%	31 93.94%
Anxiety	88	0 0.00%	0 0.00%	2 2.27%	10 11.36%	19 21.59%	53 60.23%	4 4.55%	86 97.73%
Depression	53	0 0.00%	0 0.00%	1 1.89%	8 15.09%	9 16.98%	34 64.15%	1 1.89%	52 98.11%
Stress	58	0 0.00%	0 0.00%	1 1.72%	10 17.24%	12 20.69%	33 56.90%	2 3.45%	57 98.28%
Insomnia	25	0 0.00%	2 8.00%	1 4.00%	5 20.00%	4 16.00%	9 36.00%	4 16.00%	22 88.00%
Headache	25	0 0.00%	0 0.00%	0 0.00%	3 12.00%	7 28.00%	13 52.00%	2 8.00%	25 100.00%
Muscle Tension	43	0 0.00%	1 2.33%	1 2.33%	9 20.93%	11 25.58%	19 44.19%	2 4.65%	41 95.35%

Treatment results obtained prior to use of Alpha-Stim

Prior Treatment	71	7 9.86%	12 16.90%	26 36.62%	11 15.49%	13 18.31%	2 2.82%	0 0.00%	26 36.62%

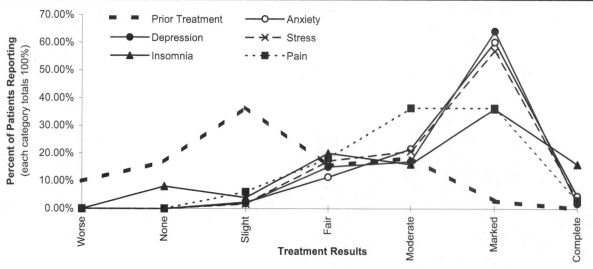

Summary for Diagnostic Category: ANXIETY

Number of Alpha-Stim treatments

# Reported	1	2	3 - 5	6 - 10	11 - 15	16 - 20	21+	Ongoing	Received in: Doctor's Office	Patient's Home
77	3	4	9	15	7	4	20	15	10	4
	3.90%	5.19%	11.69%	19.48%	9.09%	5.19%	25.97%	19.48%	71.43%	28.57%

Alpha-Stim settings used

# Reported	Intensity (µA) 100	200	300	400	500	600	Frequency (Hz) 0.5	1.5	100	Time (minutes/treatment) 0 - 10	11 - 20	21 - 60	>60
95	10	18	30	25	32	7	87	5	4	6	30	47	1
	11%	19%	32%	26%	34%	7%	91.58%	5.26%	4.21%	7.14%	35.71%	55.95%	1.19%

Alpha-Stim treatment course

# Reported	Treated With Earclips	Probes	Electrodes	Completed Satisfactory	Still Receiving	Discontinued treatment because: Not Efficacious	Side Effects	Insurance ran out	Other
95	92	5	3	43	44	3	0	2	3
	96.84%	5.26%	3.16%	45.26%	46.32%	3.16%	0.00%	2.11%	3.16%

Average residual relief received with a single Alpha-Stim treatment

	# Reported	None	Hours <1	1 - 8	9 - 23	Days 1	2	3 - 6	7+	Never Returned
Pain	7	0	0	2	0	3	1	0	0	1
		0.00%	0.00%	28.57%	0.00%	42.86%	14.29%	0.00%	0.00%	14.29%
Anxiety	15	0	0	2	0	7	1	2	3	0
		0.00%	0.00%	13.33%	0.00%	46.67%	6.67%	13.33%	20.00%	0.00%

Medication use / Other concomitant therapy received with Alpha-Stim

Medication use: Increased	No Change	Reduced	Eliminated	# Reported	None	Psycho-therapy	Chiro-practic	Acu-puncture	Bio-feedback	Physical Therapy	Other
0	7	3	3	86	18	32	12	5	6	8	14
0.00%	53.85%	23.08%	23.08%		20.93%	37.21%	13.95%	5.81%	6.98%	9.30%	16.28%

Eliminated use of these drugs: Anti-depressant (1), Anti-Convulsant (1), Narcotic (1), Lorcet (1), Amitriptyline (1), Paxil (1), Xanax (1).

Reduced use of these drugs: Floricet (1), Corcet (1), Soma (1), Valium (1), Sleeping Medications (1), Neurontin (1).

Increased use of this drug:

Side effects reported with use of Alpha-Stim

92 (94.85%) "None" reported   Specify: heavy feeling (1), metalic taste (1), little dizzy (1).

Doctor's evaluation of Alpha-Stim

# Reported	Efficacious	Safe	Reasonably Well Tolerated
94	86	85	39
	91.49%	90.43%	41.49%

Doctor's evaluation of Alpha-Stim ('98 survey only)

# Reported	Would Use Alpha-Stim Again	Most Efficacious for this Diagnosis	Other
10	10	1	0
	100.00%	10.00%	0.00%

Quality of life ('98 survey only)

Lose of Work YES	NO	Return to Work YES	NO	Work Comp YES	NO	Improve Family Life YES	NO	Improve Social Life YES	NO	Overall QOL YES	NO	Rx by: MD/ DO	PhD	DDS	DC	PT	Other	Not Specified
5	7	2	4	2	3	8	3	9	2	10	2	11	1	0	0	0	2	0
42%	58%	33%	67%	40%	60%	73%	27%	82%	18%	83%	17%							

Summary for Diagnostic Category: DENTAL ANXIETY

61 total N   19 male (age range 10-61, mean 38)   0 inpatients

                          42 female (age range 10-84, mean 42)   61 outpatients

Treatment(s) used prior to Alpha-Stim:

ECT	physical therapy	sedative-hypnotics
psychotherapy	surgery	psychostimulants
behavior modification	other non-drug	major tranquilizers
milliampere TENS	alcohol	analgesics
chiropractic	1 anxiolitics	NSAIDs
nerve blocks	1 anti-depressants	muscle relaxants
biofeedback	narcotics	1 other drugs

Reason(s) for discontinuing prior treatment:

still using	exacerbated	negative drug effects	moved
not efficacious	too expensive	uses Alpha-Stim	other

Side effects of prior treatment:

none	felt drugged	sedation
pain	drug sensitivity/allergy	GI discomfort
addiction	mental cloudiness	other

Treatment results obtained by using Alpha-Stim

Chief Complaints	# Reported	Worse (neg)	None (no change)	Slight (<24%)	Fair (25 - 49%)	Moderate (50 - 74%)	Marked (75 - 99%)	Complete (100%)	Significant Improvement (>25%)
Pain	0								
Anxiety	39	0 0.00%	0 0.00%	0 0.00%	4 10.26%	18 46.15%	17 43.59%	0 0.00%	39 100.00%
Depression	0								
Stress	34	0 0.00%	0 0.00%	1 2.94%	7 20.59%	15 44.12%	11 32.35%	0 0.00%	33 97.06%
Insomnia	0								
Headache	0								
Muscle Tension	10	0 0.00%	0 0.00%	0 0.00%	1 10.00%	1 10.00%	8 80.00%	0 0.00%	10 100.00%
Treatment results obtained prior to use of Alpha-Stim									
Prior Treatment	3	0 0.00%	0 0.00%	0 0.00%	1 33.33%	2 66.67%	0 0.00%	0 0.00%	3 100.00%

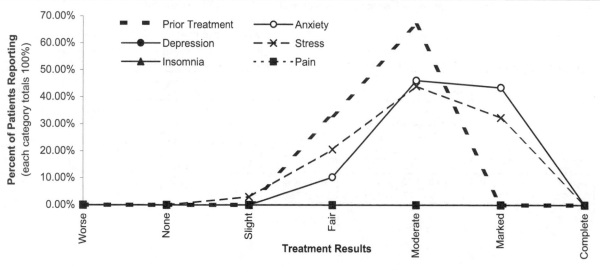

Summary for Diagnostic Category: DENTAL ANXIETY

Number of Alpha-Stim treatments

# Reported	1	2	3 - 5	6 - 10	11 - 15	16 - 20	21+	Ongoing	Received in: Doctor's Office	Received in: Patient's Home
57	32	16	9						61	
	56.14%	28.07%	15.79%	0.00%	0.00%	0.00%	0.00%	0.00%	100.00%	0.00%

Alpha-Stim settings used

# Reported	Intensity (µA)						Frequency (Hz)			Time (minutes/treatment)			
	100	200	300	400	500	600	0.5	1.5	100	0 - 10	11 - 20	21 - 60	>60
61	59	1					61					44	17
	97%	2%	0%	0%	0%	0%	100.00%	0.00%	0.00%	0.00%	0.00%	72.13%	27.87%

Alpha-Stim treatment course

# Reported	Treated With Earclips	Probes	Electrodes	Completed Satisfactory	Still Receiving	Discontinued treatment because: Not Efficacious	Side Effects	Insurance ran out	Other
61	61			57					
	100.00%	0.00%	0.00%	93.44%	0.00%	0.00%	0.00%	0.00%	0.00%

Average residual relief received with a single Alpha-Stim treatment

	# Reported	None	Hours <1	1 - 8	9 - 23	Days 1	2	3 - 6	7+	Never Returned
Pain										
Anxiety	1		1							
		0.00%	100.00%	0.00%	0.00%	0.00%	0.00%	0.00%	0.00%	0.00%

Medication use / Other concomitant therapy received with Alpha-Stim

Medication use: In-creased	No Change	Re-duced	Elimi-nated	# Reported	None	Psycho-therapy	Chiro-practic	Acu-puncture	Bio-feedback	Physical Therapy	Other
			1	58	58						
0.00%	0.00%	0.00%	100.00%		100.00%	0.00%	0.00%	0.00%	0.00%	0.00%	0.00%

Eliminated use of these drugs:

Reduced use of these drugs:

Increased use of this drug:

Side effects reported with use of Alpha-Stim

59 (96.72%) "None" reported   Specify:

Doctor's evaluation of Alpha-Stim

# Reported	Efficacious	Safe	Reasonably Well Tolerated
59	56	59	59
	94.92%	100.00%	100.00%

Doctor's evaluation of Alpha-Stim ('98 survey only)

# Reported	Would Use Alpha-Stim Again	Most Efficacious for this Diagnosis	Other
1	1		
	100.00%	0.00%	0.00%

Quality of life ('98 survey only)

Lose of Work YES	NO	Return to Work YES	NO	Work Comp YES	NO	Improve Family Life YES	NO	Improve Social Life YES	NO	Overall QOL YES	NO	Rx by: MD/ DO	PhD	DDS	DC	PT	Other	Not Specified
	1	1												61				
0%	100%	100%	0%															

Summary for Diagnostic Category: DEPRESSION

69 total N   20 male (age range 16-67, mean 42)   5 inpatients

49 female (age range 14-85, mean 44)   54 outpatients

Treatment(s) used prior to Alpha-Stim:

16 ECT	28 physical therapy	18 sedative-hypnotics
34 psychotherapy	14 surgery	3 psychostimulants
9 behavior modification	3 other non-drug	11 major tranquilizers
13 milliampere TENS	11 alcohol	10 analgesics
8 chiropractic	16 anxiolitics	31 NSAIDs
9 nerve blocks	44 anti-depressants	22 muscle relaxants
5 biofeedback	28 narcotics	1 other drugs

Reason(s) for discontinuing prior treatment:

7 still using	2 exacerbated	2 negative drug effects	moved
31 not efficacious	5 too expensive	uses Alpha-Stim	2 other

Side effects of prior treatment:

10 none	6 felt drugged	1 sedation
2 pain	4 drug sensitivity/allergy	2 GI discomfort
2 addiction	1 mental cloudiness	6 other

Treatment results obtained by using Alpha-Stim

Chief Complaints	# Reported	Worse (neg)	None (no change)	Slight (<24%)	Fair (25 - 49%)	Moderate (50 - 74%)	Marked (75 - 99%)	Complete (100%)	Significant Improvement (>25%)
Pain	49	0 0.00%	1 2.04%	4 8.16%	6 12.24%	14 28.57%	22 44.90%	2 4.08%	44 89.80%
Anxiety	57	0 0.00%	2 3.51%	1 1.75%	8 14.04%	15 26.32%	30 52.63%	1 1.75%	54 94.74%
Depression	61	0 0.00%	1 1.64%	3 4.92%	6 9.84%	16 26.23%	30 49.18%	5 8.20%	57 93.44%
Stress	46	0 0.00%	2 4.35%	0 0.00%	2 4.35%	15 32.61%	26 56.52%	1 2.17%	44 95.65%
Insomnia	30	0 0.00%	3 10.00%	4 13.33%	2 6.67%	10 33.33%	9 30.00%	2 6.67%	23 76.67%
Headache	30	1 3.33%	0 0.00%	1 3.33%	3 10.00%	5 16.67%	15 50.00%	5 16.67%	28 93.33%
Muscle Tension	43	0 0.00%	2 4.65%	1 2.33%	7 16.28%	17 39.53%	15 34.88%	1 2.33%	40 93.02%

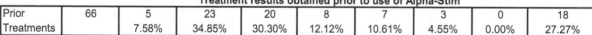

Treatment results obtained prior to use of Alpha-Stim

Prior Treatments	66	5 7.58%	23 34.85%	20 30.30%	8 12.12%	7 10.61%	3 4.55%	0 0.00%	18 27.27%

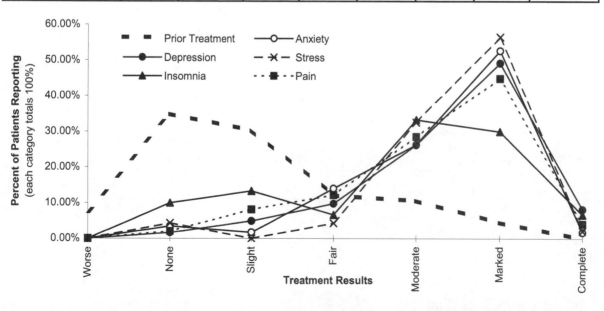

Summary for Diagnostic Category: DEPRESSION

Number of Alpha-Stim treatments

# Reported	1	2	3 - 5	6 - 10	11 - 15	16 - 20	21+	Ongoing	Received in: Doctor's Office	Received in: Patient's Home
50	1	2	11	10	6	1	4	11	27	17
	2.00%	4.00%	22.00%	20.00%	12.00%	2.00%	8.00%	22.00%	61.36%	38.64%

Alpha-Stim settings used

# Reported	Intensity (µA) 100	200	300	400	500	600	Frequency (Hz) 0.5	1.5	100	Time (minutes/treatment) 0 - 10	11 - 20	21 - 60	>60
69	11	25	9	9	7	16	68	5	0	5	15	27	3
	16%	36%	13%	13%	10%	23%	98.55%	7.25%	0.00%	10.00%	30.00%	54.00%	6.00%

Alpha-Stim treatment course

# Reported	Treated With Earclips	Probes	Electrodes	Completed Satisfactory	Still Receiving	Discontinued treatment because: Not Efficacious	Side Effects	Insurance ran out	Other
60	43	24	16	17	43	1	0	2	4
	71.67%	40.00%	26.67%	28.33%	71.67%	1.67%	0.00%	3.33%	6.67%

Average residual relief received with a single Alpha-Stim treatment

	# Reported	None	Hours <1	1 - 8	9 - 23	Days 1	2	3 - 6	7+	Never Returned
Pain	29	3	1	6	2	2	3	9	2	1
		10.34%	3.45%	20.69%	6.90%	6.90%	10.34%	31.03%	6.90%	3.45%
Anxiety	27	2	0	6	1	3	2	11	2	1
		7.41%	0.00%	22.22%	3.70%	11.11%	7.41%	40.74%	7.41%	3.70%

Medication use / Other concomitant therapy received with Alpha-Stim

Increased	No Change	Reduced	Eliminated	# Reported	None	Psychotherapy	Chiropractic	Acupuncture	Biofeedback	Physical Therapy	Other
0	17	13	4	63	16	19	8	8	2	16	3
0.00%	50.00%	38.24%	11.76%		25.40%	30.16%	12.70%	12.70%	3.17%	25.40%	4.76%

Eliminated use of these drugs: antidepressants (1), NSAIDs (1)

Reduced use of these drugs: analgesics (1), NSAIDs (4), anti-depressants (1), anxiolitics (1), muscle relaxants (1), narcotics (3), Ambion (1), Imitrex (1), Vicadin HP (1).

Increased use of this drug:

Side effects reported with use of Alpha-Stim:
66 (95.65%) "None" reported   Specify: marked decrease in food consumption of cumpulsive overeater (1), dizziness (1), heavy feeling (1).

Doctor's evaluation of Alpha-Stim

# Reported	Efficacious	Safe	Reasonably Well Tolerated
64	57	58	40
	89.06%	90.63%	62.50%

Doctor's evaluation of Alpha-Stim ('98 survey only)

# Reported	Would Use Alpha-Stim Again	Most Efficacious for this Diagnosis	Other
25	13	16	2
	52.00%	64.00%	8.00%

Quality of life ('98 survey only)

Lose of Work YES	NO	Return to Work YES	NO	Work Comp YES	NO	Improve Family Life YES	NO	Improve Social Life YES	NO	Overall QOL YES	NO	Rx by: MD/DO	PhD	DDS	DC	PT	Other	Not Specified
18	14	3	14	5	11	21	7	20	8	22	7	19						
56%	44%	18%	82%	31%	69%	75%	25%	71%	29%	76%	24%							

Summary for Diagnostic Category: MIXED ANXIETY DEPRESSIVE DISORDER

9 total N   3 male (age range 49-54, mean 51)   0 inpatients

6 female (age range 27-60, mean 44)   9 outpatients

Treatment(s) used prior to Alpha-Stim:

1 ECT	physical therapy	1 sedative-hypnotics
6 psychotherapy	3 surgery	1 psychostimulants
2 behavior modification	2 other non-drug	5 major tranquilizers
milliampere TENS	2 alcohol	analgesics
chiropractic	anxiolitics	1 NSAIDs
nerve blocks	6 anti-depressants	1 muscle relaxants
biofeedback	1 narcotics	4 other drugs

Reason(s) for discontinuing prior treatment:

1 still using	exacerbated	negative drug effects	moved
4 not efficacious	too expensive	uses Alpha-Stim	1 other

Side effects of prior treatment:

none	felt drugged	sedation
pain	drug sensitivity/allergy	GI discomfort
addiction	mental cloudiness	1 other

Treatment results obtained by using Alpha-Stim

Chief Complaints	# Reported	Worse (neg)	None (no change)	Slight (<24%)	Fair (25 - 49%)	Moderate (50 - 74%)	Marked (75 - 99%)	Complete (100%)	Significant Improvement (>25%)
Pain	7	0 0.00%	0 0.00%	0 0.00%	2 28.57%	4 57.14%	1 14.29%	0 0.00%	7 100.00%
Anxiety	8	0 0.00%	0 0.00%	0 0.00%	2 25.00%	2 25.00%	4 50.00%	0 0.00%	8 100.00%
Depression	9	0 0.00%	0 0.00%	0 0.00%	2 22.22%	2 22.22%	5 55.56%	0 0.00%	9 100.00%
Stress	7	0 0.00%	0 0.00%	0 0.00%	2 28.57%	3 42.86%	2 28.57%	0 0.00%	7 100.00%
Insomnia	6	0 0.00%	0 0.00%	0 0.00%	2 33.33%	1 16.67%	3 50.00%	0 0.00%	6 100.00%
Headache	4	0 0.00%	0 0.00%	0 0.00%	1 25.00%	0 0.00%	3 75.00%	0 0.00%	4 100.00%
Muscle Tension	5	0 0.00%	0 0.00%	0 0.00%	2 40.00%	1 20.00%	2 40.00%	0 0.00%	5 100.00%

Treatment results obtained prior to use of Alpha-Stim

Prior Treatments	9	0 0.00%	2 22.22%	3 33.33%	1 11.11%	3 33.33%	0 0.00%	0 0.00%	4 44.44%

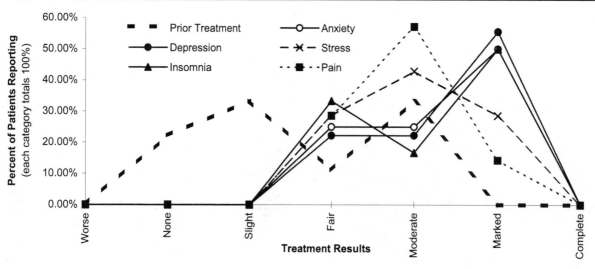

Summary for Diagnostic Category: MIXED ANXIETY DEPRESSIVE DISORDER

Number of Alpha-Stim treatments

# Reported	1	2	3 - 5	6 - 10	11 - 15	16 - 20	21+	Ongoing	Received in: Doctor's Office	Received in: Patient's Home
5	0.00%	0.00%	1 20.00%	1 20.00%	2 40.00%	1 20.00%	0.00%	0.00%		

Alpha-Stim settings used

# Reported	Intensity (µA) 100	200	300	400	500	600	Frequency (Hz) 0.5	1.5	100	Time (minutes/treatment) 0 - 10	11 - 20	21 - 60	>60
9	0%	1 11%	0%	3 33%	3 33%	5 56%	7 77.78%	3 33.33%	1 11.11%	1 12.50%	4 50.00%	3 37.50%	0.00%

Alpha-Stim treatment course

# Reported	Treated With Earclips	Probes	Electrodes	Completed Satisfactory	Still Receiving	Discontinued treatment because: Not Efficacious	Side Effects	Insurance ran out	Other
9	9 100.00%	0.00%	0.00%	0.00%	7 77.78%	0.00%	0.00%	2 22.22%	0.00%

Average residual relief received with a single Alpha-Stim treatment

	# Reported	None	Hours <1	1 - 8	9 - 23	Days 1	2	3 - 6	7+	Never Returned
Pain										
Anxiety										

Medication use / Other concomitant therapy received with Alpha-Stim

Increased	No Change	Reduced	Eliminated	# Reported	None	Psychotherapy	Chiropractic	Acupuncture	Biofeedback	Physical Therapy	Other
				7	0.00%	4 57.14%	2 28.57%	1 14.29%	0.00%	0.00%	1 14.29%

Eliminated use of these drugs:

Reduced use of these drugs:

Increased use of this drug:

Side effects reported with use of Alpha-Stim:

7 (77.78%) "None" reported   Specify: calming effect (1), better concentration (1)

Doctor's evaluation of Alpha-Stim

# Reported	Efficacious	Safe	Reasonably Well Tolerated
9	8 88.89%	9 100.00%	4 44.44%

Doctor's evaluation of Alpha-Stim ('98 survey only)

# Reported	Would Use Alpha-Stim Again	Most Efficacious for this Diagnosis	Other

Quality of life ('98 Survey Only)

Lose of Work YES	NO	Return to Work YES	NO	Work Comp YES	NO	Improve Family Life YES	NO	Improve Social Life YES	NO	Overall QOL YES	NO	Rx by: MD/DO	PhD	DDS	DC	PT	Other	Not Specified

Summary for Diagnostic Category: STRESS

40 total N

12 male (age range 5-52, mean 36)   1 inpatients

28 female (age range 28-52, mean 41)   29 outpatients

Treatment(s) used prior to Alpha-Stim:

1 ECT	4 physical therapy	1 sedative-hypnotics
8 psychotherapy	1 surgery	2 psychostimulants
8 behavior modification	9 other non-drug	5 major tranquilizers
1 milliampere TENS	10 alcohol	1 analgesics
7 chiropractic	4 anxiolitics	4 NSAIDs
nerve blocks	4 anti-depressants	3 muscle relaxants
biofeedback	6 narcotics	4 other drugs

Reason(s) for discontinuing prior treatment:

7 still using	2 exacerbated	1 negative drug effects	1 moved
14 not efficacious	4 too expensive	uses Alpha-Stim	3 other

Side effects of prior treatment:

13 none	3 felt drugged	sedation
pain	drug sensitivity/allergy	GI discomfort
2 addiction	mental cloudiness	5 other

Treatment results obtained by using Alpha-Stim

Chief Complaints	# Reported	Worse (neg)	None (no change)	Slight (<24%)	Fair (25 - 49%)	Moderate (50 - 74%)	Marked (75 - 99%)	Complete (100%)	Significant Improvement (>25%)
Pain	22	0 0.00%	0 0.00%	0 0.00%	3 13.64%	5 22.73%	11 50.00%	3 13.64%	22 100.00%
Anxiety	28	0 0.00%	0 0.00%	1 3.57%	2 7.14%	7 25.00%	16 57.14%	2 7.14%	27 96.43%
Depression	11	0 0.00%	0 0.00%	0 0.00%	1 9.09%	4 36.36%	6 54.55%	0 0.00%	11 100.00%
Stress	24	0 0.00%	0 0.00%	0 0.00%	2 8.33%	3 12.50%	17 70.83%	2 8.33%	24 100.00%
Insomnia	11	0 0.00%	0 0.00%	0 0.00%	1 9.09%	5 45.45%	5 45.45%	0 0.00%	11 100.00%
Headache	8	0 0.00%	0 0.00%	0 0.00%	1 12.50%	3 37.50%	2 25.00%	2 25.00%	8 100.00%
Muscle Tension	16	0 0.00%	0 0.00%	0 0.00%	3 18.75%	2 12.50%	10 62.50%	1 6.25%	16 100.00%

Treatment results obtained prior to use of Alpha-Stim

Prior Treatments	35	4 11.43%	7 20.00%	7 20.00%	6 17.14%	8 22.86%	3 8.57%	0 0.00%	17 48.57%

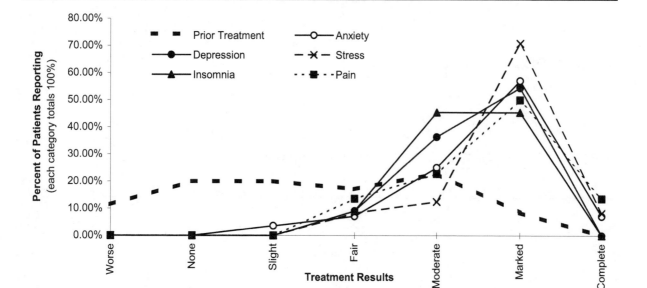

Summary for Diagnostic Category: STRESS

Number of Alpha-Stim treatments

# Reported	1	2	3 - 5	6 - 10	11 - 15	16 - 20	21+	Ongoing	Received in: Doctor's Office	Patient's Home
34	5	0	5	3	3	4	8	6	3	3
	14.71%	0.00%	14.71%	8.82%	8.82%	11.76%	23.53%	17.65%	50.00%	50.00%

Alpha-Stim settings used

# Reported	Intensity (µA)						Frequency (Hz)			Time (minutes/treatment)			
	100	200	300	400	500	600	0.5	1.5	100	0 - 10	11 - 20	21 - 60	>60
38	3	10	10	3	19	1	38	4	2	2	30	8	0
	8%	26%	26%	8%	50%	3%	100.00%	10.53%	5.26%	5.00%	75.00%	20.00%	0.00%

Alpha-Stim treatment course

# Reported	Treated With			Completed Satisfactory	Still Receiving	Discontinued treatment because:				
	Earclips	Probes	Electrodes			Not Efficacious	Side Effects	Insurance ran out	Other	
40	39	0	1	16	22	1	0	0	2	
	97.50%	0.00%	2.50%	40.00%	55.00%	2.50%	0.00%	0.00%	5.00%	

Average residual relief received with a single Alpha-Stim treatment

	# Reported	None	Hours			Days				Never Returned
			<1	1 - 8	9 - 23	1	2	3 - 6	7+	
Pain	1	0.00%	1 100.00%	0.00%	0.00%	0.00%	0.00%	0.00%	0.00%	0.00%
Anxiety	2	0.00%	0.00%	1 50.00%	0.00%	0.00%	0.00%	0.00%	0.00%	1 50.00%

Medication use / Other concomitant therapy received with Alpha-Stim

In-creased	No Change	Re-duced	Elimi-nated	# Reported	None	Psycho-therapy	Chiro-practic	Acu-puncture	Bio-feedback	Physical Therapy	Other
0	1	2	1	35	13	1	14	4	2	2	10
					37.14%	2.86%	40.00%	11.43%	5.71%	5.71%	28.57%

Eliminated use of these drugs: Paxic (1)

Reduced use of these drugs:

Increased use of this drug:

Side effects reported with use of Alpha-Stim:

36 (90.00%) "None" reported   Specify: better concentration (1), calming effect (1),
skin irritation "nothing serious" (1), heavy feeling (1), metalic taste (1).

Doctor's evaluation of Alpha-Stim

# Reported	Efficacious	Safe	Reasonably Well Tolerated
38	33	34	18
	86.84%	89.47%	47.37%

Doctor's evaluation of Alpha-Stim ('98 survey only)

# Reported	Would Use Alpha-Stim Again	Most Efficacious for this Diagnosis	Other
2	2	0	0

Quality of life ('98 survey only)

Lose of Work		Return to Work		Work Comp		Improve Family Life		Improve Social Life		Overall QOL		Rx by:					
YES	NO	YES	NO	YES	NO	YES	NO	YES	NO	YES	NO	MD/ DO	PhD	DDS	DC	PT	Other	Not Specified
	2				1	1	1	1	1	3		2						
0%	100%			0%	100%	50%	50%	50%	50%	100%	0%						

Summary for Diagnostic Category: MOOD DISORDER DUE TO MEDICAL CONDITION

60 total N

19 male (age range 23-66, mean 45)   2 inpatients

41 female (age range 14-85, mean 44)   54 outpatients

Treatment(s) used prior to Alpha-Stim:

1 ECT	4 physical therapy	6 sedative-hypnotics
15 psychotherapy	7 surgery	2 psychostimulants
8 behavior modification	6 other non-drug	7 major tranquilizers
2 milliampere TENS	6 alcohol	6 analgesics
5 chiropractic	16 anxiolitics	5 NSAIDs
1 nerve blocks	20 anti-depressants	7 muscle relaxants
1 biofeedback	7 narcotics	13 other drugs

Reason(s) for discontinuing prior treatment:

2 still using	1 exacerbated	6 negative drug effects	moved
22 not efficacious	1 too expensive	uses Alpha-Stim	3 other

Side effects of prior treatment:

5 none	1 felt drugged	6 sedation
pain	1 drug sensitivity/allergy	2 GI discomfort
2 addiction	3 mental cloudiness	4 other

Treatment results obtained by using Alpha-Stim

Chief Complaints	# Reported	Worse (neg)	None (no change)	Slight (<24%)	Fair (25 - 49%)	Moderate (50 - 74%)	Marked (75 - 99%)	Complete (100%)	Significant Improvement (>25%)
Pain	40	0	0	2	7	13	17	1	38
		0.00%	0.00%	5.00%	17.50%	32.50%	42.50%	2.50%	95.00%
Anxiety	56	0	0	1	6	15	33	1	55
		0.00%	0.00%	1.79%	10.71%	26.79%	58.93%	1.79%	98.21%
Depression	26	0	0	1	5	8	12	0	25
		0.00%	0.00%	3.85%	19.23%	30.77%	46.15%	0.00%	96.15%
Stress	26	0	0	2	0	11	12	1	24
		0.00%	0.00%	7.69%	0.00%	42.31%	46.15%	3.85%	92.31%
Insomnia	23	0	1	0	4	8	9	1	22
		0.00%	4.35%	0.00%	17.39%	34.78%	39.13%	4.35%	95.65%
Headache	16	0	1	0	2	5	7	1	15
		0.00%	6.25%	0.00%	12.50%	31.25%	43.75%	6.25%	93.75%
Muscle Tension	24	0	0	1	6	6	10	1	23
		0.00%	0.00%	4.17%	25.00%	25.00%	41.67%	4.17%	95.83%

Treatment results obtained prior to use of Alpha-Stim

Prior Treatments	50	1	11	20	12	3	3	0	18
		2.00%	22.00%	40.00%	24.00%	6.00%	6.00%	0.00%	36.00%

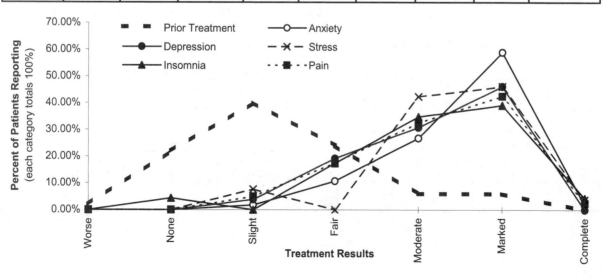

Summary for Diagnostic Category: MOOD DISORDER DUE TO MEDICAL CONDITION

Number of Alpha-Stim treatments

# Reported	1	2	3 - 5	6 - 10	11 - 15	16 - 20	21+	Ongoing	Received in: Doctor's Office	Patient's Home
49	2	3	7	10	4	7	13	3	2	5
	4.08%	6.12%	14.29%	20.41%	8.16%	14.29%	26.53%	6.12%	28.57%	71.43%

Alpha-Stim settings used

# Reported	Intensity (µA) 100	200	300	400	500	600	Frequency (Hz) 0.5	1.5	100	Time (minutes/treatment) 0 - 10	11 - 20	21 - 60	>60
58	11	19	13	7	8	4	53	5	1		34	20	
	19%	33%	22%	12%	14%	7%	91.38%	8.62%	1.72%	0.00%	62.96%	37.04%	0.00%

Alpha-Stim treatment course

# Reported	Treated With Earclips	Probes	Electrodes	Completed Satisfactory	Still Receiving	Discontinued treatment because: Not Efficacious	Side Effects	Insurance ran out	Other
60	58	1	1	14	39			1	3
	96.67%	1.67%	1.67%	23.33%	65.00%	0.00%	0.00%	1.67%	5.00%

Average residual relief received with a single Alpha-Stim treatment

	# Reported	None	<1	Hours 1 - 8	9 - 23	1	Days 2	3 - 6	7+	Never Returned
Pain	2	1				1				
		50.00%	0.00%	0.00%	0.00%	50.00%	0.00%	0.00%	0.00%	0.00%
Anxiety	5					4	1			
		0.00%	0.00%	0.00%	0.00%	80.00%	20.00%	0.00%	0.00%	0.00%

Medication use / Other concomitant therapy received with Alpha-Stim

In- creased	No Change	Re- duced	Elimi- nated	# Reported	None	Psycho- therapy	Chiro- practic	Acu- puncture	Bio- feedback	Physical Therapy	Other
	2		1	51	9	4	8	1	17	7	10
0.00%	66.67%	0.00%	33.33%		17.65%	7.84%	15.69%	1.96%	33.33%	13.73%	19.61%

Eliminated use of these drugs: anti-depressants (1)

Reduced use of these drugs:

Increased use of this drug:

Side effects reported with use of Alpha-Stim:
56 (93.33%) "None" reported   Specify: metalic taste (1)

Doctor's evaluation of Alpha-Stim

# Reported	Efficacious	Safe	Reasonably Well Tolerated
57	49	47	44
	85.96%	82.46%	77.19%

Doctor's evaluation of Alpha-Stim ('98 survey only)

# Reported	Would Use Alpha-Stim Again	Most Efficacious for this Diagnosis	Other
4	4	1	
	100.00%	25.00%	0.00%

Quality of life ('98 survey only)

Lose of Work YES	NO	Return to Work YES	NO	Work Comp YES	NO	Improve Family Life YES	NO	Improve Social Life YES	NO	Overall QOL YES	NO	Rx by: MD/ DO	PhD	DDS	DC	PT	Other	Not Specified
2	1		1		1	4		4		4		4						
67%	33%	0%	100%	0%	100%	100%	0%	100%	0%	100%	0%							

Summary for Diagnostic Category: INSOMNIA DUE TO MEDICAL CONDITION

26 total N

4 male (age range 40-55, mean 46)   0 inpatients
22 female (age range 26-86, mean 44)   23 outpatients

Treatment(s) used prior to Alpha-Stim:

ECT	4 physical therapy	5 sedative-hypnotics
6 psychotherapy	1 surgery	1 psychostimulants
5 behavior modification	6 other non-drug	1 major tranquilizers
2 milliampere TENS	4 alcohol	2 analgesics
6 chiropractic	3 anxiolitics	4 NSAIDs
nerve blocks	8 anti-depressants	4 muscle relaxants
1 biofeedback	3 narcotics	7 other drugs

Reason(s) for discontinuing prior treatment:

5 still using	exacerbated	3 negative drug effects	moved
6 not efficacious	too expensive	1 uses Alpha-Stim	1 other

Side effects of prior treatment:

9 none	2 felt drugged	sedation
pain	1 drug sensitivity/allergy	1 GI discomfort
addiction	mental cloudiness	3 other

Treatment results obtained by using Alpha-Stim

Chief Complaints	# Reported	Worse (neg)	None (no change)	Slight (<24%)	Fair (25 - 49%)	Moderate (50 - 74%)	Marked (75 - 99%)	Complete (100%)	Significant Improvement (>25%)
Pain	19	0	0	0	3	3	12	1	19
		0.00%	0.00%	0.00%	15.79%	15.79%	63.16%	5.26%	100.00%
Anxiety	16	0	0	0	1	3	11	1	16
		0.00%	0.00%	0.00%	6.25%	18.75%	68.75%	6.25%	100.00%
Depression	10	0	0	0	1	1	8	0	10
		0.00%	0.00%	0.00%	10.00%	10.00%	80.00%	0.00%	100.00%
Stress	12	0	0	0	0	6	4	2	12
		0.00%	0.00%	0.00%	0.00%	50.00%	33.33%	16.67%	100.00%
Insomnia	25	0	1	0	4	1	14	5	24
		0.00%	4.00%	0.00%	16.00%	4.00%	56.00%	20.00%	96.00%
Headache	9	0	0	0	0	1	6	2	9
		0.00%	0.00%	0.00%	0.00%	11.11%	66.67%	22.22%	100.00%
Muscle Tension	11	0	0	0	3	1	5	2	11
		0.00%	0.00%	0.00%	27.27%	9.09%	45.45%	18.18%	100.00%

Treatment results obtained prior to use of Alpha-Stim

Prior Treatments	25	0	3	10	6	5	1	0	12
		0.00%	12.00%	40.00%	24.00%	20.00%	4.00%	0.00%	48.00%

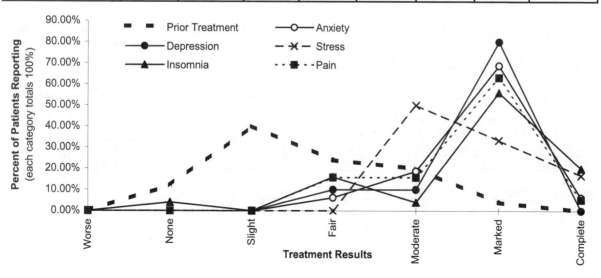

Summary for Diagnostic Category: INSOMNIA DUE TO MEDICAL CONDITION

Number of Alpha-Stim treatments

# Reported	1	2	3 - 5	6 - 10	11 - 15	16 - 20	21+	Ongoing	Received in: Doctor's Office	Patient's Home
22	1		4	2	3	3	3	6		1
	4.55%	0.00%	18.18%	9.09%	13.64%	13.64%	13.64%	27.27%	0.00%	100.00%

Alpha-Stim settings used

# Reported	Intensity (µA) 100	200	300	400	500	600	Frequency (Hz) 0.5	1.5	100	Time (minutes/treatment) 0 - 10	11 - 20	21 - 60	>60
25	1	9	8	1	5		24	2		1	17	5	
	4%	36%	32%	4%	20%	0%	96.00%	8.00%	0.00%	4.35%	73.91%	21.74%	0.00%

Alpha-Stim treatment course

# Reported	Treated With Earclips	Probes	Electrodes	Completed Satisfactory	Still Receiving	Discontinued treatment because: Not Efficacious	Side Effects	Insurance ran out	Other
26	26			5	21				
	100.00%	0.00%	0.00%	19.23%	80.77%	0.00%	0.00%	0.00%	0.00%

Average residual relief received with a single Alpha-Stim treatment

	# Reported	None	<1	Hours 1 - 8	9 - 23	1	Days 2	3 - 6	7+	Never Returned
Pain										
Anxiety	1									1
		0.00%	0.00%	0.00%	0.00%	0.00%	0.00%	0.00%	0.00%	100.00%

Medication use / Other concomitant therapy received with Alpha-Stim

In- creased	No Change	Re- duced	Elimi- nated	# Reported	None	Psycho- therapy	Chiro- practic	Acu- puncture	Bio- feedback	Physical Therapy	Other
			1	26	3		5	3	7	4	10
0.00%	0.00%	0.00%	100.00%		11.54%	0.00%	19.23%	11.54%	26.92%	15.38%	38.46%

Eliminated use of these drugs: Ambien (1), Xanax (1)

Reduced use of these drugs:

Increased use of this drug:

Side effects reported with use of Alpha-Stim:

25 (96.15%) "None" reported   Specify: heavy feeling (1)

Doctor's evaluation of Alpha-Stim

# Reported	Efficacious	Safe	Reasonably Well Tolerated
24	22	20	19
	91.67%	83.33%	79.17%

Doctor's evaluation of Alpha-Stim ('98 survey only)

# Reported	Would Use Alpha-Stim Again	Most Efficacious for this Diagnosis	Other
1		1	
	0.00%	100.00%	0.00%

Quality of life ('98 survey only)

Lose of Work YES	NO	Return to Work YES	NO	Work Comp YES	NO	Improve Family Life YES	NO	Improve Social Life YES	NO	Overall QOL YES	NO	Rx by: MD/ DO	PhD	DDS	DC	PT	Other	Not Specified
1		1				1		1		2		1			1			
100%	0%	100%	0%			100%	0%	100%	0%	100%	0%							

Summary for Diagnostic Category: SUBSTANCE ABUSE

28 total N   17 male (age range 22-50, mean 35)   13 inpatients
             11 female (age range 21-49, mean 34)   14 outpatients

Treatment(s) used prior to Alpha-Stim:

ECT	1 physical therapy	5 sedative-hypnotics
19 psychotherapy	2 surgery	3 psychostimulants
11 behavior modification	1 other non-drug	5 major tranquilizers
milliampere TENS	11 alcohol	1 analgesics
chiropractic	4 anxiolitics	NSAIDs
nerve blocks	8 anti-depressants	muscle relaxants
1 biofeedback	6 narcotics	10 other drugs

Reason(s) for discontinuing prior treatment:

1 still using	4 exacerbated	negative drug effects	moved
9 not efficacious	too expensive	uses Alpha-Stim	3 other

Side effects of prior treatment:

none	felt drugged	sedation
pain	1 drug sensitivity/allergy	1 GI discomfort
1 addiction	mental cloudiness	6 other

Treatment results obtained by using Alpha-Stim

Chief Complaints	# Reported	Worse (neg)	None (no change)	Slight (<24%)	Fair (25 - 49%)	Moderate (50 - 74%)	Marked (75 - 99%)	Complete (100%)	Significant Improvement (>25%)
Pain	12	0 0.00%	0 0.00%	1 8.33%	2 16.67%	2 16.67%	6 50.00%	1 8.33%	11 91.67%
Anxiety	23	0 0.00%	1 4.35%	0 0.00%	4 17.39%	6 26.09%	9 39.13%	3 13.04%	22 95.65%
Depression	19	0 0.00%	0 0.00%	1 5.26%	4 21.05%	6 31.58%	7 36.84%	1 5.26%	18 94.74%
Stress	18	0 0.00%	0 0.00%	2 11.11%	3 16.67%	5 27.78%	6 33.33%	2 11.11%	16 88.89%
Insomnia	11	0 0.00%	1 9.09%	0 0.00%	1 9.09%	2 18.18%	4 36.36%	3 27.27%	10 90.91%
Headache	8	0 0.00%	1 12.50%	0 0.00%	0 0.00%	2 25.00%	5 62.50%	0 0.00%	7 87.50%
Muscle Tension	12	0 0.00%	0 0.00%	1 8.33%	1 8.33%	3 25.00%	5 41.67%	2 16.67%	11 91.67%
Treatment results obtained prior to use of Alpha-Stim									
Prior Treatments	25	5 20.00%	11 44.00%	4 16.00%	4 16.00%	1 4.00%	0 0.00%	0 0.00%	5 20.00%

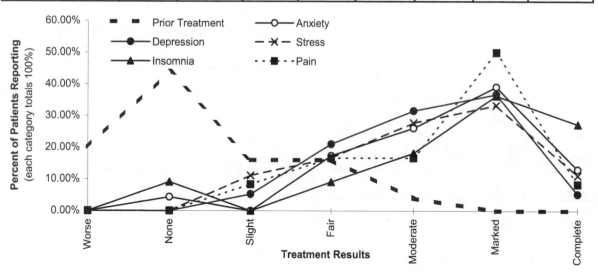

Summary for Diagnostic Category: SUBSTANCE ABUSE

Number of Alpha-Stim treatments

# Reported	1	2	3 - 5	6 - 10	11 - 15	16 - 20	21+	Ongoing	Received in: Doctor's Office	Patient's Home
24	0.00%	0.00%	5 20.83%	5 20.83%	3 12.50%	5 20.83%	7 29.17%	1 4.17%		

Alpha-Stim settings used

# Reported	Intensity (µA) 100	200	300	400	500	600	Frequency (Hz) 0.5	1.5	100	Time (minutes/treatment) 0 - 10	11 - 20	21 - 60	>60
28	7 25%	9 32%	15 54%	9 32%	15 54%	10 36%	28 100.00%	0.00%	0.00%	0.00%	10 37.04%	17 62.96%	0.00%

Alpha-Stim treatment course

# Reported	Treated With Earclips	Probes	Electrodes	Completed Satisfactory	Still Receiving	Discontinued treatment because: Not Efficacious	Side Effects	Insurance ran out	Other
28	28 100.00%	0.00%	0.00%	13 46.43%	8 28.57%	0.00%	0.00%	0.00%	4 14.29%

Average residual relief received with a single Alpha-Stim treatment

	# Reported	None	<1	Hours 1 - 8	9 - 23	1	Days 2	3 - 6	7+	Never Returned
Pain										
Anxiety										

Medication use / Other concomitant therapy received with Alpha-Stim

In- creased	No Change	Re- duced	Elimi- nated	# Reported	None	Psycho- therapy	Chiro- practic	Acu- puncture	Bio- feedback	Physical Therapy	Other
				25	1 4.00%	15 60.00%	4 16.00%	2 8.00%	2 8.00%	1 4.00%	6 24.00%

Eliminated use of these drugs:

Reduced use of these drugs:

Increased use of this drug:

Side effects reported with use of Alpha-Stim:

24 (85.71%) "None" reported   Specify: Dizziness - first two treatments (1)

Doctor's evaluation of Alpha-Stim

# Reported	Efficacious	Safe	Reasonably Well Tolerated
28	26 92.86%	23 82.14%	18 64.29%

Doctor's evaluation of Alpha-Stim ('98 survey only)

# Reported	Would Use Alpha-Stim Again	Most Efficacious for this Diagnosis	Other

Quality of life ('98 survey only)

Lose of Work YES	NO	Return to Work YES	NO	Work Comp YES	NO	Improve Family Life YES	NO	Improve Social Life YES	NO	Overall QOL YES	NO	Rx by: MD/ DO	PhD	DDS	DC	PT	Other	Not Specified

Summary for Diagnostic Category: POST TRAUMATIC STRESS DISORDER

5 total N

3 male (age range 47, mean 47)
2 female

0 inpatients
5 outpatients

Treatment(s) used prior to Alpha-Stim:

ECT	physical therapy	sedative-hypnotics
1 psychotherapy	1 surgery	psychostimulants
behavior modification	1 other non-drug	2 major tranquilizers
milliampere TENS	alcohol	analgesics
chiropractic	3 anxiolitics	3 NSAIDs
nerve blocks	3 anti-depressants	1 muscle relaxants
biofeedback	2 narcotics	2 other drugs

Reason(s) for discontinuing prior treatment:

still using	exacerbated	negative drug effects	moved
2 not efficacious	too expensive	uses Alpha-Stim	other

Side effects of prior treatment:

none	felt drugged	sedation
pain	drug sensitivity/allergy	GI discomfort
addiction	mental cloudiness	other

Treatment results obtained by using Alpha-Stim

Chief Complaints	# Reported	Worse (neg)	None (no change)	Slight (<24%)	Fair (25 - 49%)	Moderate (50 - 74%)	Marked (75 - 99%)	Complete (100%)	Significant Improvement (>25%)
Pain	1	0	0	0	0	1	0	0	1
		0.00%	0.00%	0.00%	0.00%	100.00%	0.00%	0.00%	100.00%
Anxiety	5	0	0	0	0	2	3	0	5
		0.00%	0.00%	0.00%	0.00%	40.00%	60.00%	0.00%	100.00%
Depression	4	0	0	0	1	3	0	0	4
		0.00%	0.00%	0.00%	25.00%	75.00%	0.00%	0.00%	100.00%
Stress	5	0	0	0	1	3	1	0	5
		0.00%	0.00%	0.00%	20.00%	60.00%	20.00%	0.00%	100.00%
Insomnia	1	0	0	0	0	1	0	0	1
		0.00%	0.00%	0.00%	0.00%	100.00%	0.00%	0.00%	100.00%
Headache	2	0	0	0	0	2	0	0	2
		0.00%	0.00%	0.00%	0.00%	100.00%	0.00%	0.00%	100.00%
Muscle Tension	2	0	0	0	0	2	0	0	2
		0.00%	0.00%	0.00%	0.00%	100.00%	0.00%	0.00%	100.00%

Treatment results obtained prior to use of Alpha-Stim

Prior Treatments	4	0	2	1	1	0	0	0	1
		0.00%	50.00%	25.00%	25.00%	0.00%	0.00%	0.00%	25.00%

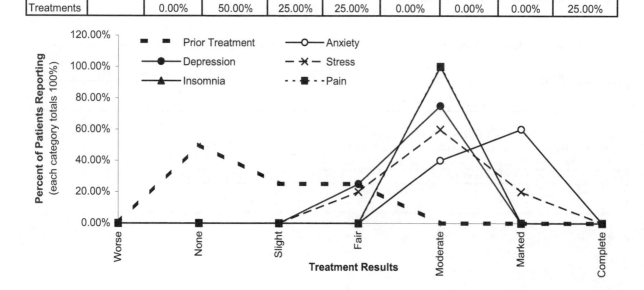

Summary for Diagnostic Category: POST TRAUMATIC STRESS DISORDER

Number of Alpha-Stim treatments

# Reported	1	2	3 - 5	6 - 10	11 - 15	16 - 20	21+	Ongoing	Received in: Doctor's Office	Patient's Home
5	0.00%	0.00%	0.00%	2 40.00%	0.00%	0.00%	1 20.00%	1 20.00%	0.00%	1 100.00%

Alpha-Stim settings used

# Reported	Intensity (µA) 100	200	300	400	500	600	Frequency (Hz) 0.5	1.5	100	Time (minutes/treatment) 0 - 10	11 - 20	21 - 60	>60
5	0%	1 20%	1 20%	3 60%	0%	1 20%	5 100.00%	0.00%	0.00%	0.00%	2 50.00%	2 50.00%	0.00%

Alpha-Stim treatment course

# Reported	Treated With Earclips	Probes	Electrodes	Completed Satisfactory	Still Receiving	Discontinued treatment because: Not Efficacious	Side Effects	Insurance ran ou	Other
4	4 100.00%	0.00%	0.00%	0.00%	4 100.00%	0.00%	0.00%	1 25.00%	0.00%

Average residual relief received with a single Alpha-Stim treatment

	# Reported	None	Hours <1	1 - 8	9 - 23	1	Days 2	3 - 6	7+	Never Returned
Pain	1	0.00%	0.00%	0.00%	0.00%	0.00%	0.00%	1 100.00%	0.00%	0.00%
Anxiety	1	0.00%	0.00%	0.00%	0.00%	0.00%	0.00%	1 100.00%	0.00%	0.00%

Medication use: / Other concomitant therapy received with Alpha-Stim

Increased	No Change	Reduced	Eliminated	# Reported	None	Psycho- therapy	Chiro- practic	Acu- puncture	Bio- feedback	Physical Therapy	Other
	1			5	0.00%	2 40.00%	0.00%	0.00%	2 40.00%	0.00%	1 20.00%

Eliminated use of these drugs:

Reduced use of these drugs:

Increased use of this drug:

Side effects reported with use of Alpha-Stim:
5 (100.00%) "None" reported   Specify:

Doctor's evaluation of Alpha-Stim

# Reported	Efficacious	Safe	Reasonably Well Tolerated
5	5 100.00%	5 100.00%	4 80.00%

Doctor's evaluation of Alpha-Stim ('98 survey only)

# Reported	Would Use Alpha-Stim Again	Most Efficacious for this Diagnosis	Other
1	0.00%	1 100.00%	0.00%

Quality of life ('98 survey only)

Lose of Work YES	NO	Return to Work YES	NO	Work Comp YES	NO	Improve Family Life YES	NO	Improve Social Life YES	NO	Overall QOL YES	NO	Rx by: MD/ DO	PhD	DDS	DC	PT	Other	Not Specified
0%	1 100%					0%	1 100%	0%	1 100%	0%	1 100%							

Summary for Diagnostic Category: ATTENTION DEFICIT DISORDER

2 total N   0 male   0 inpatients
                         2 female (age range 9-38, mean 24)   2 outpatients

Treatment(s) used prior to Alpha-Stim:

ECT	physical therapy	sedative-hypnotics
1 psychotherapy	surgery	psychostimulants
1 behavior modification	other non-drug	major tranquilizers
milliampere TENS	alcohol	analgesics
chiropractic	anxiolitics	NSAIDs
nerve blocks	anti-depressants	muscle relaxants
biofeedback	narcotics	other drugs

Reason(s) for discontinuing prior treatment:

still using	exacerbated	negative drug effects	moved
not efficacious	too expensive	uses Alpha-Stim	other

Side effects of prior treatment:

none	felt drugged	sedation
pain	drug sensitivity/allergy	GI discomfort
addiction	mental cloudiness	other

Treatment results obtained by using Alpha-Stim

Chief Complaints	# Reported	Worse (neg)	None (no change)	Slight (<24%)	Fair (25 - 49%)	Moderate (50 - 74%)	Marked (75 - 99%)	Complete (100%)	Significant Improvement (>25%)
Pain									
Anxiety	1					1			1
		0.00%	0.00%	0.00%	0.00%	100.00%	0.00%	0.00%	100.00%
Depression	1				1				1
		0.00%	0.00%	0.00%	100.00%	0.00%	0.00%	0.00%	100.00%
Stress	1				1				1
		0.00%	0.00%	0.00%	100.00%	0.00%	0.00%	0.00%	100.00%
Insomnia									
Headache									
Muscle Tension									

Treatment results obtained prior to use of Alpha-Stim

Prior Treatments	1	0	0	0	1	0	0	0	1
		0.00%	0.00%	0.00%	100.00%	0.00%	0.00%	0.00%	100.00%

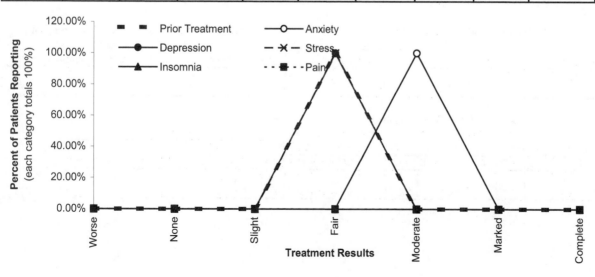

Summary for Diagnostic Category: ATTENTION DEFICIT DISORDER

Number of Alpha-Stim treatments

# Reported	1	2	3 - 5	6 - 10	11 - 15	16 - 20	21+	Ongoing	Received in: Doctor's Office	Received in: Patient's Home
2	0.00%	0.00%	1 50.00%	0.00%	0.00%	1 50.00%	0.00%	0.00%		

Alpha-Stim settings used

# Reported	Intensity (µA) 100	200	300	400	500	600	Frequency (Hz) 0.5	1.5	100	Time (minutes/treatment) 0 - 10	11 - 20	21 - 60	>60
2	0%	0%	2 100%	1 50%	0%	0%	2 100.00%	0.00%	0.00%	0.00%	2 100.00%	0.00%	0.00%

Alpha-Stim treatment course

# Reported	Treated With Earclips	Probes	Electrodes	Completed Satisfactory	Still Receiving	Discontinued treatment because: Not Efficacious	Side Effects	Insurance ran out	Other
2	1 50.00%	0.00%	0.00%	0.00%	2 100.00%	0.00%	0.00%	0.00%	0.00%

Average residual relief received with a single Alpha-Stim treatment

	# Reported	None	<1	Hours 1 - 8	9 - 23	1	2	Days 3 - 6	7+	Never Returned
Pain										
Anxiety										

Medication use / Other concomitant therapy received with Alpha-Stim

In- creased	No Change	Re- duced	Elimi- nated	# Reported	None	Psycho- therapy	Chiro- practic	Acu- puncture	Bio- feedback	Physical Therapy	Other
				1	0.00%	1 100.00%	0.00%	0.00%	0.00%	0.00%	0.00%

Eliminated use of these drugs:

Reduced use of these drugs:

Increased use of this drug:

Side effects reported with use of Alpha-Stim:

2 (100.00%) "None" reported   Specify:

Doctor's evaluation of Alpha-Stim

# Reported	Efficacious	Safe	Reasonably Well Tolerated
1	1 100.00%	1 100.00%	0.00%

Doctor's evaluation of Alpha-Stim ('98 survey only)

# Reported	Would Use Alpha-Stim Again	Most Efficacious for this Diagnosis	Other

Quality of life ('98 survey only)

Lose of Work YES	NO	Return to Work YES	NO	Work Comp YES	NO	Improve Family Life YES	NO	Improve Social Life YES	NO	Overall QOL YES	NO	Rx by: MD/ DO	PhD	DDS	DC	PT	Other	Not Specified

Survey Results for Pain and Other Indications

Summary for Diagnostic Category: BACK PAIN

62 total N   27 male (age range 24-87, mean 45)   0 inpatients
                          35 female (age range 27-92, mean 48)   56 outpatients

Treatment(s) used prior to Alpha-Stim:

ECT	38 physical therapy	11 sedative-hypnotics
10 psychotherapy	10 surgery	psychostimulants
6 behavior modification	8 other non-drug	5 major tranquilizers
20 milliampere TENS	alcohol	12 analgesics
16 chiropractic	7 anxiolitics	35 NSAIDs
12 nerve blocks	18 anti-depressants	32 muscle relaxants
3 biofeedback	24 narcotics	20 other drugs

Reason(s) for discontinuing prior treatment:

11 still using	2 exacerbated	1 negative drug effects	moved
20 not efficacious	3 too expensive	uses Alpha-Stim	5 other

Side effects of prior treatment:

16 none	6 felt drugged	5 sedation
2 pain	drug sensitivity/allergy	7 GI discomfort
addiction	mental cloudiness	4 other

Treatment results obtained by using Alpha-Stim

Chief Complaints	# Reported	Worse (neg)	None (no change)	Slight (<24%)	Fair (25 - 49%)	Moderate (50 - 74%)	Marked (75 - 99%)	Complete (100%)	Significant Improvement (>25%)
Pain	59	0	1	3	9	21	18	7	55
		0.00%	1.69%	5.08%	15.25%	35.59%	30.51%	11.86%	93.22%
Anxiety	41	0	1	4	3	7	25	1	36
		0.00%	2.44%	9.76%	7.32%	17.07%	60.98%	2.44%	87.80%
Depression	22	0	0	2	5	5	7	3	20
		0.00%	0.00%	9.09%	22.73%	22.73%	31.82%	13.64%	90.91%
Stress	39	0	0	3	3	11	21	1	36
		0.00%	0.00%	7.69%	7.69%	28.21%	53.85%	2.56%	92.31%
Insomnia	18	0	3	2	3	4	5	1	13
		0.00%	16.67%	11.11%	16.67%	22.22%	27.78%	5.56%	72.22%
Headache	15	0	1	1	5	2	2	4	13
		0.00%	6.67%	6.67%	33.33%	13.33%	13.33%	26.67%	86.67%
Muscle Tension	49	0	1	2	7	15	21	3	46
		0.00%	2.04%	4.08%	14.29%	30.61%	42.86%	6.12%	93.88%
Treatment results obtained prior to use of Alpha-Stim									
Prior Treatments	58	3	17	15	16	7	0	0	23
		5.17%	29.31%	25.86%	27.59%	12.07%	0.00%	0.00%	39.66%

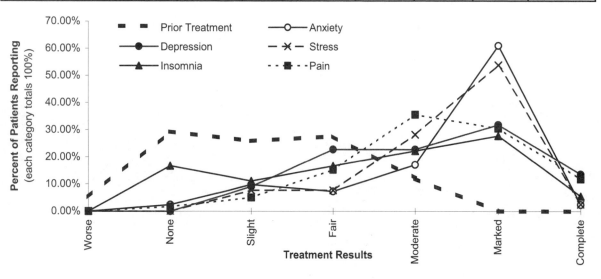

Summary for Diagnostic Category: BACK PAIN

Number of Alpha-Stim treatments

# Reported	1	2	3 - 5	6 - 10	11 - 15	16 - 20	21+	Ongoing	Received in: Doctor's Office	Received in: Patient's Home
45	1	4	8	12	1	2	11	6	40	29
	2.22%	8.89%	17.78%	26.67%	2.22%	4.44%	24.44%	13.33%	57.97%	42.03%

Alpha-Stim settings used

# Reported	Intensity (µA) 100	200	300	400	500	600	Frequency (Hz) 0.5	1.5	100	Time (minutes/treatment) 0 - 10	11 - 20	21 - 60	>60
61	6	18	5	1	6	24	51	7	5	11	10	14	4
	10%	30%	8%	2%	10%	39%	83.61%	11.48%	8.20%	28.21%	25.64%	35.90%	10.26%

Alpha-Stim treatment course

# Reported	Treated With Earclips	Probes	Electrodes	Completed Satisfactory	Still Receiving	Discontinued treatment because: Not Efficacious	Side Effects	Insurance ran out	Other
55	36	33	28	13	40	3		2	2
	65.45%	60.00%	50.91%	23.64%	72.73%	5.45%	0.00%	3.64%	3.64%

Average residual relief received with a single Alpha-Stim treatment

	# Reported	None	Hours <1	1 - 8	9 - 23	Days 1	2	3 - 6	7+	Never Returned
Pain	49	4	1	11	3	7	5	11	4	3
		8.16%	2.04%	22.45%	6.12%	14.29%	10.20%	22.45%	8.16%	6.12%
Anxiety	28	1		3		7	2	9	3	3
		3.57%	0.00%	10.71%	0.00%	25.00%	7.14%	32.14%	10.71%	10.71%

Medication use / Other concomitant therapy received with Alpha-Stim

In-creased	No Change	Re-duced	Elimi-nated	# Reported	None	Psycho-therapy	Chiro-practic	Acu-puncture	Bio-feedback	Physical Therapy	Other
	18	20	7	55	13	4	15	4	3	3	19
0.00%	40.00%	44.44%	15.56%		23.64%	7.27%	27.27%	7.27%	5.45%	5.45%	34.55%

Eliminated use of these drugs: Paxil (1), Lorcet (1), Aspirin (1), muscle relaxants (1), narcotics (1), NSAIDs (1), Relafin (1), pain killers (1)

Reduced use of these drugs: Tylenol (2), Motrin (1), Ibuprofen (2), Ambien (1), barbiturates (1), Excedrin (1), Oxycontin (1), Percocet (2), Nicotine (1), Tylenol #3 (3), Ultram (1), Demerol (1), NSAIDS (1), analgesics (2), narcotics (2), Neurontin (1), Badofin (1), Soma (1), Methadone (1), Vicadin HP (1)

Increased use of this drug:

Side effects reported with use of Alpha-Stim:

54 (87.10%) "None" reported   Specify: Dizziness (1), metalic taste (1), heavy feeling (1)

Doctor's evaluation of Alpha-Stim

# Reported	Efficacious	Safe	Reasonably Well Tolerated
58	48	49	31
	82.76%	84.48%	53.45%

Doctor's evaluation of Alpha-Stim ('98 survey only)

# Reported	Would Use Alpha-Stim Again	Most Efficacious for this Diagnosis	Other
37	26	17	2
	70.27%	45.95%	5.41%

Quality of life ('98 survey only)

Lose of Work YES	NO	Return to Work YES	NO	Work Comp YES	NO	Improve Family Life YES	NO	Improve Social Life YES	NO	Overall QOL YES	NO	Rx by: MD/DO	PhD	DDS	DC	PT	Other	Not Specified
25	15	8	21	4	4	32	7	28	8	42	5	28		1	15		3	
63%	38%	28%	72%	50%	50%	82%	18%	78%	22%	89%	11%							

Summary for Diagnostic Category: JOINT PAIN

48 total N   16 male (age range 15-68, mean 41)   1 inpatients

32 female (age range 19-76, mean 49)   44 outpatients

Treatment(s) used prior to Alpha-Stim:

ECT	32 physical therapy	4 sedative-hypnotics
5 psychotherapy	11 surgery	1 psychostimulants
4 behavior modification	3 other non-drug	3 major tranquilizers
10 milliampere TENS	alcohol	11 analgesics
1 chiropractic	2 anxiolitics	22 NSAIDs
2 nerve blocks	12 anti-depressants	14 muscle relaxants
2 biofeedback	13 narcotics	5 other drugs

Reason(s) for discontinuing prior treatment:

5 still using	exacerbated	2 negative drug effects	1 moved
20 not efficacious	too expensive	3 uses Alpha-Stim	5 other

Side effects of prior treatment:

5 none	4 felt drugged	2 sedation
1 pain	4 drug sensitivity/allergy	3 GI discomfort
addiction	mental cloudiness	2 other

Treatment results obtained by using Alpha-Stim

Chief Complaints	# Reported	Worse (neg)	None (no change)	Slight (<24%)	Fair (25 - 49%)	Moderate (50 - 74%)	Marked (75 - 99%)	Complete (100%)	Significant Improvement (>25%)
Pain	42	0	2	4	3	10	12	11	36
		0.00%	4.76%	9.52%	7.14%	23.81%	28.57%	26.19%	85.71%
Anxiety	29	0	1	2	4	4	14	4	26
		0.00%	3.45%	6.90%	13.79%	13.79%	48.28%	13.79%	89.66%
Depression	17	0	1	2	3	3	7	1	14
		0.00%	5.88%	11.76%	17.65%	17.65%	41.18%	5.88%	82.35%
Stress	19	0	1	1	3	4	10	0	17
		0.00%	5.26%	5.26%	15.79%	21.05%	52.63%	0.00%	89.47%
Insomnia	13	0	4	1	1	3	2	2	8
		0.00%	30.77%	7.69%	7.69%	23.08%	15.38%	15.38%	61.54%
Headache	8	0	1	1	1	0	2	3	6
		0.00%	12.50%	12.50%	12.50%	0.00%	25.00%	37.50%	75.00%
Muscle Tension	33	0	3	0	3	15	8	4	30
		0.00%	9.09%	0.00%	9.09%	45.45%	24.24%	12.12%	90.91%

Treatment results obtained prior to use of Alpha-Stim

Prior Treatments	45	1	11	14	6	4	9	0	19
		2.22%	24.44%	31.11%	13.33%	8.89%	20.00%	0.00%	42.22%

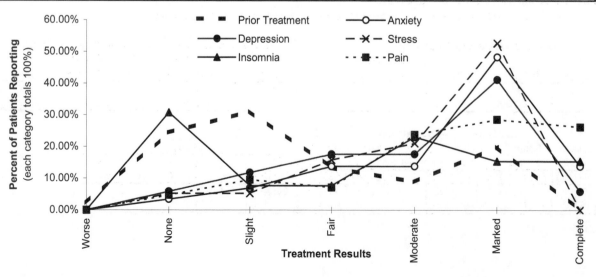

Summary for Diagnostic Category: JOINT PAIN

Number of Alpha-Stim treatments

# Reported	1	2	3 - 5	6 - 10	11 - 15	16 - 20	21+	Ongoing	Received in: Doctor's Office	Patient's Home
24	5	2	7	4	1	2	3		9	7
	20.83%	8.33%	29.17%	16.67%	4.17%	8.33%	12.50%	0.00%	56.25%	43.75%

Alpha-Stim settings used

# Reported	Intensity (µA) 100	200	300	400	500	600	Frequency (Hz) 0.5	1.5	100	Time (minutes/treatment) 0 - 10	11 - 20	21 - 60	>60
34	5	5	5	3	4	11	32	1	1	2	11	12	
	15%	15%	15%	9%	12%	32%	94.12%	2.94%	2.94%	8.00%	44.00%	48.00%	0.00%

Alpha-Stim treatment course

# Reported	Treated With Earclips	Probes	Electrodes	Completed Satisfactory	Still Receiving	Discontinued treatment because: Not Efficacious	Side Effects	Insurance ran out	Other
33	21	21	16	12	13	2			4
	63.64%	63.64%	48.48%	36.36%	39.39%	6.06%	0.00%	0.00%	12.12%

Average residual relief received with a single Alpha-Stim treatment

	# Reported	Hours None	<1	1 - 8	9 - 23	Days 1	2	3 - 6	7+	Never Returned
Pain	24	4		5	3	4	2	3	2	2
		16.67%	0.00%	20.83%	12.50%	16.67%	8.33%	12.50%	8.33%	8.33%
Anxiety	15	2		1		6	1	3	1	1
		13.33%	0.00%	6.67%	0.00%	40.00%	6.67%	20.00%	6.67%	6.67%

Medication use / Other concomitant therapy received with Alpha-Stim

In-creased	No Change	Re-duced	Elimi-nated	# Reported	None	Psycho-therapy	Chiro-practic	Acu-puncture	Bio-feedback	Physical Therapy	Other
	9	7		30	2		3	3	1	6	6
0.00%	56.25%	43.75%	0.00%		6.67%	0.00%	10.00%	10.00%	3.33%	20.00%	20.00%

Eliminated use of these drugs: Advil (3), Tylenol, (1), Aspirin (1), analgesics (3), NSAIDs (1), Lidocaine (1), Relafin (1)

Reduced use of these drugs: Ibuprofen (1), Neurontin (1), Badofin (1), Soma (1), Methadone (1)

Increased use of this drug:

Side effects reported with use of Alpha-Stim:

47 (97.92%) "None" reported   Specify: Dizziness (1)

Doctor's Evaluation of Alpha-Stim

# Reported	Efficacious	Safe	Reasonably Well Tolerated
44	32	33	23
	72.73%	75.00%	52.27%

Doctor's evaluation of Alpha-Stim ('98 survey only)

# Reported	Would Use Alpha-Stim Again	Most Efficacious for this Diagnosis	Other
31	23	16	2
	74.19%	51.61%	6.45%

Quality of life ('98 survey only)

Lose of Work YES	NO	Return to Work YES	NO	Work Comp YES	NO	Improve Family Life YES	NO	Improve Social Life YES	NO	Overall QOL YES	NO	Rx by: MD/ DO	PhD	DDS	DC	PT	Other	Not Specified
12	21	5	10	3	9	22	5	21	4	26	1	15		1	3	2		
36%	64%	33%	67%	25%	75%	81%	19%	84%	16%	96%	4%							

Summary for Diagnostic Category: CERVICAL PAIN

38 total N

13 male (age range 34-57, mean 44)
25 female (age range 15-74, mean 44)

1 inpatients
32 outpatients

Treatment(s) used prior to Alpha-Stim:

ECT
11 psychotherapy
4 behavior modification
12 milliampere TENS
10 chiropractic
5 nerve blocks
1 biofeedback

19 physical therapy
10 surgery
7 other non-drug
1 alcohol
5 anxiolitics
18 anti-depressants
10 narcotics

8 sedative-hypnotics
psychostimulants
3 major tranquilizers
12 analgesics
22 NSAIDs
17 muscle relaxants
13 other drugs

Reason(s) for discontinuing prior treatment:

3 still using
21 not efficacious

2 exacerbated
2 too expensive

1 negative drug effects
2 uses Alpha-Stim

moved
5 other

Side effects of prior treatment:

7 none
3 pain
addiction

2 felt drugged
1 drug sensitivity/allergy
1 mental cloudiness

3 sedation
6 GI discomfort
5 other

Treatment results obtained by using Alpha-Stim

Chief Complaints	# Reported	Worse (neg)	None (no change)	Slight (<24%)	Fair (25 - 49%)	Moderate (50 - 74%)	Marked (75 - 99%)	Complete (100%)	Significant Improvement (>25%)
Pain	36	0 0.00%	0 0.00%	2 5.56%	6 16.67%	10 27.78%	16 44.44%	2 5.56%	34 94.44%
Anxiety	25	0 0.00%	1 4.00%	2 8.00%	1 4.00%	8 32.00%	10 40.00%	3 12.00%	22 88.00%
Depression	17	0 0.00%	1 5.88%	0 0.00%	2 11.76%	4 23.53%	7 41.18%	3 17.65%	16 94.12%
Stress	22	0 0.00%	1 4.55%	0 0.00%	3 13.64%	8 36.36%	8 36.36%	2 9.09%	21 95.45%
Insomnia	13	0 0.00%	2 15.38%	3 23.08%	2 15.38%	3 23.08%	2 15.38%	1 7.69%	8 61.54%
Headache	22	0 0.00%	1 4.55%	1 4.55%	5 22.73%	3 13.64%	8 36.36%	4 18.18%	20 90.91%
Muscle Tension	30	0 0.00%	0 0.00%	1 3.33%	5 16.67%	12 40.00%	9 30.00%	3 10.00%	29 96.67%
Treatment results obtained prior to use of Alpha-Stim									
Prior Treatments	37	2 5.41%	10 27.03%	11 29.73%	6 16.22%	8 21.62%	0 0.00%	0 0.00%	14 37.84%

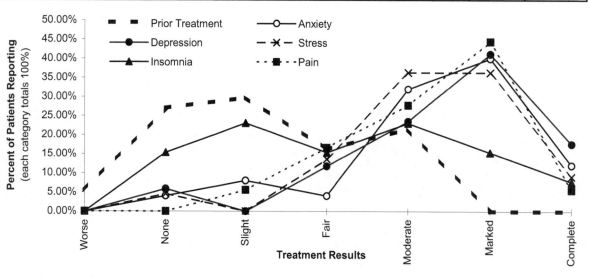

Summary for Diagnostic Category: CERVICAL PAIN

Number of Alpha-Stim treatments

# Reported	1	2	3 - 5	6 - 10	11 - 15	16 - 20	21+	Ongoing	Received in: Doctor's Office	Patient's Home
29	0.00%	5 17.24%	3 10.34%	8 27.59%	2 6.90%	3 10.34%	7 24.14%	1 3.45%	18 75.00%	6 25.00%

Alpha-Stim settings used

# Reported	Intensity (µA) 100	200	300	400	500	600	Frequency (Hz) 0.5	1.5	100	Time (minutes/treatment) 0 - 10	11 - 20	21 - 60	>60
35	2 6%	10 29%	3 9%	3 9%	4 11%	13 37%	28 80.00%	9 25.71%	2 5.71%	3 11.11%	9 33.33%	11 40.74%	4 14.81%

Alpha-Stim treatment course

# Reported	Treated With Earclips	Probes	Electrodes	Completed Satisfactory	Still Receiving	Discontinued treatment because: Not Efficacious	Side Effects	Insurance ran out	Other
28	25 89.29%	14 50.00%	11 39.29%	8 28.57%	25 89.29%	0.00%	0.00%	1 3.57%	1 3.57%

Average residual relief received with a single Alpha-Stim treatment

	# Reported	None	<1	Hours 1 - 8	9 - 23	1	Days 2	3 - 6	7+	Never Returned
Pain	29	3 10.34%	0.00%	11 37.93%	2 6.90%	2 6.90%	2 6.90%	3 10.34%	4 13.79%	2 6.90%
Anxiety	19	2 10.53%	0.00%	5 26.32%	1 5.26%	3 15.79%	1 5.26%	2 10.53%	3 15.79%	1 5.26%

Medication use / Other concomitant therapy received with Alpha-Stim

In-creased	No Change	Re-duced	Elimi-nated	# Reported	None	Psycho-therapy	Chiro-practic	Acu-puncture	Bio-feedback	Physical Therapy	Other
0.00%	12 38.71%	11 35.48%	8 25.81%	30	10 33.33%	2 6.67%	9 30.00%	1 3.33%	2 6.67%	4 13.33%	2 6.67%

Eliminated use of these drugs: analgesics (2), NSAIDs (1), narcotics (1), Amitriptyline (1), Paxil (1), anti-depressants (1), anti-convulsants (1), Stedall (1), Neurontin (1), Badofen (1), Relafin (1)

Reduced use of these drugs: Motrin (1), Flexeril (1), Ultram (1), Vicaden (1), anti-depressants (1), muscle relaxants (2), Soma (2), Amitryptaline (1), Raproxin (1), Methadone (1)

Increased use of this drug:

Side effects reported with use of Alpha-Stim:

36 (94.74%) "None" reported   Specify: heavy feeling (1), allergic to pads (1)

Doctor's evaluation of Alpha-Stim

# Reported	Efficacious	Safe	Reasonably Well Tolerated
31	24 77.42%	28 90.32%	17 54.84%

Doctor's evaluation of Alpha-Stim ('98 survey only)

# Reported	Would Use Alpha-Stim Again	Most Efficacious for this Diagnosis	Other
24	18 75.00%	11 45.83%	2 8.33%

Quality of life ('98 survey only)

Lose of Work YES	NO	Return to Work YES	NO	Work Comp YES	NO	Improve Family Life YES	NO	Improve Social Life YES	NO	Overall QOL YES	NO	Rx by: MD/DO	PhD	DDS	DC	PT	Other	Not Specified
13 54%	11 46%	5 42%	7 58%	3 30%	7 70%	19 86%	3 14%	16 80%	4 20%	20 80%	5 20%	11	2	1	7		1	

Summary for Diagnostic Category: HEADACHE (including 18 Migraines)

50 total N

15 male (age range 14-56, mean 38)   5 inpatients

35 female (age range 11-74, mean 44)   40 outpatients

Treatment(s) used prior to Alpha-Stim:

ECT	18 physical therapy	8 sedative-hypnotics
15 psychotherapy	3 surgery	psychostimulants
9 behavior modification	4 other non-drug	6 major tranquilizers
3 milliampere TENS	1 alcohol	8 analgesics
7 chiropractic	10 anxiolitics	22 NSAIDs
1 nerve blocks	26 anti-depressants	22 muscle relaxants
3 biofeedback	16 narcotics	8 other drugs

Reason(s) for discontinuing prior treatment:

11 still using	1 exacerbated	2 negative drug effects	moved
16 not efficacious	1 too expensive	1 uses Alpha-Stim	4 other

Side effects of prior treatment:

10 none	6 felt drugged	1 sedation
1 pain	1 drug sensitivity/allergy	1 GI discomfort
1 addiction	3 mental cloudiness	3 other

Treatment results obtained by using Alpha-Stim

Chief Complaints	# Reported	Worse (neg)	None (no change)	Slight (<24%)	Fair (25 - 49%)	Moderate (50 - 74%)	Marked (75 - 99%)	Complete (100%)	Significant Improvement (>25%)
Pain	34	1	0	2	7	13	10	1	31
		2.94%	0.00%	5.88%	20.59%	38.24%	29.41%	2.94%	91.18%
Anxiety	30	0	1	1	3	7	18	0	28
		0.00%	3.33%	3.33%	10.00%	23.33%	60.00%	0.00%	93.33%
Depression	14	0	0	1	3	3	7	0	13
		0.00%	0.00%	7.14%	21.43%	21.43%	50.00%	0.00%	92.86%
Stress	33	0	1	3	2	9	18	0	29
		0.00%	3.03%	9.09%	6.06%	27.27%	54.55%	0.00%	87.88%
Insomnia	17	0	1	6	2	3	5	0	10
		0.00%	5.88%	35.29%	11.76%	17.65%	29.41%	0.00%	58.82%
Headache	44	0	2	1	7	10	20	4	41
		0.00%	4.55%	2.27%	15.91%	22.73%	45.45%	9.09%	93.18%
Muscle Tension	34	0	0	0	6	10	18	0	34
		0.00%	0.00%	0.00%	17.65%	29.41%	52.94%	0.00%	100.00%

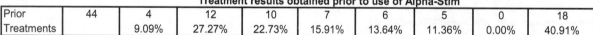

Treatment results obtained prior to use of Alpha-Stim

Prior Treatments	44	4	12	10	7	6	5	0	18
		9.09%	27.27%	22.73%	15.91%	13.64%	11.36%	0.00%	40.91%

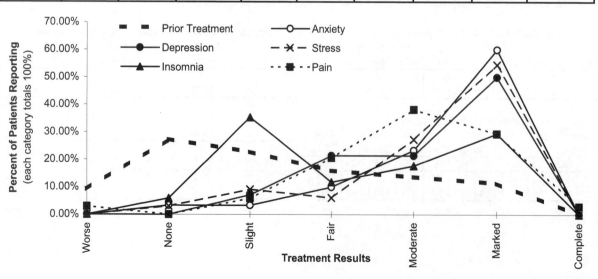

Summary for Diagnostic Category: HEADACHE (including 18 Migraines)

Number of Alpha-Stim treatments

# Reported	1	2	3 - 5	6 - 10	11 - 15	16 - 20	21+	Ongoing	Received in: Doctor's Office	Received in: Patient's Home
35	5	3	5	6	6	1	6	5	23	10
	14.29%	8.57%	14.29%	17.14%	17.14%	2.86%	17.14%	14.29%	69.70%	30.30%

Alpha-Stim settings used

# Reported	Intensity (µA) 100	200	300	400	500	600	Frequency (Hz) 0.5	1.5	100	Time (minutes/treatment) 0 - 10	11 - 20	21 - 60	>60
45	8	18	5	2	2	7	42	3	1	3	17	6	2
	18%	40%	11%	4%	4%	16%	93.33%	6.67%	2.22%	10.71%	60.71%	21.43%	7.14%

Alpha-Stim treatment course

# Reported	Treated With Earclips	Probes	Electrodes	Completed Satisfactory	Still Receiving	Discontinued treatment because: Not Efficacious	Side Effects	Insurance ran out	Other
48	43	12	7	14	27	1	3	1	2
	89.58%	25.00%	14.58%	29.17%	56.25%	2.08%	6.25%	2.08%	4.17%

Average residual relief received with a single Alpha-Stim treatment

	# Reported	None	Hours <1	1 - 8	9 - 23	Days 1	2	3 - 6	7+	Never Returned
Pain	23	4	1	6	1	1	1	5	1	2
		17.39%	4.35%	26.09%	4.35%	4.35%	4.35%	21.74%	4.35%	8.70%
Anxiety	20	3	0.00%	6	0.00%	3	0.00%	5	3	0.00%
		15.00%	0.00%	30.00%	0.00%	15.00%	0.00%	25.00%	15.00%	0.00%

Medication use: / Other concomitant therapy received with Alpha-Stim

Increased	No Change	Reduced	Eliminated	# Reported	None	Psychotherapy	Chiropractic	Acupuncture	Biofeedback	Physical Therapy	Other
	12	12	3	37	7		10	3	4	13	5
0.00%	44.44%	44.44%	11.11%		18.92%	0.00%	27.03%	8.11%	10.81%	35.14%	13.51%

Eliminated use of these drugs: Aspirin (1), anti-depressants (1), anti convulsants (1), narcotics (1), NSAIDS (1)

Reduced use of these drugs: DHE (1), Imitrex (3), Depakote (1), Xanax (1), Desril (1), Trazodone (1), Prozac (1), Inderal (1), Amitriptyline (1), anti-depressants (1), muscle relaxants (3), narcotics (2), sedatives (1), NSAIDS (1)

Increased use of this drug:

Side effects reported with use of Alpha-Stim:

45 (90.00%) "None" reported   Specify: dizziness (2), anger (1), anxiety (1), nausea (2), metal taste (1), heavy feeling (1)

Doctor's evaluation of Alpha-Stim

# Reported	Efficacious	Safe	Reasonably Well Tolerated
40	34	35	29
	85.00%	87.50%	72.50%

Doctor's evaluation of Alpha-Stim ('98 survey only)

# Reported	Would Use Alpha-Stim Again	Most Efficacious for this Diagnosis	Other
24	14	7	5
	58.33%	29.17%	20.83%

Quality of life ('98 survey only)

Lose of Work YES	NO	Return to Work YES	NO	Work Comp YES	NO	Improve Family Life YES	NO	Improve Social Life YES	NO	Overall QOL YES	NO	Rx by: MD/DO	PhD	DDS	DC	PT	Other	Not Specified
12	14	7	6	1	7	17	5	16	5	20	5	17	1		3		2	
46%	54%	54%	46%	13%	88%	77%	23%	76%	24%	80%	20%							

Summary for Diagnostic Category: FIBROMYALGIA

42 total N   3 male (age range 40-54, mean 45)   1 inpatients
                    39 female (age range 14-75, mean 45)   37 outpatients

Treatment(s) used prior to Alpha-Stim:

ECT	29 physical therapy	8 sedative-hypnotics
13 psychotherapy	6 surgery	psychostimulants
10 behavior modification	1 other non-drug	8 major tranquilizers
14 milliampere TENS	alcohol	4 analgesics
2 chiropractic	8 anxiolitics	30 NSAIDs
2 nerve blocks	29 anti-depressants	28 muscle relaxants
biofeedback	12 narcotics	3 other drugs

Reason(s) for discontinuing prior treatment:

5 still using	1 exacerbated	2 negative drug effects	moved
11 not efficacious	too expensive	2 uses Alpha-Stim	5 other

Side effects of prior treatment:

6 none	2 felt drugged	4 sedation
1 pain	2 drug sensitivity/allergy	3 GI discomfort
addiction	3 mental cloudiness	2 other

Treatment results obtained by using Alpha-Stim

Chief Complaints	# Reported	Worse (neg)	None (no change)	Slight (<24%)	Fair (25 - 49%)	Moderate (50 - 74%)	Marked (75 - 99%)	Complete (100%)	Significant Improvement (>25%)
Pain	40	0	0	6	9	9	14	2	34
		0.00%	0.00%	15.00%	22.50%	22.50%	35.00%	5.00%	85.00%
Anxiety	32	0	2	3	5	7	14	1	27
		0.00%	6.25%	9.38%	15.63%	21.88%	43.75%	3.13%	84.38%
Depression	24	0	4	3	6	2	8	1	17
		0.00%	16.67%	12.50%	25.00%	8.33%	33.33%	4.17%	70.83%
Stress	32	0	2	4	4	7	15	0	26
		0.00%	6.25%	12.50%	12.50%	21.88%	46.88%	0.00%	81.25%
Insomnia	25	0	4	4	3	6	6	2	17
		0.00%	16.00%	16.00%	12.00%	24.00%	24.00%	8.00%	68.00%
Headache	31	0	2	4	6	6	8	5	25
		0.00%	6.45%	12.90%	19.35%	19.35%	25.81%	16.13%	80.65%
Muscle Tension	38	0	0	2	8	9	17	2	36
		0.00%	0.00%	5.26%	21.05%	23.68%	44.74%	5.26%	94.74%

Treatment results obtained prior to use of Alpha-Stim

Prior Treatments	42	3	8	16	8	3	4	0	15
		7.14%	19.05%	38.10%	19.05%	7.14%	9.52%	0.00%	35.71%

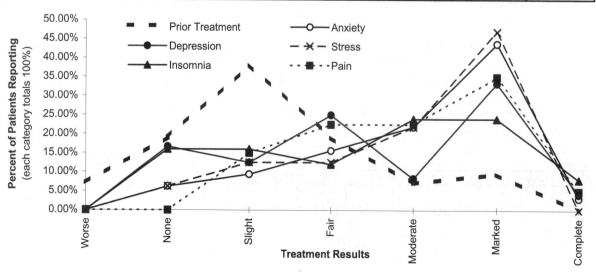

Summary for Diagnostic Category: FIBROMYALGIA

Number of Alpha-Stim treatments

# Reported	1	2	3 - 5	6 - 10	11 - 15	16 - 20	21+	Ongoing	Received in: Doctor's Office	Received in: Patient's Home
21		4	4			1	5	7	20	20
	0.00%	19.05%	19.05%	0.00%	0.00%	4.76%	23.81%	33.33%	50.00%	50.00%

Alpha-Stim settings used

# Reported	Intensity (µA) 100	200	300	400	500	600	Frequency (Hz) 0.5	1.5	100	Time (minutes/treatment) 0 - 10	11 - 20	21 - 60	>60
39	6	17	4	2	7	4	33	7	2	2	10	3	3
	15%	44%	10%	5%	18%	10%	84.62%	17.95%	5.13%	11.11%	55.56%	16.67%	16.67%

Alpha-Stim treatment course

# Reported	Treated With Earclips	Probes	Electrodes	Completed Satisfactory	Still Receiving	Discontinued treatment because: Not Efficacious	Side Effects	Insurance ran out	Other
41	37	17	17	2	33		1		1
	90.24%	41.46%	41.46%	4.88%	80.49%	0.00%	2.44%	0.00%	2.44%

Average residual relief received with a single Alpha-Stim treatment

	# Reported	None	Hours <1	1 - 8	9 - 23	Days 1	2	3 - 6	7+	Never Returned
Pain	32	2		12	1	2	2	9	3	1
		6.25%	0.00%	37.50%	3.13%	6.25%	6.25%	28.13%	9.38%	3.13%
Anxiety	19		1	6		5		7	3	
		0.00%	5.26%	31.58%	0.00%	26.32%	0.00%	36.84%	15.79%	0.00%

Medication use / Other concomitant therapy received with Alpha-Stim

In- creased	No Change	Re- duced	Elimi- nated	# Reported	None	Psycho- therapy	Chiro- practic	Acu- puncture	Bio- feedback	Physical Therapy	Other
	11	17	3	28	3		2	5		17	1
0.00%	35.48%	54.84%	9.68%		10.71%	0.00%	7.14%	17.86%	0.00%	60.71%	3.57%

Eliminated use of these drugs: NSAIDs (2), Acetaminophen (1)

Reduced use of these drugs: Soma (1), Amitriptyline (1), Methadone (1), Neurontin (1), Baclofen (1), Percocet (1), pain medication (1), Valium (1), Naproxin (2), Flexoril (1), anti-depressants (1), NSAIDs (1), muscle relaxants (4), sedatives(1)

Increased use of this drug:

Side effects reported with use of Alpha-Stim:

39 (92.86%) "None" reported   Specify: Itching/skin irritation (2), dizziness (1)

Doctor's evaluation of Alpha-Stim

# Reported	Efficacious	Safe	Reasonably Well Tolerated
35	24	25	23
	68.57%	71.43%	65.71%

Doctor's evaluation of Alpha-Stim ('98 survey only)

# Reported	Would Use Alpha-Stim Again	Most Efficacious for this Diagnosis	Other
26	17	14	3
	65.38%	53.85%	11.54%

Quality of life ('98 survey only)

Lose of Work YES	NO	Return to Work YES	NO	Work Comp YES	NO	Improve Family Life YES	NO	Improve Social Life YES	NO	Overall QOL YES	NO	Rx by: MD/ DO	PhD	DDS	DC	PT	Other	Not Specified
19	10	4	15	4	4	22	8	23	7	25	4	28	1	1				
66%	34%	21%	79%	50%	50%	73%	27%	77%	23%	86%	14%							

Summary for Diagnostic Category: COMPLEX REGIONAL PAIN SYNDROME (TYPE I)
(formerly known as Reflex Sympathetic Dystrophy)

8 total N　　　　1 male (age range 50, mean 50)　　　　0 inpatients
　　　　　　　　　7 female (age range 16-85, mean 41)　　　6 outpatients

Treatment(s) used prior to Alpha-Stim:

ECT	5 physical therapy	1 sedative-hypnotics
1 psychotherapy	1 surgery	psychostimulants
1 behavior modification	other non-drug	1 major tranquilizers
3 milliampere TENS	alcohol	1 analgesics
1 chiropractic	1 anxiolitics	6 NSAIDs
2 nerve blocks	6 anti-depressants	4 muscle relaxants
1 biofeedback	3 narcotics	1 other drugs

Reason(s) for discontinuing prior treatment:

1 still using	exacerbated	negative drug effects	moved
4 not efficacious	too expensive	uses Alpha-Stim	other

Side effects of prior treatment:

none	1 felt drugged	sedation
pain	drug sensitivity/allergy	GI discomfort
addiction	mental cloudiness	2 other

Treatment results obtained by using Alpha-Stim

Chief Complaints	# Reported	Worse (neg)	None (no change)	Slight (<24%)	Fair (25 - 49%)	Moderate (50 - 74%)	Marked (75 - 99%)	Complete (100%)	Significant Improvement (>25%)
Pain	8	0	0	2	2	1	3	0	6
		0.00%	0.00%	25.00%	25.00%	12.50%	37.50%	0.00%	75.00%
Anxiety	6	0	0	1	2	1	2	0	5
		0.00%	0.00%	16.67%	33.33%	16.67%	33.33%	0.00%	83.33%
Depression	4	0	0	0	2	1	1		4
		0.00%	0.00%	0.00%	50.00%	25.00%	25.00%	0.00%	100.00%
Stress	5	0	0	1	0	2	2	0	4
		0.00%	0.00%	20.00%	0.00%	40.00%	40.00%	0.00%	80.00%
Insomnia	2	0	0	0	0	2	0	0	2
		0.00%	0.00%	0.00%	0.00%	100.00%	0.00%	0.00%	100.00%
Headache	3	0	0	0	1	1	1	0	3
		0.00%	0.00%	0.00%	33.33%	33.33%	33.33%	0.00%	100.00%
Muscle Tension	5	0	0	0	1	2	2	0	5
		0.00%	0.00%	0.00%	20.00%	40.00%	40.00%	0.00%	100.00%
Treatment results obtained prior to use of Alpha-Stim									
Prior Treatments	44	0	40	3	1	0	0	0	1
		0.00%	90.91%	6.82%	2.27%	0.00%	0.00%	0.00%	2.27%

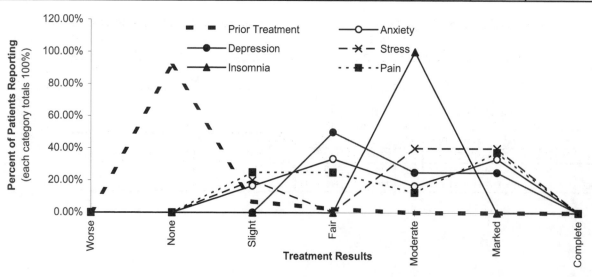

Summary for Diagnostic Category: COMPLEX REGIONAL PAIN SYNDROME (TYPE I)

(formerly known as Reflex Sympathetic Dystrophy)

Number of Alpha-Stim treatments

# Reported	1	2	3 - 5	6 - 10	11 - 15	16 - 20	21+	Ongoing	Received in: Doctor's Office	Received in: Patient's Home
3				2			1		4	2
	0.00%	0.00%	0.00%	66.67%	0.00%	0.00%	33.33%	0.00%	66.67%	33.33%

Alpha-Stim settings used

# Reported	Intensity (µA) 100	200	300	400	500	600	Frequency (Hz) 0.5	1.5	100	Time (minutes/treatment) 0 - 10	11 - 20	21 - 60	>60
7	1	4			1	1	5	2			1	2	
	14%	57%	0%	0%	14%	14%	71.43%	28.57%	0.00%	0.00%	33.33%	66.67%	0.00%

Alpha-Stim treatment course

# Reported	Treated With Earclips	Probes	Electrodes	Completed Satisfactory	Still Receiving	Discontinued treatment because: Not Efficacious	Side Effects	Insurance ran out	Other
8	7	6	4	2	5				1
	87.50%	75.00%	50.00%	25.00%	62.50%	0.00%	0.00%	0.00%	12.50%

Average residual relief received with a single Alpha-Stim treatment

	# Reported	None	Hours <1	1 - 8	9 - 23	Days 1	2	3 - 6	7+	Never Returned
Pain	4			1		1		2		
		0.00%	0.00%	25.00%	0.00%	25.00%	0.00%	50.00%	0.00%	0.00%
Anxiety	3					2		1		
		0.00%	0.00%	0.00%	0.00%	66.67%	0.00%	33.33%	0.00%	0.00%

Medication Use: In-creased	No Change	Re-duced	Elimi-nated	# Reported	None	Other Concomitant therapy received with Alpha-Stim Psycho-therapy	Chiro-practic	Acu-puncture	Bio-feedback	Physical Therapy	Other
1	1	4		6				3	1	5	
16.67%	16.67%	66.67%	0.00%		0.00%	0.00%	0.00%	50.00%	16.67%	83.33%	0.00%

Eliminated use of these drugs:

Reduced use of these drugs: Ibuprophen (2), muscle relaxants (1)

Increased use of this drug: Zoloft (1)

Side effects reported with use of Alpha-Stim:

7 (87.50%) "None" reported   Specify: ringing in ears (1)

Doctor's evaluation of Alpha-Stim

# Reported	Efficacious	Safe	Reasonably Well Tolerated
7	6	6	7
	85.71%	85.71%	100.00%

Doctor's evaluation of Alpha-Stim ('98 survey only)

# Reported	Would Use Alpha-Stim Again	Most Efficacious for this Diagnosis	Other
4	2	3	
	50.00%	75.00%	0.00%

Quality of life ('98 survey only)

Lose of Work YES	NO	Return to Work YES	NO	Work Comp YES	NO	Improve Family Life YES	NO	Improve Social Life YES	NO	Overall QOL YES	NO	Rx by: MD/DO	PhD	DDS	DC	PT	Other	Not Specified
3	2	1	3		1	3	2	3	2	6		4					1	
60%	40%	25%	75%	0%	100%	60%	40%	60%	40%	100%	0%							

Summary for Diagnostic Category: CLOSED HEAD INJURIES

6 total N

1 male (age range 46, mean 46)
5 female (age range 38-52, mean 45)

0 inpatients
5 outpatients

Treatment(s) used prior to Alpha-Stim:

ECT	2 physical therapy	2 sedative-hypnotics
4 psychotherapy	surgery	psychostimulants
2 behavior modification	other non-drug	3 major tranquilizers
2 milliampere TENS	1 alcohol	analgesics
2 chiropractic	3 anxiolitics	3 NSAIDs
nerve blocks	5 anti-depressants	3 muscle relaxants
biofeedback	2 narcotics	other drugs

Reason(s) for discontinuing prior treatment:

still using	exacerbated	negative drug effects	moved
3 not efficacious	too expensive	uses Alpha-Stim	2 other

Side effects of prior treatment:

none	felt drugged	sedation
pain	drug sensitivity/allergy	GI discomfort
addiction	mental cloudiness	2 other

Treatment results obtained by using Alpha-Stim

Chief Complaints	# Reported	Worse (neg)	None (no change)	Slight (<24%)	Fair (25 - 49%)	Moderate (50 - 74%)	Marked (75 - 99%)	Complete (100%)	Significant Improvement (>25%)
Pain	4	0	0	1	0	1	2	0	3
		0.00%	0.00%	25.00%	0.00%	25.00%	50.00%	0.00%	75.00%
Anxiety	6	0	0	0	2	1	3	0	6
		0.00%	0.00%	0.00%	33.33%	16.67%	50.00%	0.00%	100.00%
Depression	3	0	0	0	0	1	2	0	3
		0.00%	0.00%	0.00%	0.00%	33.33%	66.67%	0.00%	100.00%
Stress	5	0	0	0	0	1	4	0	5
		0.00%	0.00%	0.00%	0.00%	20.00%	80.00%	0.00%	100.00%
Insomnia	4	0	0	0	0	2	2	0	4
		0.00%	0.00%	0.00%	0.00%	50.00%	50.00%	0.00%	100.00%
Headache	5	0	0	0	0	2	3	0	5
		0.00%	0.00%	0.00%	0.00%	40.00%	60.00%	0.00%	100.00%
Muscle Tension	6	0	0	0	1	3	2	0	6
		0.00%	0.00%	0.00%	16.67%	50.00%	33.33%	0.00%	100.00%
Treatment results obtained prior to use of Alpha-Stim									
Prior Treatments	6	0	2	2	1	0	1	0	2
		0.00%	33.33%	33.33%	16.67%	0.00%	16.67%	0.00%	33.33%

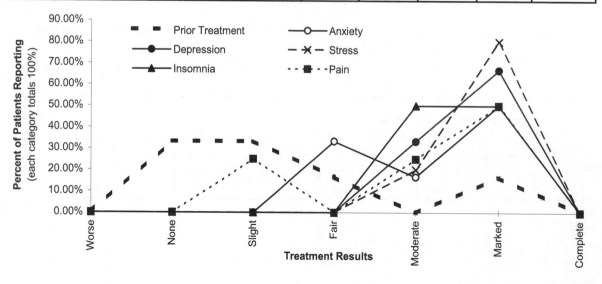

Summary for Diagnostic Category: CLOSED HEAD INJURIES

Number of Alpha-Stim treatments | **Received in:**

# Reported	1	2	3 - 5	6 - 10	11 - 15	16 - 20	21+	Ongoing	Doctor's Office	Patient's Home
3	1				1			1	2	3
	33.33%	0.00%	0.00%	0.00%	33.33%	0.00%	0.00%	33.33%	40.00%	60.00%

Alpha-Stim settings used

# Reported	Intensity (µA)						Frequency (Hz)			Time (minutes/treatment)			
	100	200	300	400	500	600	0.5	1.5	100	0 - 10	11 - 20	21 - 60	>60
5		3		2	2	1	6	2			1	1	
	0%	60%	0%	40%	40%	20%	120.00%	40.00%	0.00%	0.00%	50.00%	50.00%	0.00%

Alpha-Stim treatment course

# Reported	Treated With			Completed Satisfactory	Still Receiving	Discontinued treatment because:			
	Earclips	Probes	Electrodes			Not Efficacious	Side Effects	Insurance ran out	Other
5	4	1	1	1	4			1	
	80.00%	20.00%	20.00%	20.00%	80.00%	0.00%	0.00%	20.00%	0.00%

Average residual relief received with a single Alpha-Stim treatment

	# Reported	None	<1	Hours 1 - 8	9 - 23	1	2	Days 3 - 6	7+	Never Returned
Pain	3					1		2		
		0.00%	0.00%	0.00%	0.00%	33.33%	0.00%	66.67%	0.00%	0.00%
Anxiety	3					1		2		
		0.00%	0.00%	0.00%	0.00%	33.33%	0.00%	66.67%	0.00%	0.00%

Medication use: | Other concomitant therapy received with Alpha-Stim

Increased	No Change	Reduced	Eliminated	# Reported	None	Psycho-therapy	Chiro-practic	Acu-puncture	Bio-feedback	Physical Therapy	Other
		2		3		1	1	1		1	
0.00%	0.00%	100.00%	0.00%		0.00%	33.33%	33.33%	33.33%	0.00%	33.33%	0.00%

Eliminated use of these drugs:

Reduced use of these drugs: narcotics (1), Ibuprofen (1)

Increased use of this drug:

Side effects reported with use of Alpha-Stim:

5 (83.33%) "None" reported   Specify: ringing in the ears intensified (1)

Doctor's evaluation of Alpha-Stim

# Reported	Efficacious	Safe	Reasonably Well Tolerated
5	5	5	2
	100.00%	100.00%	40.00%

Doctor's evaluation of Alpha-Stim ('98 survey only)

# Reported	Would Use Alpha-Stim Again	Most Efficacious for this Diagnosis	Other
2	1	2	
	50.00%	100.00%	0.00%

Quality of life ('98 survey only)

Lose of Work		Return to Work		Work Comp		Improve Family Life		Improve Social Life		Overall QOL		Rx by:						
YES	NO	YES	NO	YES	NO	YES	NO	YES	NO	YES	NO	MD/ DO	PhD	DDS	DC	PT	Other	Not Specified
1	1		1				2		2	1	1	2						
50%	50%	0%	100%			0%	100%	0%	100%	50%	50%							

Summary for Diagnostic Category: TEMPOROMANDIBULAR DISORDER

7 total N   1 male (age range 35, mean 35)   0 inpatients

6 female (age range 32-57, mean 44)   5 outpatients

Treatment(s) used prior to Alpha-Stim:

ECT	3 physical therapy	2 sedative-hypnotics
1 psychotherapy	2 surgery	psychostimulants
1 behavior modification	1 other non-drug	2 major tranquilizers
4 milliampere TENS	alcohol	2 analgesics
chiropractic	anxiolitics	2 NSAIDs
1 nerve blocks	2 anti-depressants	3 muscle relaxants
1 biofeedback	3 narcotics	other drugs

Reason(s) for discontinuing prior treatment:

still using	exacerbated	negative drug effects	moved
5 not efficacious	too expensive	1 uses Alpha-Stim	1 other

Side effects of prior treatment:

2 none	felt drugged	sedation
pain	2 drug sensitivity/allergy	2 GI discomfort
addiction	mental cloudiness	1 other

Treatment results obtained by using Alpha-Stim

Chief Complaints	# Reported	Worse (neg)	None (no change)	Slight (<24%)	Fair (25 - 49%)	Moderate (50 - 74%)	Marked (75 - 99%)	Complete (100%)	Significant Improvement (>25%)
Pain	6	0	1	0	0	2	3	0	5
		0.00%	16.67%	0.00%	0.00%	33.33%	50.00%	0.00%	83.33%
Anxiety	6	0	0	0	1	1	1	3	6
		0.00%	0.00%	0.00%	16.67%	16.67%	16.67%	50.00%	100.00%
Depression	2	0	0	0	0	1	0	1	2
		0.00%	0.00%	0.00%	0.00%	50.00%	0.00%	50.00%	100.00%
Stress	3	0	0	0	0	1	2	0	3
		0.00%	0.00%	0.00%	0.00%	33.33%	66.67%	0.00%	100.00%
Insomnia	2	0	0	0	0	1	0	1	2
		0.00%	0.00%	0.00%	0.00%	50.00%	0.00%	50.00%	100.00%
Headache	4	1	0	0	0	0	2	1	3
		25.00%	0.00%	0.00%	0.00%	0.00%	50.00%	25.00%	75.00%
Muscle Tension	6	0	1	0	0	2	3	0	5
		0.00%	16.67%	0.00%	0.00%	33.33%	50.00%	0.00%	83.33%

Treatment results obtained prior to use of Alpha-Stim

Prior Treatments	7	1	0	4	1	1	0	0	2
		14.29%	0.00%	57.14%	14.29%	14.29%	0.00%	0.00%	28.57%

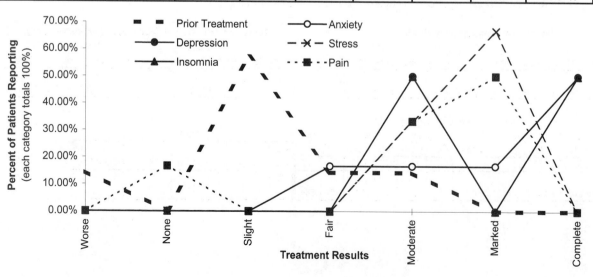

Summary for Diagnostic Category: TEMPOROMANDIBULAR DISORDER

Number of Alpha-Stim treatments

# Reported	1	2	3 - 5	6 - 10	11 - 15	16 - 20	21+	Ongoing	Received in: Doctor's Office	Received in: Patient's Home
7	1	1	2				2	1	3	3
	14.29%	14.29%	28.57%	0.00%	0.00%	0.00%	28.57%	14.29%	50.00%	50.00%

Alpha-Stim settings used

# Reported	Intensity (µA) 100	200	300	400	500	600	Frequency (Hz) 0.5	1.5	100	Time (minutes/treatment) 0 - 10	11 - 20	21 - 60	>60
6		1	1	1	2		4	2			2	2	1
	0%	17%	17%	17%	33%	0%	66.67%	33.33%	0.00%	0.00%	40.00%	40.00%	20.00%

Alpha-Stim treatment course

# Reported	Treated With Earclips	Probes	Electrodes	Completed Satisfactory	Still Receiving	Discontinued treatment because: Not Efficacious	Side Effects	Insurance ran out	Other
7	7	2	3	4	2	1			1
	100.00%	28.57%	42.86%	57.14%	28.57%	14.29%	0.00%	0.00%	14.29%

Average residual relief received with a single Alpha-Stim treatment

	# Reported	Hours None	<1	1 - 8	9 - 23	Days 1	2	3 - 6	7+	Never Returned
Pain	5	2		2						1
		40.00%	0.00%	40.00%	0.00%	0.00%	0.00%	0.00%	0.00%	20.00%
Anxiety	1			1						
		0.00%	0.00%	100.00%	0.00%	0.00%	0.00%	0.00%	0.00%	0.00%

Medication use / Other concomitant therapy received with Alpha-Stim

Increased	No Change	Reduced	Eliminated	# Reported	None	Psycho-therapy	Chiro-practic	Acu-puncture	Bio-feedback	Physical Therapy	Other
	2	2		6	4					1	1
0.00%	50.00%	50.00%	0.00%		66.67%	0.00%	0.00%	0.00%	0.00%	16.67%	16.67%

Eliminated use of these drugs: Neurontin (1), Badofen (1), Relafen (1)

Reduced use of these drugs: Valium (1), Percocet (1), Soma (1), Methadone (1)

Increased use of this drug:

Side effects reported with use of Alpha-Stim:

7 (100.00%) "None" reported   Specify:

Doctor's evaluation of Alpha-Stim

# Reported	Efficacious	Safe	Reasonably Well Tolerated
6	1	4	3
	16.67%	66.67%	50.00%

Doctor's evaluation of Alpha-Stim ('98 survey only)

# Reported	Would Use Alpha-Stim Again	Most Efficacious for this Diagnosis	Other
4	2		2
	50.00%	0.00%	50.00%

Quality of life ('98 survey only)

Lose of Work YES	NO	Return to Work YES	NO	Work Comp YES	NO	Improve Family Life YES	NO	Improve Social Life YES	NO	Overall QOL YES	NO	Rx by: MD/DO	PhD	DDS	DC	PT	Other	Not Specified
4	1	1	4		2	3	2	3	2	3	2	2		2				
80%	20%	20%	80%	0%	100%	60%	40%	60%	40%	60%	40%							

Summary for Diagnostic Category: CARPAL TUNNEL SYNDROME

4 total N

1 male (age range 34, mean 34)
3 female (age range 38-44, mean 40)

0 inpatients
4 outpatients

Treatment(s) used prior to Alpha-Stim:

ECT	1 physical therapy	sedative-hypnotics
1 psychotherapy	2 surgery	psychostimulants
behavior modification	1 other non-drug	major tranquilizers
1 milliampere TENS	alcohol	analgesics
chiropractic	anxiolitics	2 NSAIDs
nerve blocks	2 anti-depressants	muscle relaxants
biofeedback	1 narcotics	1 other drugs

Reason(s) for discontinuing prior treatment:

still using	exacerbated	negative drug effects	moved
2 not efficacious	too expensive	uses Alpha-Stim	1 other

Side effects of prior treatment:

none	felt drugged	sedation
pain	drug sensitivity/allergy	1 GI discomfort
addiction	mental cloudiness	other

Treatment results obtained by using Alpha-Stim

Chief Complaints	# Reported	Worse (neg)	None (no change)	Slight (<24%)	Fair (25 - 49%)	Moderate (50 - 74%)	Marked (75 - 99%)	Complete (100%)	Significant Improvement (>25%)
Pain	4	0 0.00%	0 0.00%	1 25.00%	1 25.00%	1 25.00%	1 25.00%	0 0.00%	3 75.00%
Anxiety	4	0 0.00%	0 0.00%	0 0.00%	1 25.00%	2 50.00%	0 0.00%	1 25.00%	4 100.00%
Depression	3	0 0.00%	0 0.00%	1 33.33%	0 0.00%	1 33.33%	1 33.33%	0 0.00%	2 66.67%
Stress	1	0.00%	0.00%	0.00%	0.00%	1 100.00%	0.00%	0.00%	1 100.00%
Insomnia	0								
Headache	0								
Muscle Tension	5	2 40.00%	0 0.00%	0 0.00%	0 0.00%	2 40.00%	1 20.00%	0 0.00%	3 60.00%

Treatment results obtained prior to use of Alpha-Stim

Prior Treatments	3	1 33.33%	2 66.67%	0 0.00%	0 0.00%	0 0.00%	0 0.00%	0 0.00%	0 0.00%

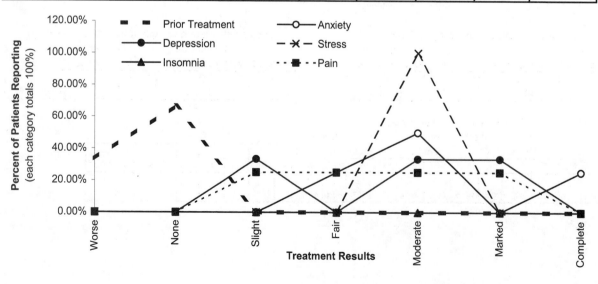

Summary for Diagnostic Category: CARPAL TUNNEL SYNDROME

Number of Alpha-Stim treatments

# Reported	1	2	3 - 5	6 - 10	11 - 15	16 - 20	21+	Ongoing	Received in: Doctor's Office	Patient's Home
2		1	1						4	2
	0.00%	50.00%	50.00%	0.00%	0.00%	0.00%	0.00%	0.00%	66.67%	33.33%

Alpha-Stim settings used

# Reported	Intensity (µA) 100	200	300	400	500	600	Frequency (Hz) 0.5	1.5	100	Time (minutes/treatment) 0 - 10	11 - 20	21 - 60	>60
4		2	2			1	3	1			1	1	
	0%	50%	50%	0%	0%	25%	75.00%	25.00%	0.00%	0.00%	50.00%	50.00%	0.00%

Alpha-Stim treatment course

# Reported	Treated With Earclips	Probes	Electrodes	Completed Satisfactory	Still Receiving	Discontinued treatment because: Not Efficacious	Side Effects	Insurance ran out	Other
4	3	2	2	1	1	1			
	75.00%	50.00%	50.00%	25.00%	25.00%	25.00%	0.00%	0.00%	0.00%

Average residual relief received with a single Alpha-Stim treatment

	# Reported	None	<1	Hours 1 - 8	9 - 23	1	Days 2	3 - 6	7+	Never Returned
Pain	2	1		1						
		50.00%	0.00%	50.00%	0.00%	0.00%	0.00%	0.00%	0.00%	0.00%
Anxiety										

Medication use / Other concomitant therapy received with Alpha-Stim

In-creased	No Change	Re-duced	Elimi-nated	# Reported	None	Psycho-therapy	Chiro-practic	Acu-puncture	Bio-feedback	Physical Therapy	Other
	2			4	2				1	1	1
0.00%	100.00%	0.00%	0.00%		50.00%	0.00%	0.00%	0.00%	25.00%	25.00%	25.00%

Eliminated use of these drugs:

Reduced use of these drugs:

Increased use of this drug:

Side effects reported with use of Alpha-Stim:

4 (100.00%) "None" reported   Specify:

Doctor's evaluation of Alpha-Stim

# Reported	Efficacious	Safe	Reasonably Well Tolerated
4	2	2	2
	50.00%	50.00%	50.00%

Doctor's evaluation of Alpha-Stim ('98 survey only)

# Reported	Would Use Alpha-Stim Again	Most Efficacious for this Diagnosis	Other
2	1	1	
	50.00%	50.00%	0.00%

Quality of Life ('98 Survey Only)

Lose of Work YES	NO	Return to Work YES	NO	Work Comp YES	NO	Improve Family Life YES	NO	Improve Social Life YES	NO	Overall QOL YES	NO	Rx by: MD/ DO	PhD	DDS	DC	PT	Other	Not Specified
2	1		3	2	2	1	3	1	3	1	3	3						
67%	33%	0%	100%	50%	50%	25%	75%	25%	75%	25%	75%							

Summary for Diagnostic Category: CHRONIC PAIN & PAIN NOT OTHERWISE SPECIFIED

37 total N   11 male (age range 5-60, mean 38)   0 inpatients

26 female (age range 26-77, mean 50)   34 outpatients

Treatment(s) used prior to Alpha-Stim:

1 ECT	11 physical therapy	4 sedative-hypnotics
8 psychotherapy	5 surgery	1 psychostimulants
2 behavior modification	4 other non-drug	3 major tranquilizers
3 milliampere TENS	1 alcohol	2 analgesics
4 chiropractic	4 anxiolitics	8 NSAIDs
nerve blocks	6 anti-depressants	9 muscle relaxants
1 biofeedback	8 narcotics	3 other drugs

Reason(s) for discontinuing prior treatment:

5 still using	exacerbated	1 negative drug effects	1 moved
13 not efficacious	too expensive	1 uses Alpha-Stim	6 other

Side effects of prior treatment:

6 none	4 felt drugged	1 sedation
2 pain	2 drug sensitivity/allergy	1 GI discomfort
addiction	2 mental cloudiness	5 other

Treatment results obtained by using Alpha-Stim

Chief Complaints	# Reported	Worse (neg)	None (no change)	Slight (<24%)	Fair (25 - 49%)	Moderate (50 - 74%)	Marked (75 - 99%)	Complete (100%)	Significant Improvement (>25%)
Pain	34	1	1	1	1	9	19	2	31
		2.94%	2.94%	2.94%	2.94%	26.47%	55.88%	5.88%	91.18%
Anxiety	27	0	1	1	0	8	15	2	25
		0.00%	3.70%	3.70%	0.00%	29.63%	55.56%	7.41%	92.59%
Depression	9	0	1	0	0	2	6	0	8
		0.00%	11.11%	0.00%	0.00%	22.22%	66.67%	0.00%	88.89%
Stress	13	0	1	0	1	7	4	0	12
		0.00%	7.69%	0.00%	7.69%	53.85%	30.77%	0.00%	92.31%
Insomnia	10	0	1	0	1	1	6	1	9
		0.00%	10.00%	0.00%	10.00%	10.00%	60.00%	10.00%	90.00%
Headache	4	0	1	0	0	1	1	1	3
		0.00%	25.00%	0.00%	0.00%	25.00%	25.00%	25.00%	75.00%
Muscle Tension	17	0	1	0	2	5	8	1	16
		0.00%	5.88%	0.00%	11.76%	29.41%	47.06%	5.88%	94.12%

Treatment results obtained prior to use of Alpha-Stim

	# Reported	Worse	None	Slight	Fair	Moderate	Marked	Complete	Significant Improvement
	31	1	9	11	6	4	0	0	10
		3.23%	29.03%	35.48%	19.35%	12.90%	0.00%	0.00%	32.26%

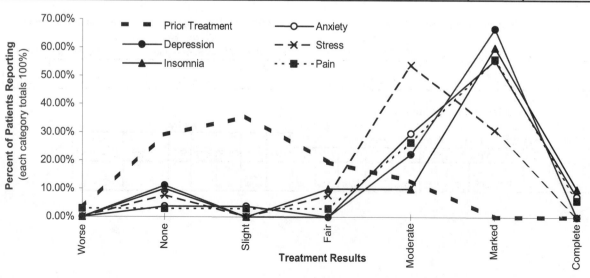

Summary for Diagnostic Category: CHRONIC PAIN & PAIN NOT OTHERWISE SPECIFIED

Number of Alpha-Stim treatments

# Reported	1	2	3 - 5	6 - 10	11 - 15	16 - 20	21+	Ongoing	Received in: Doctor's Office	Patient's Home
29	3	3	1	4	4	4	6	2	8	8
	10.34%	10.34%	3.45%	13.79%	13.79%	13.79%	20.69%	6.90%	50.00%	50.00%

Alpha-Stim settings used

# Reported	Intensity (µA)						Frequency (Hz)			Time (minutes/treatment)			
	100	200	300	400	500	600	0.5	1.5	100	0 - 10	11 - 20	21 - 60	>60
35	3	12	10	3	2	6	33	3		6	17	5	
	9%	34%	29%	9%	6%	17%	94.29%	8.57%	0.00%	21.43%	60.71%	17.86%	0.00%

Alpha-Stim treatment course

# Reported	Treated With			Completed Satisfactory	Still Receiving	Discontinued treatment because:			
	Earclips	Probes	Electrodes			Not Efficacious	Side Effects	Insurance ran out	Other
35	28	8	4	14	27	2	1		2
	80.00%	22.86%	11.43%	40.00%	77.14%	5.71%	2.86%	0.00%	5.71%

Average residual relief received with a single Alpha-Stim treatment

	# Reported	None	Hours <1	1 - 8	9 - 23	Days 1	2	3 - 6	7+	Never Returned
Pain	9	2			1	1	1	3	1	
		22.22%	0.00%	0.00%	11.11%	11.11%	11.11%	33.33%	11.11%	0.00%
Anxiety	4							2	1	1
		0.00%	0.00%	0.00%	0.00%	0.00%	0.00%	50.00%	25.00%	25.00%

Medication use: / Other concomitant therapy received with Alpha-Stim

In-creased	No Change	Re-duced	Elimi-nated	# Reported	None	Psycho-therapy	Chiro-practic	Acu-puncture	Bio-feedback	Physical Therapy	Other
	3	5	2	34	6	2	5	3	12	77	4
0.00%	30.00%	50.00%	20.00%		17.65%	5.88%	14.71%	8.82%	35.29%	226.47%	11.76%

Eliminated use of these drugs: Excedrin (1), Flexeril (1)

Reduced use of these drugs: Soma (1), NSAIDs (1), narcotics (1), analgesics (1), anti-depressants (1), muscle relaxants (1)

Increased use of this drug:

Side effects reported with use of Alpha-Stim:

35 (94.59%) "None" reported   Specify: heavy feeling (1), anger (1)

Doctor's evaluation of Alpha-Stim

# Reported	Efficacious	Safe	Reasonably Well Tolerated
34	31	31	24
	91.18%	91.18%	70.59%

Doctor's evaluation of Alpha-Stim ('98 survey only)

# Reported	Would Use Alpha-Stim Again	Most Efficacious for this Diagnosis	Other
8	5	4	2
	62.50%	50.00%	25.00%

Quality of life ('98 survey only)

Lose of Work		Return to Work		Work Comp		Improve Family Life		Improve Social Life		Overall QOL		Rx by:						
YES	NO	YES	NO	YES	NO	YES	NO	YES	NO	YES	NO	MD/DO	PhD	DDS	DC	PT	Other	Not Specified
2	8	1	3	2	3	8	2	8	2	9	2	10	1	1	2			
20%	80%	25%	75%	40%	60%	80%	20%	80%	20%	82%	18%							

Summary for Diagnostic Category: OTHER

(including Bell's Palsey, Meniere's Syndrome, Intermittent Explosive Disorder, Mercury Poisening in a Dentist)

10 total N   3 male (age range 35-46, mean 41)   0 inpatients

7 female   10 outpatients

Treatment(s) used prior to Alpha-Stim:

ECT	4 physical therapy	2 sedative-hypnotics
2 psychotherapy	1 surgery	psychostimulants
2 behavior modification	2 other non-drug	2 major tranquilizers
1 milliampere TENS	1 alcohol	1 analgesics
chiropractic	4 anxiolitics	3 NSAIDs
nerve blocks	5 anti-depressants	3 muscle relaxants
biofeedback	3 narcotics	other drugs

Reason(s) for discontinuing prior treatment:

1 still using	exacerbated	1 negative drug effects	moved
4 not efficacious	too expensive	uses Alpha-Stim	2 other

Side effects of prior treatment:

3 none	1 felt drugged	sedation
pain	1 drug sensitivity/allergy	GI discomfort
addiction	1 mental cloudiness	1 other

Treatment results obtained by using Alpha-Stim

Chief Complaints	# Reported	Worse (neg)	None (no change)	Slight (<24%)	Fair (25 - 49%)	Moderate (50 - 74%)	Marked (75 - 99%)	Complete (100%)	Significant Improvement (>25%)
Pain	7	0 0.00%	0 0.00%	0 0.00%	1 14.29%	1 14.29%	5 71.43%	0 0.00%	7 100.00%
Anxiety	9	0 0.00%	0 0.00%	0 0.00%	0 0.00%	3 33.33%	5 55.56%	1 11.11%	9 100.00%
Depression	6	0 0.00%	0 0.00%	0 0.00%	0 0.00%	1 16.67%	4 66.67%	1 16.67%	6 100.00%
Stress	8	0 0.00%	0 0.00%	0 0.00%	0 0.00%	1 12.50%	6 75.00%	1 12.50%	8 100.00%
Insomnia	5	0 0.00%	0 0.00%	0 0.00%	0 0.00%	2 40.00%	3 60.00%	0 0.00%	5 100.00%
Headache	4	0 0.00%	0 0.00%	1 25.00%	0 0.00%	1 25.00%	2 50.00%	0 0.00%	3 75.00%
Muscle Tension	4	0 0.00%	0 0.00%	0 0.00%	1 25.00%	0 0.00%	3 75.00%	0 0.00%	4 100.00%

Treatment results obtained prior to use of Alpha-Stim

Prior Treatments	9	0 0.00%	4 44.44%	1 11.11%	1 11.11%	0 0.00%	3 33.33%	0 0.00%	4 44.44%

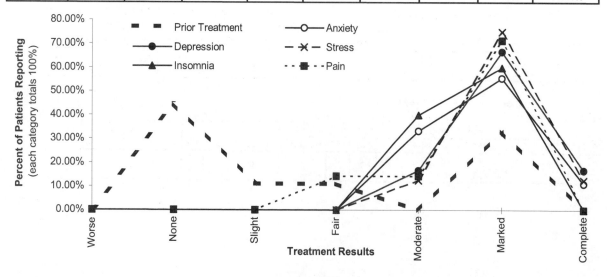

Summary for Diagnostic Category: OTHER

(including Bell's Palsey, Meniere's Syndrome, Intermittent Explosive Disorder, Mercury Poisening in a Dentist)

Number of Alpha-Stim treatments

# Reported	1	2	3 - 5	6 - 10	11 - 15	16 - 20	21+	Ongoing	Received in: Doctor's Office	Patient's Home
7	0.00%	0.00%	1 14.29%	4 57.14%	0.00%	0.00%	2 28.57%	0.00%	3 75.00%	1 25.00%

Alpha-Stim settings used

# Reported	Intensity (µA) 100	200	300	400	500	600	Frequency (Hz) 0.5	1.5	100	Time (minutes/treatment) 0 - 10	11 - 20	21 - 60	>60
10	2 20%	4 40%	1 10%	1 10%	2 20%	2 20%	9 90.00%	1 10.00%	0.00%	1 14.29%	3 42.86%	3 42.86%	0.00%

Alpha-Stim treatment course

# Reported	Treated With Earclips	Probes	Electrodes	Completed Satisfactory	Still Receiving	Discontinued treatment because: Not Efficacious	Side Effects	Insurance ran out	Other
9	9 100.00%	2 22.22%	2 22.22%	3 33.33%	5 55.56%	0.00%	0.00%	1 11.11%	1 11.11%

Average residual relief received with a single Alpha-Stim treatment

	# Reported	None	Hours <1	1 - 8	9 - 23	1	Days 2	3 - 6	7+	Never Returned
Pain	4	0.00%	0.00%	0.00%	0.00%	0.00%	2 50.00%	1 25.00%	0.00%	0.00%
Anxiety	3	0.00%	0.00%	0.00%	0.00%	0.00%	1 33.33%	1 33.33%	0.00%	0.00%

Medication use: / **Other concomitant therapy received with Alpha-Stim**

Increased	No Change	Reduced	Eliminated	# Reported	None	Psychotherapy	Chiropractic	Acupuncture	Biofeedback	Physical Therapy	Other
0.00%	1 100.00%	0.00%	0.00%	3	2 66.67%	1 33.33%	0.00%	0.00%	0.00%	0.00%	0.00%

Eliminated use of these drugs:

Reduced use of these drugs: anxiolitics (1)

Increased use of this drug:

Side effects reported with use of Alpha-Stim:

9 (90.00%) "None" reported   Specify:

Doctor's evaluation of Alpha-Stim

# Reported	Efficacious	Safe	Reasonably Well Tolerated
10	8 80.00%	8 80.00%	5 50.00%

Doctor's evaluation of Alpha-Stim ('98 survey only)

# Reported	Would Use Alpha-Stim Again	Most Efficacious for this Diagnosis	Other
4	3 75.00%	1 25.00%	0.00%

Quality of life ('98 survey only)

Lose of Work YES	NO	Return to Work YES	NO	Work Comp YES	NO	Improve Family Life YES	NO	Improve Social Life YES	NO	Overall QOL YES	NO	Rx by: MD/DO	PhD	DDS	DC	PT	Other	Not Specified
3 75%	1 25%	1 33%	2 67%	0%	2 100%	3 75%	1 25%	3 75%	1 25%	3 75%	1 25%	3					1	

Summary for Diagnostic Category: NOT SPECIFIED

19 total N   5 male (age range 44-71, mean 55)   0 inpatients
                  14 female (age range 22-53, mean 40)   10 outpatients

Treatment(s) used prior to Alpha-Stim:

ECT	physical therapy	sedative-hypnotics
3 psychotherapy	surgery	psychostimulants
behavior modification	3 other non-drug	major tranquilizers
milliampere TENS	1 alcohol	3 analgesics
2 chiropractic	anxiolitics	NSAIDs
nerve blocks	2 anti-depressants	muscle relaxants
1 biofeedback	1 narcotics	2 other drugs

Reason(s) for discontinuing prior treatment:

2 still using	exacerbated	1 negative drug effects	moved
4 not efficacious	too expensive	uses Alpha-Stim	3 other

Side effects of prior treatment:

4 none	felt drugged	sedation
pain	drug sensitivity/allergy	GI discomfort
addiction	mental cloudiness	other

Treatment results obtained by using Alpha-Stim

Chief Complaints	# Reported	Worse (neg)	None (no change)	Slight (<24%)	Fair (25 - 49%)	Moderate (50 - 74%)	Marked (75 - 99%)	Complete (100%)	Significant Improvement (>25%)
Pain	10	0 0.00%	0 0.00%	0 0.00%	1 10.00%	3 30.00%	6 60.00%	0 0.00%	10 100.00%
Anxiety	8	0 0.00%	0 0.00%	0 0.00%	2 25.00%	2 25.00%	4 50.00%	0 0.00%	8 100.00%
Depression	2	0 0.00%	0 0.00%	0 0.00%	2 100.00%	0 0.00%	0 0.00%	0 0.00%	2 100.00%
Stress	13	0 0.00%	0 0.00%	0 0.00%	3 23.08%	7 53.85%	3 23.08%	0 0.00%	13 100.00%
Insomnia	1	0 0.00%	0 0.00%	0 0.00%	1 100.00%	0 0.00%	0 0.00%	0 0.00%	1 100.00%
Headache	2	0 0.00%	0 0.00%	0 0.00%	1 50.00%	0 0.00%	1 50.00%	0 0.00%	2 100.00%
Muscle Tension	8	0 0.00%	0 0.00%	0 0.00%	1 12.50%	3 37.50%	4 50.00%	0 0.00%	8 100.00%

Treatment results obtained prior to use of Alpha-Stim

Prior Treatments	13	1 7.69%	1 7.69%	4 30.77%	4 30.77%	1 7.69%	2 15.38%	0 0.00%	7 53.85%

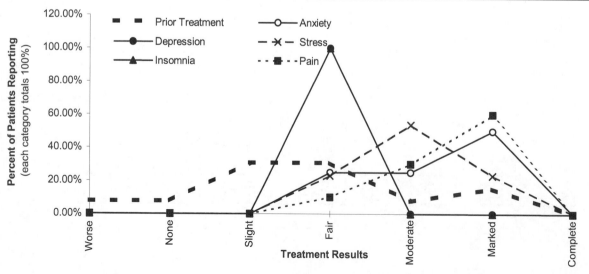

Summary for Diagnostic Category: NOT SPECIFIED

Number of Alpha-Stim treatments

# Reported	1	2	3 - 5	6 - 10	11 - 15	16 - 20	21+	Ongoing	Received in: Doctor's Office	Received in: Patient's Home
8	1 0.00%	1 12.50%	5 62.50%	1 12.50%	0.00%	0.00%	0.00%	1 12.50%	#DIV/0!	#DIV/0!

Alpha-Stim settings used

# Reported	Intensity (µA) 100	200	300	400	500	600	Frequency (Hz) 0.5	1.5	100	Time (minutes/treatment) 0 - 10	11 - 20	21 - 60	>60
13	0%	1 8%	0%	1 8%	8 62%	0%	13 100.00%	0.00%	0.00%	3 23.08%	7 53.85%	3 23.08%	0.00%

Alpha-Stim treatment course

# Reported	Treated With Earclips	Probes	Electrodes	Completed Satisfactory	Still Receiving	Discontinued treatment because: Not Efficacious	Side Effects	Insurance ran out	Other
19	19 100.00%	0.00%	0.00%	8 42.11%	7 36.84%	0.00%	0.00%	0.00%	0.00%

Average residual relief received with a single Alpha-Stim treatment

	# Reported	None	<1	Hours 1 - 8	9 - 23	1	Days 2	3 - 6	7+	Never Returned
Pain										
Anxiety										

Medication use / Other concomitant therapy received with Alpha-Stim

In-creased	No Change	Re-duced	Elimi-nated	# Reported	None	Psycho-therapy	Chiro-practic	Acu-puncture	Bio-feedback	Physical Therapy	Other
				17	9 52.94%	0.00%	4 23.53%	2 11.76%	1 5.88%	1 5.88%	3 17.65%

Eliminated use of these drugs:

Reduced use of these drugs:

Increased use of this drug:

Side effects reported with use of Alpha-Stim:

18 (94.74%) "None" reported   Specify:

Doctor's evaluation of Alpha-Stim

# Reported	Efficacious	Safe	Reasonably Well Tolerated
18	17 94.44%	18 100.00%	10 55.56%

Doctor's evaluation of Alpha-Stim ('98 survey only)

# Reported	Would Use Alpha-Stim Again	Most Efficacious for this Diagnosis	Other

Quality of life ('98 survey only)

Lose of Work YES	NO	Return to Work YES	NO	Work Comp YES	NO	Improve Family Life YES	NO	Improve Social Life YES	NO	Overall QOL YES	NO	Rx by: MD/ DO	PhD	DDS	DC	PT	Other	Not Specified

14

EPILOGUE

We have reviewed an eclectic compilation of medical progress that spans nearly four decades. While searching for a rational solution to the classic philosophical Cartesian mind-body problem and attempting to advance a unified theory, we have focused on the elusive psychosomatic problem to answer the age old question, why is there pain and suffering? The authors have striven to contribute and to bring us closer to a unified explanation for this dilemma.

Dr. Daniel L. Kirsch has contributed enormously to this effort by this publication based on global scientific contributions, many of which initially appeared unrelated, but all of which are now collated towards a better understanding of the neurophysiology of pain and suffering.

We have moved from receptor, to peripheral nerve, to spinal thalamic tract, and finally to thalamocortical pathways, providing the rational basis for clinical management of the distressed patient.

To the iconoclasts and critics, the authors invite constructive commentary. Res ipsiloquetor.

Pierre L. LeRoy, M.D., F.A.C.S., C.C.E.
Director, Delaware Pain Clinic
Neurosurgical Associates, P.A.
Newark, Delaware, USA

15

ABOUT THE AUTHORS

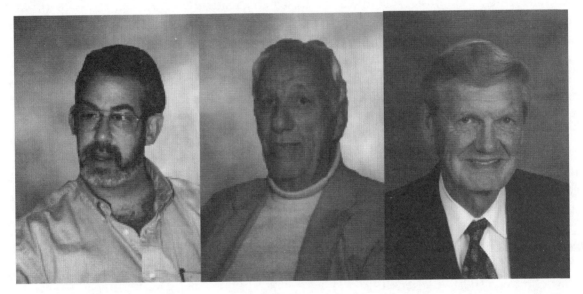

Daniel L. Kirsch, Ph.D.   Pierre L. LeRoy, M.D.   Ray B. Smith, Ph.D.

Daniel L. Kirsch, Ph.D., D.A.A.P.M., F.A.I.S.

Dr. Daniel L. Kirsch has 30 years of experience in the electromedical field, including extensive clinical practice experience.

He served as Clinical Director of three medical centers: The Center and Laboratory for Pain and Stress-Related Disorders at Columbia-Presbyterian Medical Center in New York in association with the late Kenneth Greenspan, M.D., the Sports Medicine Group in Santa Monica, California in association with Karlis Ullis, M.D., and of the Electro-Acutherapy Medical Group in Laguna Beach in association with F. P. Meyer, M.D.

In 1981, he founded Electromedical Products International, Inc. to design, manufacture, and market Alpha-Stim technology.

Dr. Kirsch graduated with a doctorate in neurobiology from City University Los Angeles in 1981, and was a professor of electromedical sciences at CULA from 1985 until he moved to Texas in 1994. In 1990 he was board certified in pain management by the American Academy of Pain Management. In 1997 he was recognized as a Fellow of the American Institute of Stress. He is also a member of the American Preventive Medical Association, American Academy of Clinical Neurophysiology, Medical Device Manufacturers Association, and the only American member of Inter-Pain, the German-Swiss organization for pain management physicians.

He was the First Editor of the *American Journal of Electromedicine*, and served on the Board of Directors of two non-profit organizations in the field: the National Institute of Electromedical Information in New York City which he cofounded, and the International Society of Bioelectricity in Shreveport. He was also a Patron Member of the National Chronic Pain Outreach Association and currently serves on the Advisory Boards of *The Canadian Journal of Clinical Medicine* and *Practical Pain Management.*

Dr. Kirsch has been on the faculty of several medical specialty boards annual relicensing conferences including the American Academy of Orthopedic Medicine, American Academy of Pain Management, Clinical Electromedical Research Academy, American Institute of Stress, American Academy of Anti-Aging Medicine, and Inter-Pain. He also lectures at and gives Grand Rounds at hospitals worldwide.

In 1992 he was a guest of His Excellency the Minister of Public Health, Dr. A. Wahab Al-Fawzan of Kuwait, where he presented a three day post-traumatic stress and pain management program to 400 health care professionals. While in Kuwait, Dr. Kirsch also gave multiple grand rounds at eight hospitals.

Dr. Kirsch is listed in *Who's Who in the World, Who's Who of Emerging Leaders in America, Two Thousand Notable Americans, The International Directory of Distinguished Leadership (UK), Men of Achievement* and other biographical reference books. The author of several scientific articles, he is frequently interviewed for television, newspapers and magazines, and has been a guest on over 200 radio programs.

He authors the chapters, *A Practical Protocol for Electromedical Treatment of Pain,* and *Electromedicine: The Other Side of Physiology,* in the American Academy of Pain Management's textbook, Pain Management: A Practical Guide for Clinicians (CRC Press, Boca Raton, Florida, 1990, revised 1991, 1994, 1998, 2002). Dr. Kirsch's most recent book, coauthored with Christian Thuile, M.D., is Schmerzen lindern ohne Chemie: CES, die Revolution in der Schmerztherapie (Internationale Ärztegesellschaft für Energiemedizin, Austria 2000; in German).

He can be reached at 2201 Garrett Morris Parkway, Mineral Wells, TX 76067-9484 USA Tel: (940) 328-0788, Fax: (940) 328-0888, email: dan@epii.com.

Pierre L. LeRoy, M.D., F.A.C.S.

Dr. Pierre L. LeRoy is an internationally renowned neurosurgeon and Director, Delaware Pain Clinic and Neurosurgical Associates, P.A. He is also a Senior Attending Neurosurgeon at the Wilmington Hospital and Chief, Department of Surgery, Section of Neurological Surgery at St. Francis Hospital. He has been a Principal Research Investigator at the Research Laboratory of the Veterans Administration Hospital. He is a Certified Clinical Engineer and holds many patents in bioengineering devices.

Dr. LeRoy is past President of the Delaware Chapter of the American College of Surgeons and the Delaware Association of Neurological Surgeons (DANS). He is a member of the Thomas Jefferson University Health Care Forum, and of the Cost Containment and Historical Committees for the American Association of Neurological Surgeons.

He is a co-founder of the American Academy of Pain Management (AAPM) and past President of the AAPM Medical Advisory Board which deals with health policy and scientific as well as socio-economic issues concerning healthcare. He is also a Founding Member of the American Pain Society.

A graduate of Jefferson Medical College in 1956, Dr. LeRoy specialized in neurological surgery at the University of Pennsylvania and was awarded a Fellowship in neuroanatomy and neurophysiology at New York University. He was board certified in neurosurgery in 1965.

Ray B. Smith, Ph.D., M.P.A.

Dr. Ray B. Smith earned his M.P.A. from the University of Southern California where he served an internship in President Carter's White House in which he co-chaired an interagency task force for the President's Office of Management and Budget. He graduated from the University of Texas in 1967 with a Ph.D. in physiological psychology.

During his graduate work, Dr. Smith's major interest was cognitive dysfunction. He had earlier served as a psychotherapist and medical administrator in the U.S. Army, following his MA degree in Counseling and Guidance at the University of Texas in 1957. He received special medical training at Ft. Sam Houston in San Antonio and was designated one of the U.S. Army's first three "Field Medical Officers", possibly the forerunner of today's physician assistant programs. In that capacity he served as acting Medical Officer for a 500 man artillery unit in Germany during his final year in the Military.

Upon completion of his doctorate, Dr. Smith taught research students at the State University of New York at Courtland for one year prior to joining American University as a senior scientist in their Center for Research in Social Systems.

In 1969 he received a grant from NIH for the study of alcoholism and drug addiction in the District of Columbia. The grant was attached to the D.C. Government's Department of Human Resources, Mental Health Administration. During his 13 years in that position, he began to study the remarkable effects of CES on the cognitive dysfunction of that subject population. It was during this time that he found upon repeated studies that CES could bring back to normal within three weeks, the short term memory loss and other cognitive dysfunctions of addicted persons, which ordinarily take from two to three years of continuous sobriety.

Since that time, he has researched CES in places as various as Washington, D.C., Ft. Worth, Texas, Santa Barbara, California, Los Angeles, California, and Salt Lake City, Utah, among others. His subject populations have been as varied as alcoholics, drug abusers, people with eating disorders, phobias, anxiety and depression, attention deficit disorder, and chronic pain.

All of his studies have been at least single-blind, and most have been double-blind, with the psychometrist and statisticians also blind to the treatment condition in each case. His studies have involved well over 1,500 subjects to date.

Since his research has covered a wide spectrum of medical and socio/psychological disorders, he has been asked to present in-depth lectures on CES to medical school faculty, the professional staff in numerous inpatient and outpatient treatment programs, and business and professional leaders associated with medical treatment programs, including major American medical insurance companies. In addition he has provided inservices, in both English and Spanish, on CES treatment in medical facilities nationwide.

After working as research consultant to various CES firms from 1980 to 1998, Dr. Smith joined Electromedical Products International, Inc. in 1998 where he currently serves as Vice President of Science where he continues to bring his in-depth knowledge of the scientific aspects of CES plus his considerable clinical skills into play in his writings and on the professional lecture circuit.

Dr. Smith was elected to membership in the University of Texas Leadership Society in the summer of 2000. The University of Texas at Austin is the nation's largest university, and the Leadership Society is comprised of former students, faculty, and administrators, selected for this special honor.

On May 4, 2001, Dr. Smith was formally installed as a member of the Chancellor's Council of the 15 campus University of Texas System. While each campus has a president and administrative officers, under Texas State law the chancellor presides over the entire system. The council interacts with the chancellor's office via an elected executive committee that meets on a regularly scheduled basis to provide input from the members of the council.

In the Spring of 2001 he was also selected to become a member of the University of Texas' Littlefield Society, another honorary group who are especially interested in the history and development of the UT campus at Austin, as well as national and international issues in which the University currently plays a role. Its members come from many walks of life, with current or former state and national academic and political leaders represented in large numbers.

Dr. Smith can be reached via email at ray@epii.com.